COMMUNICABLE DISEASE
EPIDEMIOLOGY AND CONTROL

Communicable Disease Epidemiology and Control

ROGER WEBBER

*London School of Hygiene
and Tropical Medicine*

CAB INTERNATIONAL

CAB INTERNATIONAL
Wallingford
Oxon OX10 8DE
UK

Tel: +44 (0)1491 832111
Fax: +44 (0)1491 833508
E-mail: cabi@cabi.org
Telex: 847964 (COMAGG G)

A catalogue record for this book is available from the British Library.

ISBN 0 85199 138 6

Typeset in Melior by Solidus (Bristol) Limited
Printed and bound in the UK at the University Press, Cambridge

Contents

Introduction

Diseases can be communicable or non-communicable and further sub-divided as follows:

- Epidemic ⎫
- Endemic ⎬ Communicable
- Acute ⎫
- Chronic ⎬ Non-communicable

Examples would be, in the first category, measles, in the second, malaria, in the third, accidents and, in the fourth, coronary heart disease. All of them can occur at the same time and in the same place, but communicable diseases are more common in developing countries.

Epidemic diseases devastate whole populations, as when measles ravaged Fiji, killing adults as well as children. Populations then have to start again from the survivors and recover their former strength. These are essentially young and growing populations. With endemic diseases it is children that are particularly vulnerable, so there is a high birth rate to compensate. With so many young people in the population, chronic non-communicable diseases are uncommon, but as people live longer they become more frequent. Chronic non-communicable diseases are the problem of older-aged populations as seen in the Western world.

The division between communicable and non-communicable was quite clear-cut. Where there was an organism, it was communicable; otherwise it was non-communicable. This strict boundary is becoming less well defined as new suspect organisms are discovered or diseases, by their very nature, suggest a communicable origin. Various cancers are good examples; the link between hepatitis B virus and liver-cell cancer is well established, and a preventive vaccination campaign will test its validity.

Communicable diseases tend to behave in a similar pattern. Such generalizations determine the first chapters of the book, which look at communicable disease theory, formulating common principles in both epidemiology and control.

Classifying communicable disease can be by organism, clinical presentation or system of the body attacked. These classifications are valuable for the clinician, microbiologist or parasitologist. The epidemiologist is interested in causation and methods of control, so a classification based on these criteria is used here.

Trying to find similarities can often be useful, well shown by grouping respiratory diseases into acute respiratory infections (ARI), which has produced an important advancement in the control of this common problem. Every effort has therefore been made to find common themes to make the understanding and learning of communicable diseases easier. Using control methods relevant to one infection will often be applicable to others similarly grouped, so that much can be done using epidemiological principles. Knowing the organism is not always necessary in an epidemiological approach.

The range of communicable diseases occurring throughout the world is considerable. A comprehensive list is given in Section 19.1, but only those of importance are covered in detail in the main part of the book. Emphasis is placed on developing countries as this is where most communicable diseases are found. It is hoped this selection of diseases provides a more representative perspective of the world situation (see Table I.1).

While communicable diseases mainly affect the developing world, new and emergent diseases, such as human immunodeficiency virus (HIV) infection, have reawakened developed countries to the importance of these infections. Although most communicable diseases arise within the country, there is also an international importance as more people travel to different countries and exotic diseases are imported. So it is hoped that there will be much of interest in this book for those in developed as well as the developing countries.

This book is mainly designed for the doctor in rural areas and persons working in the control of communicable diseases, often in remote areas where there is no access to a reference library. References have therefore been left out, but a list of books for further reading, which would make the basis of a small library, are given at the end. Essential entomology and parasitology have been included, as in many cases they are an integral part of the disease process, rather than kept as separate disciplines. Clinical details have been kept to the minimum required for control and prevention, as it is not intended that this book should be used for the management of individual patients.

Many of the examples are taken from my personal experience of working in Solomon Islands, Tanzania and, latterly, various Asian countries, but it is hoped they will be found relevant to other parts of the world. Much of what I have learnt has come from the many people who have helped and worked with me in these countries and I am extremely grateful to them for their wisdom and assistance.

Table I.1. Disability and mortality of communicable diseases in the world. Data from the World Bank (*World Development Report*, 1993).

Disease	DALYs (hundreds of thousands)	Deaths (thousands)
Respiratory infections (lower)	1147.5	4,251
Respiratory infections (upper)	29.2	12
Tuberculosis	464.5	2,016
Otitis media	51.2	52
Diarrhoea (acute)	543.8	1,553
Diarrhoea (chronic)	290.8	872
Dysentery	156.5	448
Measles	341.1	1,006
Tetanus	164.9	505
Pertussis	119.5	321
Polio	48.1	24
Diphtheria	2.3	4
Meningitis	80.9	242
Malaria	257.3	926
Schistosomiasis	45.3	38
Trypanosomiasis	17.8	55
Chagas' disease	27.4	23
Leishmaniasis	20.6	54
Lymphatic filariasis	8.5	0
Onchocerciasis	6.4	30
Ascaris	105.2	13
Trichuris	63.1	9
Hookworm	11.4	6
Leprosy	10.2	3
Trachoma	33.0	0
HIV infection	302.1	291
Hepatitis	19.3	77
Syphilis	63.2	186
Chlamydia	15.5	1
Gonorrhoea	4.1	3
Pelvic inflammatory disease	128.0	2
Total	4665.5	13,381

DALY, disability-adjusted life year.

The DALY is a calculation of the morbidity and mortality of the particular disease averaged out over the expected life of a person, so it reflects the prevalence of the disease and the disability it produces. For example a common disease such as respiratory infection, by its prevalence will contribute a large number of DALYs, whereas HIV infection contributes a proportionally higher number due to the high fatality rate.

Experience is invaluable, but organizing one's thoughts and developing a critical judgement comes from working in an academic environment, and many people in the London School of Hygiene and Tropical Medicine (LSHTM) have helped me in the various drafts of this manuscript. I wish to thank particularly John Ackers, David Bradley, Sandy Cairncross, Michael Colbourne (who sadly died before this was published), Janette Costello, Felicity Cutts, Paul Fine and Peter Smith. Andrew Tomkins of the Institute of Child Health and William Cutting of the University of Edinburgh kindly read through sections on the childhood infections. Maurice King gave me considerable help in the layout of the book and encouragement to persevere with it. Sameen Siddiqi from the Pakistan Institute of Medical Sciences reviewed the text for use in Asia and wrote the section on rheumatic fever. Julie Cliff, who has spent most of her working life in Africa and teaches at the University of Maputo, Mozambique, gave me much valuable advice as the manuscript was made ready for publication. But one person to whom I owe special thanks is Brian Southgate, who has been my mentor and friend over many years. He introduced me to many original concepts and has been a kindly guide to being more scientific.

Many organizations allowed me to reproduce illustrations and I am especially grateful to the World Health Organization for supplying print-quality copies of their many figures. The Overseas Development Administration (ODA) has been my employer in Solomon Islands, Tanzania and currently as a member of the Tropical Diseases Control Programme at LSHTM. They have given me considerable assistance in this entire endeavour and I would particularly like to thank the Health and Population Division Low-cost Book Programme for a generous grant towards publishing costs.

In these days of rising prices and commercial competition, it is becoming increasingly difficult to produce books that are affordable in developing countries. Every effort has been made to produce this book as cheaply as possible, without sacrificing quality, by forgoing commission and raising additional funding. As well as the support from ODA, mentioned above, I would also like to thank 3M Health Care for their generous financial help towards the production of this book. They have done much to encourage doctors to gain wider experience with their medical-student elective prize for the best report on an elective period spent in a developing country.

Despite all this help, the copy price is still higher than I would like it to be and it will only come down further if there is sufficient demand.

Any illustrations or examples that would improve a subsequent edition will be most welcome. Please send them to the London School of Hygiene and Tropical Medicine, Keppel Street, London WCIE 7HT, UK.

Part I

Theory and Methods

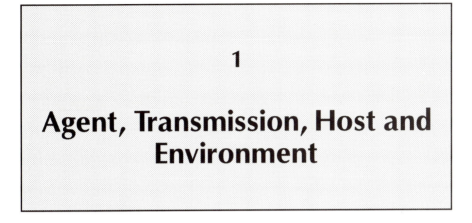

1

Agent, Transmission, Host and Environment

The key to any infectious disease is to think of it in terms of *agent, transmission, host* and *environment*. These components are illustrated in Fig. 1.1, which will be used as a framework for the description in this chapter. There needs to be a causative agent, which requires a means of transmission from one host to another, but the outcome will be influenced by the environment. These will be looked at separately, before bringing them together in determining a strategy for control.

1.1 THE AGENT

The agent can be an organism (virus, bacteria, rickettsia, protozoan, helminth, fungus or arthropod) or a physical or chemical agent (toxin or poison). If an organism, the agent needs to *multiply*, find a means of *transmission* and *survive*.

1.1.1 Multiplication

Two methods of multiplication occur, *asexual* and *sexual* reproduction, which have different advantages. In asexual reproduction, a succession of exact or almost exact replicas are produced, so that any natural selection will act on batches or strains, rather than on individuals. In contrast, sexual reproduction offers great scope for variety, both within the cells of the single organism and from one organism to another. This means that natural selection acts on individuals, and variations of vigour and adaptability occur.

There are different consequences of these methods of reproduction.

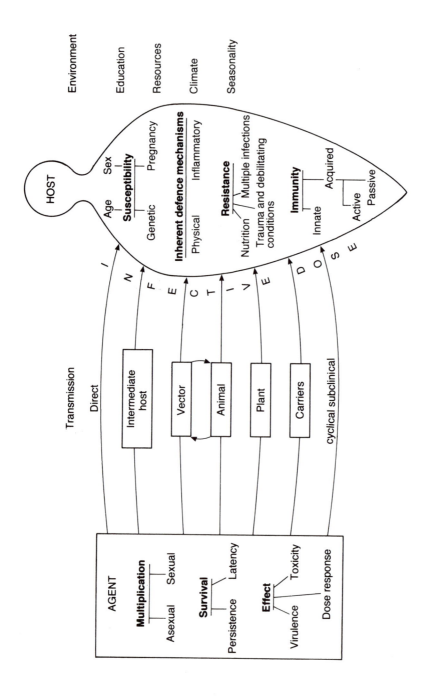

Fig. 1.1. Agent, transmission, host and environment.

With asexual organisms the strain of the organism is either successful or unsuccessful in invading the host, whereas in sexual organisms certain individuals may succeed while others do not. This is relevant in treatment.

In continuing its existence, only one organism of the asexual parasite requires to be transmitted, whereas with the sexual parasite male and female adults must meet before reproduction can take place. Some parasites seem at a tremendous disadvantage, e.g. in the filarial worm *Wuchereria bancrofti* both male and female individuals go through long migrations in the body to find an individual of the opposite sex, but despite all these problems they are one of the most successful of all parasites.

1.1.2 Survival

Agents survive by finding a suitable host within a certain period of time. They have been able to improve their chances of finding a new host or prolonging the period of time by a number of different methods.

Reservoirs

A reservoir is a storage place for water but serves as an appropriate description for a suitable place to store agents of infection. Reservoirs can be humans, animals, vectors or the inanimate environment (e.g soil, water). From a reservoir the parasites can attack new hosts of the same species or attempt to colonize different species.

Persistence

Another mechanism used by parasites to survive is the development of special stages that resist destruction in an adverse environment. Examples are the cysts of protozoa, e.g. *Entamoeba histolytica* and the eggs of nematodes, e.g. *Ascaris*. Bacteria can utilize persistence, as with spore-forming anthrax and tetanus bacilli (Fig. 1.2).

Latency

A developmental stage in the environment that is not infective to a new host is called latency. This allows the parasite time for suitable conditions to develop before changing into the infective form. *Strongyloides* exhibits latency.

Vectors

By using the services of an arthropod that comes into close proximity with the host, an agent can be transported direct from one host to another.

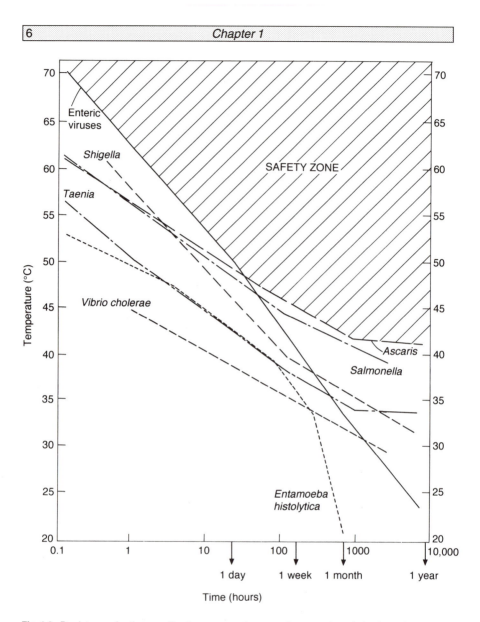

Fig. 1.2. Persistence of pathogens. The lines represent conservative upper boundaries for pathogen death – that is, estimates of the time–temperature combinations required for pathogen inactivation. Organisms can survive for long periods at low temperatures, so a composting process must be maintained at a temperature above 43°C for at least a month to effectively kill all pathogens likely to be found in human excreta. From Feachem, R.G., Bradley, D.J., Garelick, H. and Mara, D.D. (1983) *Sanitation and Disease: Health Aspects of Excreta and Wastewater Management*, World Bank, Washington, p. 79. Reprinted by permission of John Wiley & Sons Ltd.

The vector can either be part of the transmission process, such as a mosquito, which pierces the skin of the host directly and facilitates the passage of the parasite, or it can be mechanical such as the housefly, which inadvertently transmits organisms to the host on its feet and mouth-parts.

Intermediate host

Some parasites need to go through a developmental stage in an intermediate host before they can subsequently invade the final host. *Schistosoma* uses a molluscan intermediate host, whereas some parasites, e.g. *Opisthorchis*, need two intermediate hosts. Humans can either be the final host, as with the beef tapeworm, an intermediate host, as in *Echinococcus*, or both, as in the pork tapeworm.

1.1.3 The Effect of the Agent on the Host

If enough agents survive to infect a new host, they will produce a reaction or illness. The reaction will depend upon the response of the host and the agent. The effect of the agent is determined by its virulence, toxicity and dose.

Virulence

Some agents have a very marked effect on their host, while others have a mild one.

1. Subspecies, e.g. *Trypanosoma brucei gambiense* produces a milder illness then *T. b. rhodesiense*.
2. Strains of the same species, e.g. the influenza virus strains have marked differences in virulence.

Toxicity

Infectious agents elicit a host reaction, both as foreign organisms and by virtue of their toxic proteins. For example, tetanus bacilli, from their site of infection in the skin, produce toxin effects totally out of proportion to the insignificant primary focus of skin infection.

Some organisms produce toxins when they grow in food, and these toxins cause illness at a distance from themselves. An example is *Clostridium botulinum*. Some toxic chemicals can contaminate food, e.g. adulterated cooking oil, and produce an illness that has all the appearances of an epidemic.

Dose response

For each infectious agent, a minimum number of organisms is required to overcome the defences of the host and cause the disease. A large dose of organisms may be required, such as in cholera, or very few, e.g. *E. histolytica*. With some diseases, once this number is surpassed, the severity of the disease is the same whether a few or a large number of organisms are introduced. In others there is a correlation between dose and severity of illness. An example is food poisoning, where the severity of the illness is determined by the quantity of the infected food item that is consumed. On the beneficial side, a low dose of organisms may produce no symptoms of disease but be sufficient to induce immunity. Poliomyelitis is one of many examples.

1.2 TRANSMISSION

Communicable diseases fall into a number of transmission patterns, illustrated in Fig. 1.3.

1.2.1 Direct

Direct transmission includes human-to-human contact, as from dirty fingers or via food and water in the diarrhoeal diseases, or through droplet infection in the respiratory diseases. Variations of direct transmission, particularly in the environmental diseases, are as follows.

- *Autoinfection*, where humans contaminate themselves directly from their external orifices. Examples are transmission of *Enterobius* from anal scratching or infection of skin abrasions with bacteria from nose-picking.
- *Person to person following development in soil*. The hookworms and *Strongyloides* are not infective until they have undergone a developmental stage in the soil, following which they can penetrate unbroken skin, whereas *Ascaris* must develop in the soil before the swallowed eggs will infect humans.

1.2.2 Snail, Fish or Crustacean as Intermediate Host (Water-based)

This group includes schistosomiasis, in which a snail is intermediate host, and Guinea worm, where it is a copepod. In *Opisthorchis*, *Paragonimus* and *Diphyllobothrium* more than one kind of intermediate host is required.

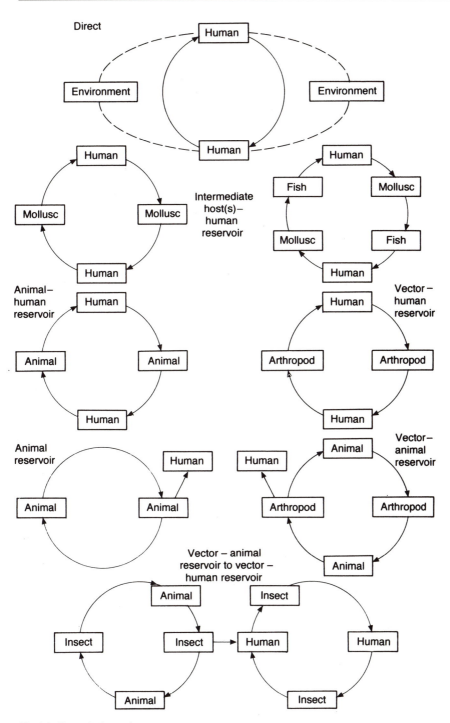

Fig. 1.3. Transmission cycles.

1.2.3 Animal as Intermediate Host (Land-based)

Taenia saginata and *T. solium* can only infect humans after they have developed into cystocerci in the animal muscle.

1.2.4 Animal Reservoir

An animal reservoir implies that the cycle is normally from one animal to another, but when humans accidentally interfere they become infected. Rabies and anthrax are examples.

1.2.5 Vector

A vector is an arthropod which carries the infection from one host to another. Infection may occur due to the feeding of the arthropod or as a result of its habits. The cycle may be:

- direct insect to human, as in malaria;
- arthropod to animal with a human entering the cycle as an abnormal host, e.g. bubonic plague;
- insect to animal including humans, from whom it is transmitted to other humans by the same or another insect vector; examples are yellow fever and East African sleeping sickness (*T. b. rhodesiense*).

Snails, especially in descriptions of schistosomiasis, are often called vectors, but they are actually intermediate hosts.

1.2.6 Zoonosis

In the classification by transmission cycle, diseases fall into two main groups, the diseases where only humans are involved and those in which there is an animal reservoir. *Zoonoses* are infections that are naturally transmitted between vertebrate animals and humans. They can be grouped according to the intimacy of the animal to human beings.

- *Domestic*, those invited animals which live in close proximity to humans, e.g. pets and farm animals.
- *Synanthropic*, animals that live in close association with humans, but are not invited, e.g. rats.
- *Exoanthropic*, animals that are not in close association with humans, e.g. monkeys.

The importance of this type of classification is that it indicates the *focality* of the disease. As domestic animals are universally distributed, domestic zoonotic diseases are cosmopolitan. At the other extreme, in an exoanthropic zoonosis, such as scrub typhus or jungle yellow fever (where monkeys are the reservoir), it is quite possible for humans to live in the same locality but separately from the disease area; humans have no part in the disease cycle but come into contact with it when they accidentally enter the affected place (focus).

In zoonoses the animal reservoir is all-important in control. In some diseases, such as the beef and pork tapeworms, good hygienic practice and inspection of the animal carcass may be all that is required to interrupt transmission. At the opposite extreme, a disease such as yellow fever can never be eradicated from the population, even if every man, woman and child are immunized, because the reservoir of disease remains in the monkey population. In a zoonosis, the animal reservoir is of prime importance and only by studying the ecology of the animal population can any rational attempt be made to control it.

1.2.7 Plants

Vegetable material that is eaten by the host can serve as a method of transmission. This can either be a specific plant, such as water calthrop, on which the cercariae of *Fasciolopsis buski* encyst, or non-specific, such as any salad vegetable that might be carrying cysts of *E. histolytica*.

1.2.8 Carriers and Subclinical Transmission

Diseases in which there is an animal reservoir, intermediate host or vector are complex and difficult to control, but, even in the simplified transmission cycle of direct spread from human to human, complications occur with the *carrier* state. A carrier is a person that is not manifesting the disease, but can transmit the infective agent. There are several types of carriers.

- Asymptomatic carriers, who remain well throughout the infection.
- Incubating or prodromal carriers, who are infectious but unaware that they are in the early stages of the disease.
- Convalescent carriers, who continue to be infectious after the clinical disease has passed.

The carrier state can be either *transient* or *chronic*.

The important features of carriers are as follows.

- The number of carriers may be far greater than the number of those who are sick.
- Carriers are not manifest so they and others are unaware that they can transmit the disease.

- As carriers are not sick, they are not restricted and therefore disseminate the disease widely.
- Chronic carriers may produce repeated outbreaks over a considerable period of time.

Identification of carriers is a singularly difficult and generally unsuccessful exercise. If the carrier is asymptomatic, the organisms are often in such reduced numbers or excreted at such infrequent intervals that routine culture techniques will not detect them. The investigation has to be repeated many times and is probably only successful at specific instances, e.g. during a minor diarrhoeal episode in a suspected typhoid carrier. A further difficulty is that clinically well people object to having investigations performed on them, so coverage is incomplete. Examples of diseases in which the carrier state is important are typhoid, amoebiasis, poliomyelitis, meningococcal meningitis, diphtheria and hepatitis B. Cholera can produce more transient carriers than the number sick. More on carriers will be found in the sections on these diseases.

In some diseases the carrier state appears to be prolonged or the disease is perpetuated when there are no carriers. This may be due to *cyclical subclinical transmission*, when infection is transmitted within a family or throughout a community, without the subjects being aware of any particular symptoms. One member of a family passes on the disease to another and becomes free of it him/herself. It is then passed on to other family members and eventually back again, so that it is maintained in a subclinical cycle. When someone who is susceptible to the disease accidentally enters this cycle or the organism is more widely disseminated, then a clinical outbreaks occurs. This is a mechanism by which poliomyelitis is maintained in the community.

1.2.9 Excreted Load

The number of organisms excreted can vary considerably according to the type of infection, the stage of the disease or other physiological conditions of the host. In diseases such as cholera, there may be vast numbers of organisms excreted (10^6–10^{12} vibrios g^{-1} of faeces), whereas in hookworm infection the number of eggs may be comparatively few. In *Schistosoma mansoni* the largest number of eggs are excreted by asymptomatic children, whereas the older case exhibiting severe manifestations may be almost non-infectious. In the otherwise harmless typhoid carrier, a bout of diarrhoea can cause the passage of a sufficient number of organisms to initiate an epidemic.

1.2.10 Infective Dose

The infective dose is the number of organisms required to produce the disease in an individual. Estimates of doses have been attempted in cholera and typhoid using healthy volunteers, but variables such as host susceptibility prevent any degree of precision. For other diseases, there are few data. Even so, grouping diseases together into those with high and those with low infective doses leads to an understanding of the mechanisms of transmission.

Infections with a low infective dose (such as enteric viruses and *E. histolytica*) can spread by person-to-person contact. This means that the provision of a safe water supply or sanitation is unlikely to have much effect. At the other extreme are organisms like typhoid and cholera, when a high infective dose (of the order of 10^6 organisms ml^{-1} of water) is required to produce the disease. Improving water quality and the reduction of pathogens in the sewage will be beneficial to the community.

1.3 HOST FACTORS

If the agent is transmitted to a new host, its successful invasion and persistence will depend upon a number of host factors.

1.3.1 Susceptibility

Genetic

Certain diseases can only affect animals, and when they are transmitted to humans they are not able to establish themselves. An example is *Plasmodium berghei*, the rodent malaria parasite, which cannot produce disease in humans although it is closely related to the human malaria parasites. Genetic disposition also determines the host's response to infecting organisms. Mycobacteria are common in the environment but only certain people develop tuberculosis or leprosy. The type of disease, e.g. tuberculoid or lepromatous leprosy, is also determined by the genetic make-up.

Age

During the course of life, different diseases affect particular age-groups. The childhood diseases of measles, chickenpox and diphtheria are found at one end of the lifespan, with the degenerative diseases and neoplasms predominating at the other.

Sex

Genetic sex-linked diseases, such as Duchenne muscular dystrophy, are restricted to one sex (in this case males), whereas poliomyelitis and goitre are more commonly found in females than males. Occupation can determine which sex is more likely to be involved, such as in sleeping sickness (discussed later), or social habits may be the determinant, such as the custom of women eating the brains of the recently dead in the highlands of Papua New Guinea making kuru predominantly a disease of women.

Pregnancy

When a woman is pregnant, her physiological mechanisms are altered and she becomes more susceptible to infections. Chickenpox is a severe disease in pregnancy and malaria attacks the pregnant woman as though she had little acquired immunity.

1.3.2 Inherent Defence Mechanisms

Any infecting organism must be able to overcome the body's *inherent defence mechanisms*. These can either be:

- *physical*, such as the skin, mucus-secreting membranes or acidity of the stomach; or
- *inflammatory*, the localized reaction which includes increased blood flow, the attraction of phagocytes and isolation of the site of inoculation.

1.3.3 Resistance

The person's susceptibility and defence mechanisms may be altered by the *resistance* of the individual. This may be lowered by the following.

- *Nutrition.* Where the nutritional status is decreased, the susceptibility to a disease is increased or the clinical illness is more severe.
- *Trauma and debilitating conditions.* Poliomyelitis may be a mild or unapparent infection, but, if associated with trauma, such as an intramuscular injection, then paralytic disease can result. The appearance of shingles or fungal infections in debilitated people is often seen.
- *Multiple infections.* The presence of one disease may make it easier for other infecting organisms. Secondary respiratory infections commonly occur in measles. Yaws has been noticed to increase and

spread more rapidly following an outbreak of chickenpox.

Immunity

Experience of previous infection by a host can lead to the development of *immunity*. This can either be *cellular*, conferred by T-lymphocyte sensitization, or *humoral*, from the B-lymphocyte response. Immunity can be either *acquired* or *passive*.

Acquired

Acquired (both cellular and humoral) immunity follows an infection or vaccination of attenuated (live or dead) organisms. This will induce the body to develop an immune response in a number of diseases. Immunity is most completely developed against the viral infections and may be permanent. With protozoal infections, e.g. malaria, it may only be maintained by repeated attacks of the organism.

Passive

Passive (humoral only) immunity is the transfer of antibodies from a mother to her child via the placenta. Passive immunity is short-lived, as in the protection of the young infant against measles for the first 6 months of life. Passive immunity can also be introduced, e.g. in rabies immune serum.

1.4 THE ENVIRONMENT

The transmission cycle used by the agent to reach the host takes place within an environment which determines the success and severity of the infection. Environmental factors are subtle, diffuse and wide-ranging. A few of the more important ones are mentioned in this section.

1.4.1 Education

Sufficient is known about most of the communicable diseases for them to be prevented, if only people were taught how. Education is a complex process; it is not just teaching people – they must understand to such an extent that they are able to modify their lives. This is not a sudden process. Changes made by one generation are used as the starting-point for improvements or modifications in the following. Change is always opposed, and steps that seem easy to the educated are mountains for the uneducated to climb. Also, education is not just the adding of new knowledge, but the rational appraisal of traditional customs.

An improvement in the level of education and understanding was probably the most important reason why endemic communicable diseases largely disappeared from the developed world. As education improved, there was a demand for improved living standards. Good water and proper sewage disposal were provided, personal hygiene became a normal rather than abnormal practice and cleanliness was sanctioned as a desirable attribute. These changes all occurred before the advent of antibiotics. The decline of tuberculosis in England and Wales (see Fig. 13.6) is a classic example of how a major communicable disease decreased as living standards rose.

1.4.2 Resources

The lack of resources leads to *poverty*, which reduces the ability to combat disease. By resources are meant everything that people have to enable them to carry out their livelihood. Perhaps the most important resource is land, which is used by the family for living on and growing crops. Alternatively this land can be used to produce commodities that can be sold as part of a manufacturing process. As the society develops, education, or the ability to perform a service, becomes a resource.

Resources are required to enact the preventive methods or raise the standards that have come to be demanded by education. At its simplest, food is required to build up body processes and prevent malnutrition. But with a little extra money a water supply can be built or a better house constructed.

Resources, *education* and *disease* are inextricably linked. Diseases are best prevented by educating people to overcome them, but resources are required by the educated to achieve this. Greater resources allow increased education, and improved education the greater utilization of resources. These both act in reducing communicable diseases.

1.4.3 Climate

Climate can be divided into different components – *temperature, rainfall* (humidity) and, less importantly, *wind*. These attributes of the climate have a marked influence on where diseases are found and the ways in which they are to be controlled.

Temperature

Temperature varies according to distance from the equator, altitude, prevailing winds and size of land masses. A number of diseases are found only in the tropics, which is the main area for communicable diseases. Temperature decreases with altitude, so that malaria will be found at the lower hot altitude, while respiratory diseases are commoner in the colder hills. At the fringe of the mosquitoes' range, exceptional conditions of temperature and humidity can produce epidemic malaria.

Temperature not only affects the presence or absence of disease, but often regulates the amount. The malaria parasite has a shorter developmental cycle as the temperature rises and so permits an increased rate of transmission. Many insect vectors have a more rapid development in the tropics, making them difficult to control. The life cycle of a number of parasites is directly related to the temperature.

Rainfall

Rainfall is perhaps the most essential element in human livelihood. Rainfall must be sufficient and regular (Fig. 1.4). This allows for crops to be planted and ensures that they come to fruition. An irregular rainfall can be as disastrous as a low rainfall, leading to failed crops, malnutrition and a reduction of resistance to infection.

Rainfall also has a direct effect on certain diseases. Moderate rainfall creates fresh breeding sites for *Anopheles* mosquitoes, but excessive rain can wash out larvae and cause a reduction in the number of mosquitoes. Some diseases, such as trachoma, favour dry arid regions.

Wind

Winds produce local alterations in the weather. A major wind system is the monsoon, which brings rainfall to the Indian subcontinent and South-East Asia. In West Africa the hot dry harmattan blows down from the Sahara, reducing humidity and increasing dust. It is these secondary effects on rainfall and temperature that determine the disease patterns.

The winds are appreciated by humans in the warm moist areas of the world, where they improve their living conditions, and avoided in the hot dry zones. However, excess wind in hurricane areas or the localized tornado causes destruction and loss of life (Fig. 1.5), exposing the population to epidemic diseases.

1.4.4 Seasonality

Temperature and rainfall together determine the best time to grow crops and the seasonal patterns of a number of diseases. In areas of almost constant rain there is very little seasonal variation, but in the drier regions seasonality can be quite marked. These areas are illustrated in Fig. 1.4.

The pattern of life determined by seasonality can be generalized as follows.

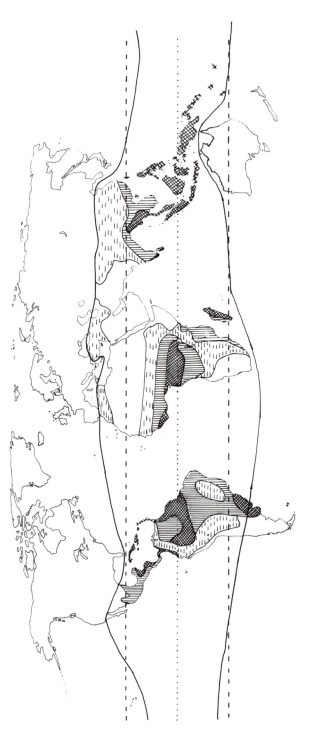
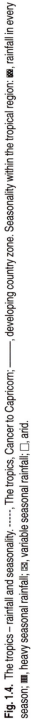

Fig. 1.4. The tropics – rainfall and seasonality. ----, The tropics, Cancer to Capricorn; ——, developing country zone. Seasonality within the tropical region: ▨, rainfall in every season; ▥, heavy seasonal rainfall; ▨, variable seasonal rainfall; ☐, arid.

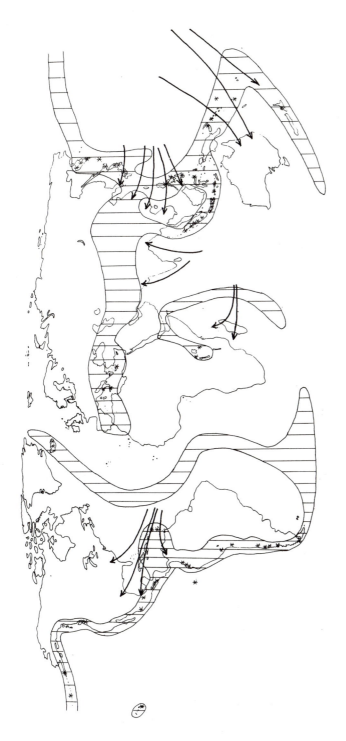

Fig. 1.5. Natural disaster zones. ▥, Earthquake areas; *, active volcanoes; ←, revolving tropical storms (tornadoes, hurricanes, cyclones).

- Food stores are low or absent during the rains as it is the longest time since the harvest.
- When the rains come, people are required to work their hardest when they have the least amount of food.
- The rains bring seasonal illnesses, especially malaria, which debilitate just when complete fitness is required.
- The time of the rains may coincide with late pregnancy, conception having taken place during harvest. Since all members of the family are required to work in the fields and much of the burden of cultivating falls on the woman, the increased strain threatens her pregnancy, while her physical reserves are stretched even further.
- Once harvest comes, body weight is restored, excess crops are stored or sold and some respite is taken before the cycle repeats itself.

This pattern leads to the following observations.

1. Attendance for treatment at medical institutions and admission to hospital often follow a cyclical pattern. This is illustrated in Fig. 1.6 where it will be seen that the reporting of ill health is least during the dry months and increases as the rains come.

2. Knowledge of the seasonality of disease can be used in health planning, the deployment of manpower, the ordering of supplies, the best time to take preventive action, etc.

3. Many illnesses show a marked seasonal pattern. Mosquitoes require

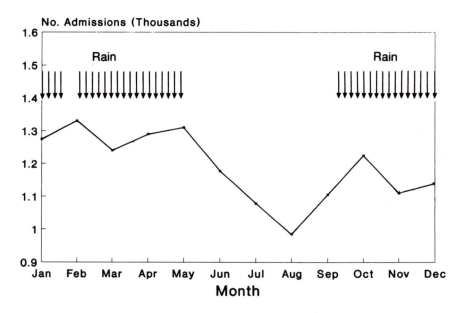

Fig. 1.6. Seasonality of admissions to Mbeya hospital, Tanzania, 1980–1983.

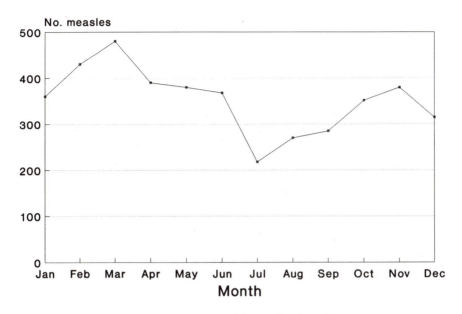

Fig. 1.7. Mean monthly measles cases, 1977–1981, Mbeya region, Tanzania.

water to breed so rainfall will determine a seasonal pattern for many of the vector-borne diseases. The massive contamination of rivers caused by the first rains washing in accumulated pollutants from the many dry months makes this a period of diarrhoeal diseases. The seasonality of cholera allows a warning system to be implemented and prevention initiated (see Section 8.6).

4. A different pattern of seasonal diseases occurs with the viral infections, measles (see Fig. 13.2) being a good example. As measles confers lifelong immunity, the only way that sufficient susceptibles can accumulate for another epidemic to occur is by immigration or reproduction. If the birth rate is high, a critical number of susceptibles will soon be produced and annual epidemics will occur. If the birth rate is low, the interval may be every 2–3 years.

5. Knowledge of the seasonality of disease allows planned preventive services. If a mobile or mass vaccination campaign is used to combat measles, then timing it in the few months before an expected epidemic is the most cost-effective. In Tanzania measles outbreaks often occur in the rainy season (Fig. 1.7), a time of shortages, malnutrition and difficult communications – the worst possible time to have to do emergency vaccination to contain the epidemic. Just a few months before, there was little ill health, nutritional status was high, road conditions were good and medical staff were at their slackest. This would have been the best time to ensure that every child was vaccinated.

2

Communicable Disease Theory

The previous chapter attempted to unify communicable diseases into basic units, the *agent*, a route of *transmission* to a *host* and the way the *environment* influences the outcome. Generalizations have been made in attempting to limit and clarify all the alternatives and variations that are possible. Developing principles, not discovering exceptions, has been the objective. A stage is now reached where interactions between these various elements can be suggested and tried. The approach can be either intuitive, a method used with reasonable success in earlier attempts at explaining disease dynamics, or analytical, where the precision, ease of modification and extrapolation are considerably greater.

2.1 FORCE OF INFECTION

In a communicable disease, the number of new cases occurring in a period of time is dependent on the number of infectious persons within a susceptible population and the degree of contact between them. Persons, whether infectious or susceptible and a period of time are all quantifiable factors, but the degree of contact can depend upon very many variables (some of which have been covered above). Such things as proximity (density) of populations, carriers, reservoirs, climate and seasonality will all have separate effects. To single these out and ascribe values to them will involve considerable and generally unnecessary complexity. In some disease patterns, certain factors have sufficient influence for them to require to be given values, but for the time being it is best to consider these all together as a *force of infection*.

The force of infection = Number of infectious individuals × transmission rate

Therefore:

Number of	=	Force of infection	×	Number of susceptible
newly infected				individuals in the
individuals				population

If the susceptible population is sufficiently large to maintain a permanent pool of susceptibles (as would happen in a disease where there is little or no immunity) and the force of infection is constant, then newly infected individuals will continue to be produced while infectious individuals remain in the population. One healthy carrier might continue to infect a large number of individuals over a long period of time, or a brief devastating epidemic, with a short period of infectiousness, may infect a large number of people over a short period of time. Parasitic infections, such as hookworm, would be an example of the former and measles of the latter. Of course, measles produces immunity, which will alter the size of the susceptible population.

The proportion of susceptible individuals can be either reduced by mortality, immunity or emigration or increased by birth or immigration. After a certain period of time a sufficient number of non–immune persons will have entered the population for a new *epidemic* of the disease to occur.

2.2 EPIDEMIC THEORY AND INVESTIGATION

Epidemics can occur unexpectedly or regularly at certain times of the year.

Endemic means the continuous presence of an infection in the community. *Epidemic* means an excess of cases in the community from that normally expected or the appearance of a new infection. The point at which an endemic disease becomes epidemic depends on the usual presence of the disease and its rate. With an unusual disease two cases could be an epidemic, whereas with a common disease (such as gastroenteritis) an epidemic is when the usual rate of the disease is substantially exceeded.

Characteristics of an epidemic disease (Fig. 2.1) are as follows.

● *Latent period*, the time interval from initial infection until start of infectiousness.
● *Incubation period*, the time interval from initial infection until the onset of clinical disease. The incubation period varies from disease to disease and for a particular disease has a *range*. This range extends from a *minimum* incubation period to a *maximum* incubation period (see Section 19.1).
● *Period of communicability*, the period during which an individual is infectious. The infectious period can start before the disease process commences (e.g. hepatitis) or after (e.g. sleeping sickness). In some

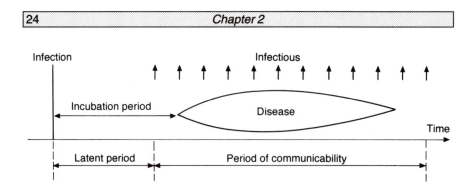

Fig. 2.1. Parameters of an infection (see text for definitions).

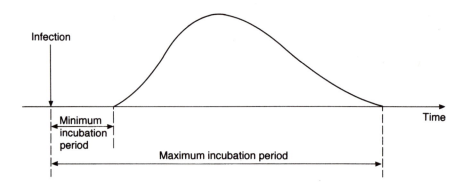

Fig. 2.2. Distribution curve of incubation times (the epidemic curve).

diseases, such as diphtheria and streptococcal infections, infectiousness starts from the date of first exposure.

Various factors modify the incubation period so that if it is plotted on a time-scale the graph rises rapidly to a peak and then tails off over a longer period (Fig. 2.2). The infecting dose, the portal of entry, the immune response of the host and a number of other factors modify the normal distribution to extend the tail of the graph. By using a log time-scale this skewed curve can be converted to a normal distribution and the mean incubation period can be measured.

An epidemic can be either a *common-source* or a *propagated-source* epidemic (Fig. 2.3).

● Common-source epidemics can further be divided into a *point-source* epidemic resulting from a single exposure, such as a food-poisoning episode, or an *extended* epidemic resulting from repeated multiple exposures over a period of time (e.g. a contaminated well).

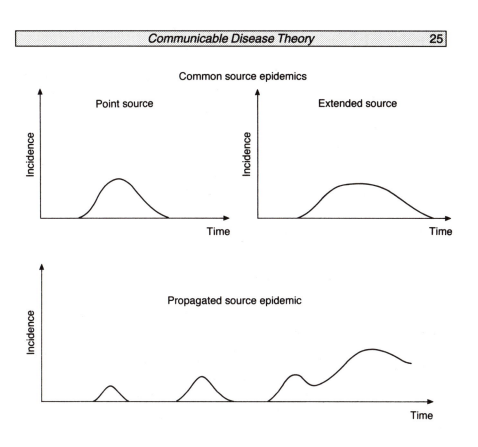

Fig. 2.3. Epidemic types.

● In a propagated–source epidemic the agent is spread through serial transfer from host to host. With a disease having a reasonably long incubation period, the initial peaks will be separated by the median incubation periods. Chickenpox (varicella) can start as an epidemic in one school; then mingling of children will lead to transfer to another school, leading to a series of propagated epidemics.

2.2.1 Investigation of a Common-source Epidemic

In the investigation of any outbreak of a disease the basic approach is to gather information on the following.

1. *Persons*: age, sex, occupation, ethnic group, etc., comparing the number infected with the population at risk.
2. *Place*: country, district, town, village, household and relationship to geographical features, such as roads, rivers, forests, etc. – conveniently marked on a map.

3. *Time*: annual, monthly (seasonal), day and hour (nocturnal/diurnal). The number of cases occurring within each time-period is plotted on a graph. These aspects will be covered in greater detail later.

In a *point-source* epidemic the number of cases of the disease occurring each day is plotted on a graph to produce an epidemic curve. The earliest cases will be those with the minimum incubation period and the last those with the maximum incubation period if all were infected at a single point in time, as illustrated in Fig. 2.4. So knowing the incubation period can indicate the time of infection and indicate the possible source.

Three factors describe a point-source epidemic.

- The epidemic curve.
- The incubation period of the disease.
- The time of infection.

If only two of these factors are known, the third can be deduced. From the epidemic curve, the median (or geometric mean) of the incubation periods is determined. If the disease is known from its clinical features, the incubation period will also be known (Section 19.1). So, measuring this known incubation period back in time from the median incubation period on the curve or the minimum incubation period from the beginning of the curve, the time of infection can be calculated. The source, now localized to a restricted period of time, can be more easily investigated.

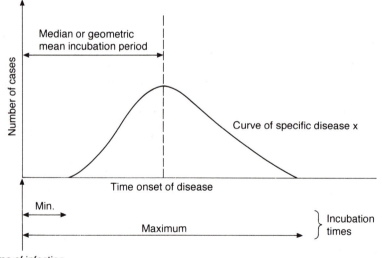

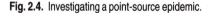

Fig. 2.4. Investigating a point-source epidemic.

If the disease is unknown but there is evidence of the time of infection (e.g. a particular event in time that brought all the cases together or linked them by a common phenomenon), the incubation period can be calculated and a disease (or aetiological agent producing a disease) with this incubation period suspected. This method was used to work out the incubation period for the first epidemic of ebola haemorrhagic fever, as there were a large number of fatal cases that occurred in one hospital at the same time.

In an *extended*-source epidemic, the time of infection can be deduced by measuring back in time from the first case on the rising epidemic curve to the maximum and minimum incubation periods of the diagnosed disease. Search within this defined period of time can elucidate the source.

Epidemics are suitably described by expressing them in *attack rates*. In a common-source epidemic, the *overall attack rate* is used.

$$\text{Overall attack rate} = \frac{\text{Number of individuals affected during an epidemic}}{\text{Number (of susceptible) exposed to the risk}}$$

2.2.2 Investigation of Propagated-source Epidemics

With a propagated-source epidemic, phases of infection occur at regular intervals. The time-period between these phases is called the *serial*

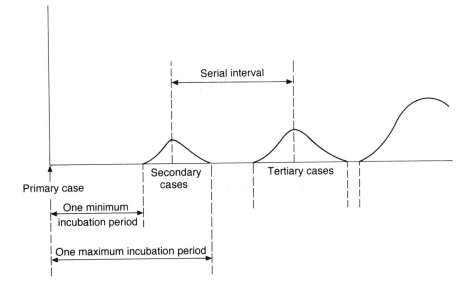

Fig. 2.5. Investigation of a propagated-source epidemic.

interval (Fig. 2.5). Contagiousness or the probability that an exposure will lead to a transmission is measured by:

$$\text{Secondary attack rate} = \frac{\begin{array}{c}\text{Number of cases within one minimum}\\ \text{and one maximum incubation period}\\ \text{(secondary cases) from the primary case}\end{array}}{\text{Number (of susceptible) exposed to the risk}}$$

2.2.3 Dynamics of Epidemics

The increase in cases in an epidemic has given rise to a measure called the *basic reproduction rate*. This measures the mean number of subsequent cases of an infection from a single case in an unlimited, wholly susceptible population. For example, if one case gave rise to two and these two to four, etc., as illustrated in Fig. 2.6, the basic reproduction rate would be 2. This is the most extreme situation. In reality the epidemic is modified by immunity, or the population limited by people having

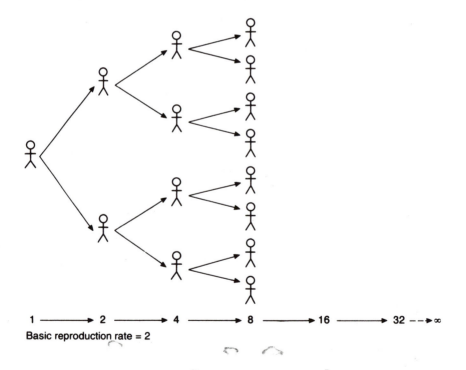

1 ──────▶ 2 ──────▶ 4 ──────▶ 8 ──────▶ 16 ──────▶ 32 --▶ ∞

Basic reproduction rate = 2

Fig. 2.6. Basic reproduction rate increasing – i.e. > 1. Maximal transmission: every infection produces a new case.

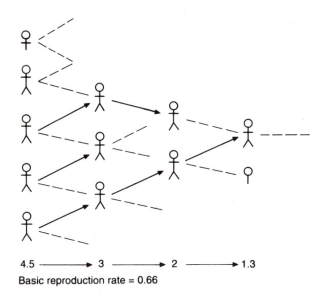

4.5 ──────► 3 ──────► 2 ──────► 1.3

Basic reproduction rate = 0.66

Fig. 2.7. Basic reproduction rate decreasing – i.e. < 1. Unsustained transmission: each transmission gives rise to less than one new case and the infection dies out.

already become infected, so such a rapid rate of increase does not occur. If the basic reproduction rate is less than 1, as illustrated in Fig. 2.7, the epidemic will not take off. The importance of this concept is in control, whereby, if the case reproduction rate can be reduced below 1 the disease will die out.

2.2.4 Population Size

As mentioned above, the continuation of an epidemic is determined by the number of susceptibles remaining in the population. Once an individual has experienced an episode of the disease (whether manifest or not), he/she may develop immunity (either temporary or permanent) or die. When a certain number of individuals have developed immunity, there are insufficient susceptibles and the infection dies out. This collective permanent immunity (as occurs in viral infections) is called the *herd immunity*. After a period of time, depending on the size of the population, this herd immunity becomes diluted by new individuals being born (or by immigration) and a new epidemic can take place. This is called the *critical population* (the theoretical minimum host population size required to maintain an infecting agent). It depends upon the infectious agent, the demographic structure and the conditions (hygiene, etc.) of the host population. In Third World countries with their high birth rates, the critical population is less than in developed countries. Examples of the critical human population size are for measles 500,000 and varicella 10,000.

If the population is less than the critical size, regular epidemics will occur at intervals related to the population size. An example is given in Fig. 13.2 of a measles epidemic which occurred regularly every 3 years in a well-defined community. These regular epidemics can be analysed in the same way as a propagated-source epidemic, from which it has been shown that the smaller the community, the longer is the interval between epidemics.

An extension of the concept of herd immunity shows that not everyone in a population needs to be vaccinated to prevent an epidemic. On the same principle as calculating the critical population, the *critical rate of vaccination coverage* can also be worked out, in other words the population that will need to be successfully vaccinated to reduce the population at risk below the epidemic threshold. It can similarly be shown that even if this target is not reached, the epidemic will be put off until a future date when the susceptible unvaccinated children will have grown older and therefore be able to cope with the infection better. This is illustrated in Fig. 13.2.

2.2.5 Investigating Food- and Water-borne Outbreaks

Case–control and cohort study methods can be used to investigate food- and water-borne outbreaks.

Case–control studies

An example of the use of a case–control study in a cholera investigation is given where fish were suspected to contain the aetiological agent. In this community people preferred to eat fish marinated but uncooked. Cases were interviewed as to whether they ate raw fish and compared with a similar group who had not had the disease. The results are set out in a two-by-two table. There was a significant finding: χ^2 50.47; $P < 0.001$.

A reasonable estimate of the *relative risk* can be arrived at (as the incidence rates are not known) from the two-by-two table, using the odds ratio: *ad/cb*. In the example, the relative risk of contracting cholera after eating raw fish is:

$$\frac{31 \times 60}{3 \times 8} = 77.5$$

	Cases	Controls	Total
Ate raw fish	31	8	39
Did not eat raw fish	3	60	63
Total	34	68	102

Suspected cause	Cases	Controls
Present	a	b
Absent	c	d

Cohort studies

A cohort is a group of people exposed to an aetiological agent. By following this group over time, the risk of developing disease can be measured. A modification of the technique can be used in outbreak investigation, particularly food poisoning. This compares the attack rate in the persons exposed to the factor with the attack rate in those not exposed to the factor. In a food-poisoning outbreak where various foods are suspected, the attack rates in those eating and not eating the range of foods can be compared. This is best illustrated by using an example. In Table 2.1, most of the relative risk values are about 1, but there is over four times the risk of becoming ill if you ate fish, so the

Table 2.1. Food-specific attack rates and the relative risks of eating different foods. Meal eaten by 152 persons.

Food item	Ate			Did not eat			
	Ill	Well	Attack rate (%)	Ill	Well	Attack rate (%)	Relative risk
Rice	115	28	80.4	45	4	55.5	1.4
Potatoes	111	31	78.2	9	1	90.0	0.9
Fish	93	22	80.9	17	30	18.9	4.3
Beans	101	29	77.7	16	6	72.7	1.1
Coconut	86	22	79.6	24	20	54.5	1.5
Bananas	109	32	77.3	10	1	90.9	0.8

investigator would suspect fish as being the most likely cause. (For a fuller description of epidemiological methods see Vaughan and Morrow (1989) *Manual of Epidemiology for District Health Management.*)

2.3 ENDEMICITY

An endemic disease implies that there is a constant rate of infection occurring in the community. As new individuals are born, they become infected, either retaining the infection for life, being cured (including self-cure) or becoming immune. Prevalence rates will measure the level of endemicity as it applies to the community.

While it is useful to compare prevalence from one community to another, on more careful investigation it will be found that within a community prevalence rates vary. These areas of increased prevalence within a community are called foci. Two types of foci occur.

- *Host focality*, where some individuals have more severe infection than others, e.g. worm load in schistosomiasis.
- *Geographical focality*, where certain localities have a higher prevalence rate than others. Malaria exhibits geographical focality.

These concepts are important in control strategy. When a control method is applied equally to a community, the overall decrease in disease will leave the foci to maintain infection. However, if the foci are identified and treated, the infectious source is contained (Fig. 2.8).

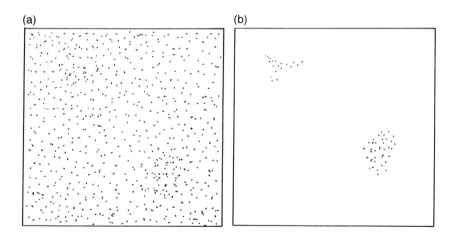

Fig. 2.8. The focality of endemic disease. (a) A universally homogeneous prevalence rate is measured in an area. (b) Once control measures have been implemented, foci of persistent transmission are revealed.

2.4 QUANTITATIVE DYNAMICS

Estimates of the magnitude of the infectious process or the degree of control likely to be achieved can be calculated. As an introduction to quantitative dynamics, examples of helminth infections are used.

2.4.1 Hookworm

Consider a family of five people, with four out of the five infected with hookworms producing on average some 4000 eggs g^{-1} of faeces. Approximately 200 g of faeces are voided by the average person per day so the four people are excreting $4 \times 4000 \times 200 = 3.2 \times 10^6$ eggs per day. If each of these eggs resulted in a viable larva, the potential for infection would be astronomical.

If the head of the household is now persuaded to install a latrine and encourages his/her family to use it, hopefully there should be no further contamination of the surroundings and infection will decrease as the worms die off. Unfortunately the youngest child does not understand how to use a latrine and, despite being taken to it by the mother, half of the stools are still deposited indiscriminately around the neighbourhood. This results in 100 (g) × 4000 (eggs) = 4×10^5 eggs deposited, which means that the potential for infecting the rest of the family has hardly altered. (This is a simplistic example implying that the eggs will still be concentrated where infection is most likely to occur.)

2.4.2 Schistosomiasis

An idealized situation is illustrated in Fig. 2.9. Ten people with schistosomiasis are all potential polluters of a body of water. Each gram of faeces might contain 80 eggs, but if only half of them reach the water there are still 40×200 (an average stool specimen is 200 g) = 8×10^3 eggs per person or 8×10^4 eggs from all ten people reaching the water every day. The miracidium that hatches from the egg needs to find a host snail to complete its development. Snails can reproduce rapidly so that one snail can produce a colony in 40 days and be infective in 60. The numbers of cercaria liberated from a snail are immense, but because they need to find a human host within 24 hours (generally less) few are successful. The ten people entering the water at the other side of the picture could all become infected, but in reality only a proportion are likely to be so.

When control is considered, there is the choice of preventing pollution of the water, destroying the snails or preventing water contact. (There is also mass treatment of the population which will reduce the total egg load, but for the present argument it will not be discussed here.)

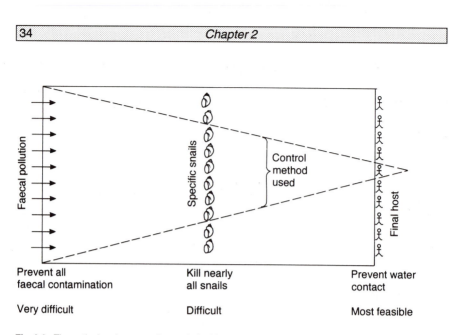

Faecal pollution

Specific snails

Control
method
used

Final host

| Prevent all
faecal contamination | Kill nearly
all snails | Prevent water
contact |
| Very difficult | Difficult | Most feasible |

Fig. 2.9. Theoretical environmental control of schistosomiasis.

If latrines were provided and nine out of the ten people used them, there would still be 8×10^3 eggs from the tenth person going into the water, sufficient to maintain almost the same level of snail infections. If all the snails were destroyed except a few, within 60 days the situation would return to what it was before. However, if any one of the ten people could be prevented from making contact with the water, his/her freedom from infection would be absolute.

Of course, the situation is never as clear-cut as this, but the illustration is made to show that a sanitation or molluscicide programme needs to be virtually perfect, whereas prevention from water contact can provide protection for the individual. This is a simplified example, but a more realistic situation can be simulated by the use of mathematical models.

Mathematical models will not be covered in any more detail, but some examples will be found in Part II, where they have been valuable for certain diseases. They are especially useful in determining control strategy, which is the subject of the next few chapters.

3

Control Principles and Strategy*

3.1 CONTROL PRINCIPLES

Control can be directed at either the agent, the transmission route, the host or the environment. Sometimes it is necessary to use several control strategies. The general methods of control are summarized in Fig. 3.1.

3.1.1 The Agent

Destruction of the agent can be by specific treatment, using drugs that kill the agent *in vivo*, or, if it is outside the body, by the use of antiseptics, sterilization, incineration or radiation.

3.1.2 Transmission Route

When the agent is attempting to travel to a host, it is more easily prevented, so more methods of control have been developed to interrupt transmission.

Quarantine or isolation

Keeping the agent at a sufficient distance and for a sufficient length of time away from the host until it dies or becomes inactive can be effective in preventing transmission. Quarantine or isolation can be used for animals as well as humans, more effective in the former because they can be forcibly restrained. Because it is difficult to quarantine humans, it is not widely practised as a method of control, except where the disease is

*For more details on reporting and surveillance see Vaughan, J.P. and Morrow, R. (1989), *Manual of Epidemiology for District Health Management*.

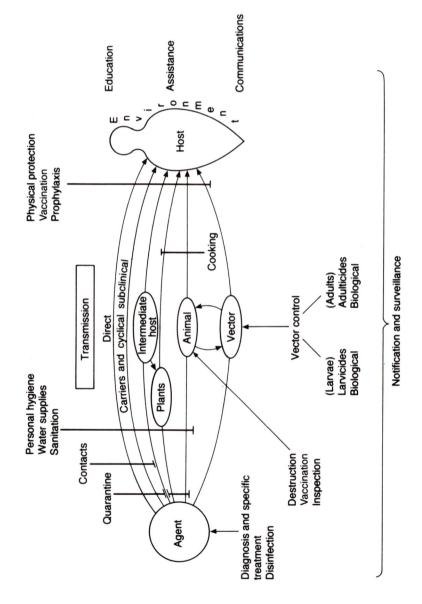

Fig. 3.1. Control principles.

very infectious or the patient can be restrained easily, e.g. in hospital (Lassa fever).

Contacts

People who might have become infected because of their close proximity to a case are called contacts. They can be isolated, given prophylactic treatment or kept under surveillance.

Environmental health

Methods of personal hygiene, water–supplies and sanitation are particularly effective against all agents transmitted by the faecal–oral route, whether by direct transmission or complex parasitic cycles involving intermediate hosts.

Animals

Whether they act as reservoirs or intermediate hosts, animals can be controlled by *destruction* or *vaccination* (e.g. against rabies). If animals are to be eaten, their carcasses can be *inspected* to make sure they are free of parasitic stages.

Cooking

Proper cooking renders plant and animal produce safe for consumption, but some toxins are heat-resistant.

Vector

Vector control is one of the most highly developed methods of interrupting transmission. This is because the parasite utilizes a vulnerable stage for development and transport. Attack on vectors can either be on their larval stage by using *larvicides* and methods of biological control or while they are adults with insecticides.

3.1.3 Host

The host can be protected by physical methods (mosquito nets, clothing, housing, etc.), by immunization against specific diseases, or by taking regular prophylaxis.

3.1.4 Environment

The environment of the host can be improved by education, assistance (agricultural advice, subsidies, loans, etc.) and improvement in communications (to market produce, reach health facilities, attend school, etc.). In time these will be the most effective methods of preventing continuation of the transmission cycle.

3.2 CONTROL STRATEGY

In any communicable disease outbreak the following sequence of events will need to be gone through.

- Identification of the cause (diagnosis).
- Notification.
- Treatment of cases.
- Interruption of transmission.
- Prevention of recurrence.
- Analysis and writing of a report.
- Surveillance.

These are not mutually exclusive stages and, although they are in order of action, several can be carried out at the same time. The cause must be identified and notified as soon as possible, but judgement needs to be used in spending time making an accurate diagnosis or starting treatment with the information that is available. There will be great pressure to treat cases, which is a necessary humanitarian action, but, until transmission is interrupted, more cases will occur. Once the disease is under control, methods must be implemented to prevent recurrence. Finally the outbreak is analysed and written up. A surveillance system is on the lookout for the first indications of the communicable disease starting again. These stages will be considered in more detail.

3.2.1 Identification and Investigation

Confirmation of diagnosis

As the agents of most communicable diseases are now known, a provisional diagnosis will probably have been made by the person reporting the illness. This must be confirmed by laboratory methods or by careful clinical judgement (e.g. measles). Relevant specimen containers and transport media will need to be taken by the investigator.

Normally the confirmation of diagnosis is a relatively easy matter, but several specimens may be required and restraint exercised in rushing to a diagnosis (e.g. in typhoid). Alternatively, it may be a unique and rare disease in which the aetiology and transmission have not been worked out. If this is the case, expert assistance is sought, while general principles of control are carried out.

Extent of infected cases

Enquiry and search is made to determine whether this is a unique case or there is an outbreak. Cases may be hidden or an exaggeration made to attract medical attention.

Progress

Is this the first case, or have there been several cases over a period of time? Have the cases come from another administrative area or country and is there a risk that they might infect other areas? Was notification received and should notification be given?

The epidemiological investigation

Collecting information on 'cause' and method of transmission utilizes the three pillars of epidemiology, *persons*, *place* and *time*. Information should be collected from as many angles and from as wide a field as possible. The more pointers there are to a method of transmission, the stronger will be the case.

It will generally not be possible to complete a detailed epidemiological investigation before starting some control methods, e.g. if it is diarrhoeal disease, emergency boiling of drinking-water can be started. However, the full investigation must be made and completed, as quite often different factors come to light. A full investigation will help prevent a recurrence.

The method used in an epidemiological search is as follows.

- Look for a common event that is shared by all the cases.
- Study exceptions to see if there are rational explanations.
- Base these findings on the population at risk.
- Elucidate changes that have occurred in the environment which may have favoured the outbreak (seasonal, population movements, etc.).
- Make a hypothesis of cause, route of transmission and method of control.

3.2.2 Treatment of Cases

The priority is to organize the treatment of cases rather than become involved in the clinical management. The important task is to investigate the outbreak and instigate control. This should be by the following means.

- Setting up emergency treatment centres or arranging transport of cases to hospital.
- Mobilization of staff, medicines and equipment according to need.
- Formulation of a standard treatment schedule.
- Making rules on period of quarantine, management of contacts, prevention of carriers and disposal of the dead.

3.2.3. Interruption of Transmission

Once a hypothesis of causation is made from the epidemiological investigation, a method of control is commenced. This can be in three different phases.

- Emergency.
- Specific.
- Long-term prevention.

If the communicable disease is in epidemic form and threatening a large number of people, emergency methods must be started as soon as possible. These are often non-specific and commenced before the detailed investigation has been finished. As an illustration of these three different strategies, an epidemic of dengue can be used. The emergency method would be a knock-down spray, such as fogging, which kills all adult mosquitoes indiscriminately. This will control the immediate problem but, once the number of adult mosquitoes builds up again, the epidemic might recommence. The specific method will be a programme selectively against the *Aedes* mosquito vector, by destroying all temporary breeding places and using larvicides in water containers. Long-term prevention will be by permanently altering breeding places, placing mosquito netting over essential water tanks, repairing broken guttering and all the techniques that are available for removing the mosquito permanently.

3.2.4 Analysis

A communicable-disease outbreak should be analysed in detail and written down as a report. This will be based on the investigations made, the control methods used and the outcome. Number of cases and deaths are items of information that authorities are particularly interested in. The functions of a report are:

- Inform planning and organizing authorities what has happened.
- Notify other workers who are or might soon be participating in a similar outbreak.
- Make a record to be referred to in future outbreaks.
- Provide information for the general public.
- Elicit funds for more permanent preventive measures.
- As an illustration for teaching purposes.
- If of an original nature, for the advancement of science.

3.2.5 Surveillance

Surveillance is the watching of the environment for any new diseases to appear and the monitoring of change in known diseases.

The key to surveillance is reporting, developed in such a way that an active watch is kept, not the desperate call of an established epidemic. Surveillance methods can be emergency, routine, passive or active.

Emergency

Emergency surveillance is set up during an outbreak to monitor special-risk areas such as contacts, bacteria counts, etc. Suspect cases or contacts should be kept under observation. Monitoring of treatment can detect the appearance of resistant organisms or an imbalance in the treatment regime. Utilization of staff and equipment can also be built into an emergency surveillance system.

Routine or passive

This can be most easily considered in the communicable disease model of *agent, transmission, host* and *environment.* Here are some examples.

- Antibiotic resistance patterns of agents. Checking the sensitivity of organisms to the antibiotics being used for treatment will indicate when resistance is occurring and the treatment regime needs to be changed.
- In transmission, the incidence of diarrhoea can indicate an impending outbreak or an increase in mortality the possibility that cholera might be present (see further in Section 8.6). With yellow fever the *Aedes aegypti* indexes will indicate whether transmission is likely to occur.
- Vaccine utilization will give an idea of the number of people

protected, but this can be improved by measuring the immune status of a sample of those vaccinated.

- Rainfall and temperature records will give information on seasonality and other environmental factors.

Active

This implies a deliberate activity to secure data. An example is active case detection in malaria surveillance, where a technician searches out malaria cases (see Fig. 4.2).

Reporting can be through:

- the basic health services;
- special sentinel units, e.g. public health laboratories;
- unipurpose workers, e.g. active case detection (ACD) technicians in malaria or leprosy field workers.
- statutory bodies, e.g. notification of births and deaths;
- allied disciplines, e.g. veterinary and entomology services;
- persons in authority, village leaders, schoolteachers, etc.

4

Control Organization

4.1 CONTROL AND ERADICATION

A communicable disease can be *controlled* or *eradicated*. By controlling a disease it is kept at such a minimum endemicity that it is no longer a health hazard. Eradication on the other hand sets out to eliminate the disease completely. The difference between control and eradication can be summarized as follows.

	Control	Eradication
Objective	Minimal incidence	Complete elimination
Duration	Indefinitely	Limited
Coverage	Areas of high incidence	Entire area
Method	Effective	Faultless
Reservoir	Animal or environment	Human only
Organization	Good	Perfect
Costs	Moderate for a long time	High for limited period
Complications	Acceptable	Extremely serious
Imported cases	Not important	Very important
Surveillance	Reasonable	Very good

Putting the entire health effort, funded by international support, into the eradication of a disease requires organization of the very highest order. During this century there have been three global eradication efforts, one successful, one almost successful and one not successful. The eradication of smallpox from the world has been one of public health's greatest triumphs against disease. This was only possible because the vaccine was extremely effective, there was no other reservoir but humans and the organization was very good. The global yaws campaign eradicated yaws from large areas of the world, but it is still endemic in some places and on the increase in others. The tremendous progress of the malaria eradication campaign only to be followed by an equally impressive resurgence of the disease has been a devastating set-back to the doctrine of eradication. (There have been other localized eradication programmes, such as *Anopheles gambiae* from South America, while poliomyelitis is being eradicated at this time.) With eradication it is an all-or-none process; if it is not completed, the disease can return to its former levels and all is wasted. In these circumstances, it is preferable to choose the alternative target of control, which will be the method used in the majority of infections.

4.2 CAMPAIGNS AND GENERAL PROGRAMMES

Communicable diseases can be controlled by special campaigns or made a function of the general health services. Special campaigns have the attraction of putting all the effort into one particular disease, often with considerable initial success, but over the long term they can break down. Integrating the control method with the general health services often gives a more consistent result. The advantages and disadvantages are as follows.

	Campaigns	General health services
Effectiveness	Initially very good	Only moderate
Continuation	Poor	Moderate
Duration	Short	Long
Staff	Special required	General health workers
Salary	Inflated	Average
Staff problems	No career structure	Addition to routine duties
Cost	High	Low
Integration	Low	High

It is the lack of integration of the campaign into the general health services that destroys the good progress made. There are difficulties over emphasis, staff absorption and resentment by the multipurpose worker. Campaign workers are often specially recruited for the task, probably from non-medical backgrounds, and are paid an inflated salary to offset the time-limited nature of the operation. The general health services are not used to dealing with the special disease and feel they are being given extra work, while still being paid the same. An alternative might be to use the general health services for a brief special effort, which can continue to be maintained in their routine services. An example is given in Section 5.1.6, where, knowing the epidemic pattern, the general health services were mobilized to do mass vaccination before the peak was expected. In the rest of the year they continued with the routine immunization programme.

4.3 CAMPAIGN PROGRAMME STAGES

During the malaria eradication campaigns, a high level of organizational methodology was developed, and it is useful to review this for developing a communicable-disease control service. The four stages are as follows.

- Preparatory.
- Attack phase.
- Consolidation.
- Maintenance.

4.3.1 Preparatory Stage

The preparatory stage is perhaps the most important and time spent on collecting baseline data, trying to forecast problems and assessing the feasibility of the proposal is always time well spent. A detailed survey of the disease endemicity will be required, perhaps preceded by a census. Maps are essential and if suitable ones are not available then they need to be drawn. They must contain up-to-date village locations, preferably with the population marked on them. Figure 4.1 is an example of a map prepared in this way.

Every level of society must be committed, from the senior administrative head, through divisional chiefs and influential people, to the established health worker. It is the people that are troubled by the disease and it is ultimately they who will decide what is to be done about it. Without their complete and continued cooperation, any special effort is doomed to failure.

Logistic planning of persons, money and materials is often the easiest part to initiate, but one of the most difficult to maintain. Utilizing existing staff, who retain all their usual functions and continue in an established pattern of service, is preferable to recruiting special staff. No disease control programme has remained within estimates; it nearly always costs more than expected. There are additions that were not foreseen, inflation increases faster than allowed for and the programme takes longer than planned. If adequate finances cannot be secured and the programme has to be abandoned, the net result is worse than doing nothing in the first

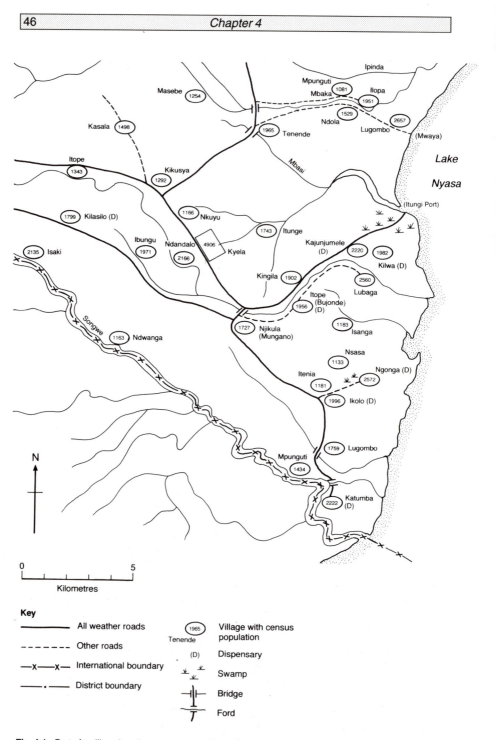

Fig. 4.1. Part of a village location map prepared for a disease control programme.

place. It is more serious to damage the existing health services by diverting funds from them.

Included in the preparatory stage is a *pilot programme* to try out the techniques and organization in a limited area. The pilot programme is a scaled-down version of the full programme, not a special effort to show what can be done. The area chosen should be fully representative of the larger area to be covered. If there are marked variations, several different pilot studies may be required.

The pilot programme can be for a set period of time or continued into the full programme after it has been assessed. If there are major difficulties, it should not proceed further until the whole strategy has been rethought. If there are minor problems, these are indicators of major problems in the future.

4.3.2 Attack Phase

In the attack phase, the method that was found to be effective in the pilot programme is extended to the whole area. Alternatively, it can be planned to cover the area in sequence, but this may not be possible if

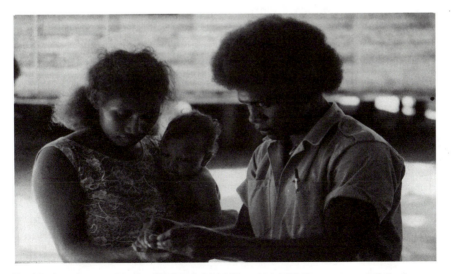

Fig. 4.2. An active case detection (ACD) technician taking a blood slide from a woman suffering from fever in a malaria eradication programme (St Isabel, Solomon Islands).

reinfection is likely to occur. Timetables and procedures are required to ensure that separate teams cover the area in a regular manner. Realistic targets are set and organization developed to make sure they are kept. The delay of one part will cause delay of everything else.

During the attack phase, the progress of the control method is assessed by making serial surveys. A randomizing technique similar to that of the baseline survey is used and the results are compared.

As control proceeds successfully, cases of the disease will become fewer, so an *active surveillance* system is required to search for the remaining cases (Fig. 4.2). A routine or passive surveillance system will have been established in the planning phase. Active surveillance is not a substitute for it, but the two systems should work closely together.

The attack phase is the most expensive part of the programme, so a definite target is set to signal completion. The objective is to reduce the number of cases to such a low level that, when the control method is removed, the disease will not recur. Once this stage has been reached, the control method is stopped and reliance placed on the surveillance services to detect remaining cases. The programme now enters the stage of consolidation.

4.3.3 Consolidation

In the consolidation phase, the full apparatus of disease reduction is disbanded and reliance placed on small specialist teams, who can rapidly respond to the active surveillance system. If a focus of malaria is found, focal spraying and radical treatment of cases are implemented. If yaws is suspected, mass penicillin injections are given in the surrounding area. The essence of the consolidation phase is speed and efficiency. If rapid remedial action cannot be carried out, the disease is liable to return.

4.4 CONTROL PROGRAMMES

In *control* the disease is reduced by the amount that funds and staff availability permit. This means that substantial reduction is not even attempted and no time-limit is set. This should not be regarded as an inferior technique, as a failed eradication programme would have wasted vast sums of money and would probably have left the population in a more vulnerable state. A limited control programme may be sufficient to reduce the burden of disease to allow a rise in the standard of living, which in the long term will have the most sustained effect on controlling the disease.

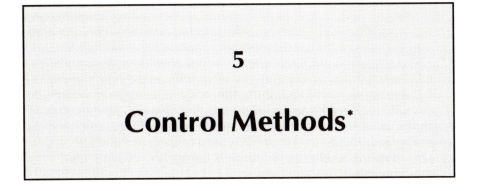

5

Control Methods*

The main methods of communicable disease control are *immunization, environmental methods* and *vector control.*

5.1 VACCINATION

5.1.1 Vaccines

The newborn baby carries antibodies transmitted from its mother across the placenta and from early breast-feeding, so protecting it at a very vulnerable stage in life. The effects of these antibodies wear off after 6 weeks to 6 months, so the baby starts making its own from natural or artificial infections that it acquires.

The immune system of the full-term newborn is capable of producing antibodies and mobilizing cellular defences. Bacillus Calmette–Guérin (BCG) and polio can be given shortly after birth and killed antigen vaccines can also work from the first month. Some live vaccines, such as measles, do not provide protection if given early because of circulating maternal antibodies.

Vaccines can be of four different kinds.

● *Live attenuated organisms* give the body an actual infection, inducing antibody production. This is the best kind of vaccine as it generates maximal response from a single dose and as a consequence immunity

*For details on the various methods of protecting and improving water-supplies, the reader is referred to Cairncross, S. and Feachem, R. (1978) *Small Water Supplies,* Ross Institute, London. Further details on the construction and siting of sanitary facilities will be found in Cairncross, S. (1988) *Small Scale Sanitation,* Ross Institute, London.

is long-lasting. The danger with live attenuated vaccines is that the organisms could revert to the virulent strain. Examples are measles and oral poliomyelitis (polio), which are attenuated virus infections, and BCG, which is an attenuated bacterium.

- *Killed organisms* are used when it is not possible to produce a live attenuated strain. Immunity does not develop so well and the vaccine has to be repeated to induce the body defence mechanisms to increase their response. An example is pertussis (whooping cough).
- *Active components* can be separated from organisms and vaccines made from these. Good immunity is produced, but they are expensive to manufacture. An example is hepatitis B vaccine, which is a viral antigen (HBsAg).
- *Toxoids* are detoxified bacterial exotoxins and are an important way of producing antibodies to bacterial toxins. They do not prevent the infection, but they counteract the dangerous effects of the toxin. Like killed organisms, several doses have to be given to induce a sufficient antibody response and booster doses repeated from time to time to maintain the level. Diphtheria and tetanus toxoid are two vaccines in this category.

5.1.2 Vaccine Schedules

The type of vaccine and the age of risk of developing the target disease determine the optimum time and schedule for giving each vaccine. The characteristics of the principal vaccine-preventable diseases (included in the EPI (Expanded Programme of Immunization) programme in most developing countries) are as follows.

Tetanus

Tetanus can enter the neonate through an infected umbilical cord, producing a high mortality. Protection is by immunizing women with tetanus toxoid. This protection is short-lived and the child should be given tetanus toxoid early in infancy (diphtheria, pertussis and tetanus (DPT)). Toxoid is also given to adults as a course of three immunizations to prevent tetanus or, if not so protected, when there is a wound which could possibly be infected with *Clostridium tetani*. The World Health Organization (WHO) policy is to vaccinate all women of childbearing age, with a lifetime total of five doses of tetanus toxoid.

Tuberculosis

The maximum age risk of tuberculosis depends on the prevalence of active infection in the community. Where there are many open cases, even small children are at risk, but, in a society where most cases are in older people and individuals do not contact many others until they start work in young adulthood, the period of greatest risk is adolescence. In many developing countries open tuberculosis is widespread, and old and young mix more in large joint families. Early protection is given by immunization at birth, preferably with repeat doses at school entry.

Whooping cough

Whooping-cough (pertussis) is a serious disease of young children, with often a fatal outcome in those less than 6 months. Vaccination must start before this time, preferably at 1 month or soon after, to produce a sufficient level of antibodies.

Diphtheria

Diphtheria, is a dangerous disease at any age, so it is preferable to start protection early. Diphtheria, pertussis and tetanus are normally combined in a triple vaccine (DPT), given at monthly intervals in early childhood, after the first month of age.

Poliomyelitis

Poliomyelitis infection is by three different strains of virus. The oral vaccine (OPV) contains all three attenuated strains of the virus, but the gut may not be infected by three strains at the same time and three doses are required to ensure protection. In developing countries, where wild polio virus is circulating, the first dose is given as soon after birth as possible, followed by three other doses at the same time as DPT. In the WHO global eradication programme, mass immunization, regardless of previous immunization, is given to all children under 5 (two doses at an interval of 4 weeks), followed by 'mopping up' in areas of low coverage or where continuing transmission is identified. Inactivated polio vaccine (IPV) is favoured in many developed countries, but is more expensive and produces less herd immunity.

Measles

Measles is one of the most important causes of childhood death and disability in the tropics. It reaches maximal prevalence by the end of the first year of life, but many children will already have been infected by 6 months. Maternal antibodies do not diminish sufficiently until 6 months for the attenuated virus to be effective, so the optimal time for immunization is 9 months.

Different vaccines can be combined, such as DPT, or can be given together, e.g. DPT and polio. A sufficient interval must be left between doses to allow time for the antibody response to take place. One month is normally sufficient. All these factors and the national characteristics of a country will determine the immunization pattern to be followed. A suggested regime is as follows.

Before birth	Tetanus toxoid to all women of childbearing age
Birth	BCG plus polio
1–2 months	DPT plus polio
2–3 months	DPT plus polio
3–6 months	DPT plus polio
9 months	Measles

DPT and polio vaccine can be given even if the child has a mild illness. Measles vaccine can also be given if the child has a mild illness, as it does not have any effect for several days, by which time the minor illness will have finished. Vaccination should always be given to the malnourished child, who is at particular risk from infection. Protective response is good except in cases of severe kwashiorkor.

5.1.3 Operational Factors

In planning vaccination programmes, cultural, logistic and other operational factors largely determine the coverage. Some of these are as follows.

- The strongest motivation to attend maternal and child health (MCH) clinics is immediately after the child has been born, so the shorter the interval between birth and vaccination, the more likely is it that children will be brought by their mothers.
- A range of ages, days and combinations should be available so that the time of attendance is always the right time for vaccination. If a mother is told to bring her child back at a set time or at a specific age of the child, she probably will not bother.
- Admission to hospital is an ideal opportunity to check that the vaccination schedule is up to date. Measles vaccination is particularly important as many children contract serious measles when admitted to hospital for another complaint.
- A primary course need never be repeated, even if the booster dose is long delayed.
- An interrupted course can be resumed whenever feasible without starting from the beginning again.
- If the interval between doses ends up being longer than planned,

the immunological effect will not be reduced. The only disadvantage to long-drawn-out schedules is that the individual is not rapidly protected.

5.1.4 The Cold Chain

The cold chain is a descriptive term for the whole sequence of links that must be maintained in transporting the vaccine in a viable condition from the manufacturer to the person to be immunized. Vaccines will only survive when they are maintained at the correct temperature. There are certain limits when the vaccine can be allowed to depart from the optimal temperature, but the range and time are very short and vaccines rapidly lose their potency. To immunize with non-potent vaccine is not only a waste of time and money but also brings discredit upon the vaccination programme.

Some vaccines are stored at freezing temperature (poliomyelitis, BCG and measles), while others are at the standard refrigerator temperature of 4–8°C, (DPT and tetanus). If stored at the wrong temperature, the vaccine will be destroyed. The two elements of the cold chain are speed of transport and maintenance of a steady temperature. The fastest means of getting a vaccine from one place to another is used. It is collected as soon as it arrives at its destination and placed in a refrigerator. Most vaccine batches are accompanied by a temperature-sensitive strip, which changes colour if they have become too warm. The viability of the vaccine can then be checked and the problem link in the cold chain detected.

Cold boxes are very well insulated containers lined with freezer packs, in which vaccines can be transported or stored for up to 7 days. They are valuable for mobile vaccination teams. For the individual vaccinator, a hand-held vacuum flask will store vaccines for 1–2 days, depending on the outside temperature.

Certain vaccines, such as measles and BCG, are sensitive to light and need to be protected while they are being diluted, stored and given to the person. Special dark glass syringes can be obtained, but covering with a cloth is just as efficient. Many potent vaccines are destroyed by being drawn up into syringes that are still warm from the sterilizing process, a sad end to a long cold chain.

5.1.5 Mobile and Static Clinics

Vaccination can be from static and/or mobile clinics. Their various advantages and disadvantages are as follows.

	Static	Mobile
Coverage	Limited to 10 km radius	Large areas
Availability	Always	Occasional
Transport	Not required	Required
Costs	High capital, low recurrent costs	Moderate capital, high recurrent costs
Vaccine supplies	Often erratic	Good

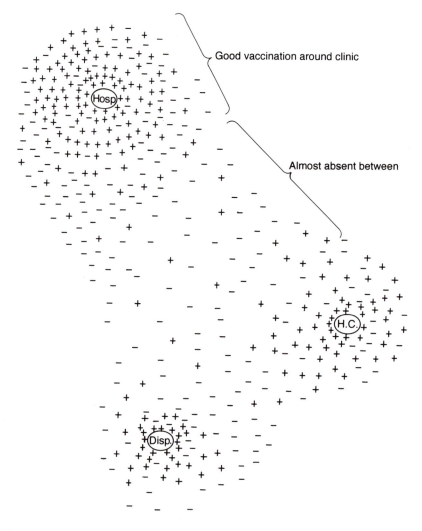

Good vaccination around clinic

Almost absent between

Fig. 5.1. Unequal vaccination coverage from static clinics. +, Vaccinated child; –, non-vaccinated child; HOSP., hospital; H.C., health centre; DISP., dispensary.

A static clinic responsible for providing primary care services (including delivery) for both the mother and the child is the most effective. A child stands a greater chance of receiving all its vaccines from a static health unit. However, as the distance from a clinic increases, the probability of a mother bringing her child to the clinic decreases for every kilometre to be walked. Coverage is best closest to the clinic and decreases further away, with often large gaps between clinics, as shown in Fig. 5.1. It is the inadequately covered areas between the static clinics where an epidemic is likely to occur. Outreach services or mobile clinics then become valuable in vaccinating the in-between areas.

Mobile clinics are easier to organize where only one dose of vaccine is required (e.g. measles), but have a special place in poliomyelitis vaccination programmes, where a mass campaign can reduce wild virus.

5.1.6 Seasonality and Vaccination Campaigns

Many infections follow a seasonal pattern with sufficient regularity for peaks of incidence to be forecast. If these are known, the epidemic can be averted by carrying out a mass vaccination before it is expected (see Fig. 1.7).

5.1.7 Ring Vaccination

If an epidemic is spreading, it can be contained by vaccinating everyone in a ring round the site of the epidemic. Villages should be chosen where cases have not yet been reported and an attempt made to vaccinate as many people as possible. If the ring is too close to the epidemic, the disease may already have affected some people outside the defensive ring and then another will need to be started even further away.

5.1.8 Economies of Vaccination

Vaccination coverage is often poor because of constraints put on staff about the cost of vaccines. Vaccines should be supplied in small dose quantities so that a vial can be opened even if there is only one child to be vaccinated. Spare vaccine can often be used up on other children attending the health centre for other reasons. The cost of vaccination is not just the price of the actual vial of vaccine but includes the whole cold chain and the salary of the vaccinator. To have a vaccinator sitting around not vaccinating because there are not enough children to warrant opening a vial is a false economy. Proportional costs have been calculated as follows.

Capital	12–15%	Transport	20%
Salaries	45%	Vaccine	5%
Training	2–3%	Other	12–16%

5.1.9 Vaccine Efficacy

Vaccine efficacy is calculated by:

$$\text{Vaccine efficacy (VE)} = \frac{(\text{Attack rate in unvaccinated} - \text{attack rate in vaccinated})}{\text{Attack rate in unvaccinated}} \times 100\%$$

(Attack rate is discussed in Section 2.2.1.) The vaccine efficacy indicates the maximum achievable level, but poor vaccination technique or storage can reduce this. Also, the more people that are vaccinated, the greater the number of apparent vaccine failures. The above equation can be rewritten to express the percentage of cases vaccinated (PCV) in terms of the percentage of the population vaccinated (PPV) and vaccine efficacy (VE);

$$PCV = \frac{PPV - (PPV \times VE)}{1 - (PPV \times VE)}$$

By knowing two of these variables, the third can be calculated. Figure 5.2 shows three curves generated from the equation, each for a different vaccine efficacy. These curves predict the theoretical proportion of cases with a vaccine history. For example, if a measles epidemic is observed in a population with homogeneous measles exposure where 90% of the individuals are vaccinated (PPV = 90%) with a 90% effective vaccine (VE = 90%), the expected percentage of measles cases with a history of being vaccinated would be 47% (PCV = 47%; Example A). However, if only 50% were vaccinated, then 9% of the cases would be found to have been vaccinated (Example B). This is not to say that there is anything wrong with the vaccination programme, but explains why there may appear to be an unexpected number of vaccinated among the cases.

More details on vaccination will be found under the relevant disease in Part II.

5.2 ENVIRONMENTAL CONTROL METHODS

Many diseases result from contamination of the environment. Transmission can be direct (e.g. by fingers) or via food and water. The

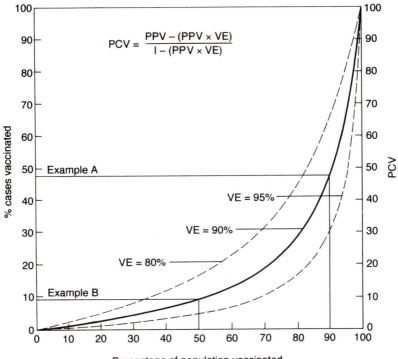

$$PCV = \frac{PPV - (PPV \times VE)}{1 - (PPV \times VE)}$$

Fig. 5.2. Percentage of cases vaccinated (PCV) per percentage of population vaccinated (PPV), for three values of vaccine efficacy (VE). Reproduced by permission from *Weekly Epidemiological Record* 7, 20 February 1981. World Health Organization, Geneva.

mechanisms are schematically illustrated in Fig. 5.3. The various control methods available are as follows.

- Personal and domestic hygiene.
- The proper preparation, cooking and storage of food.
- Use of water supplies.
- Proper disposal of excreta and waste.
- Miscellaneous methods, including meat inspection and protection from insects.

Classifying the water- and sanitation-related diseases into well-defined categories allows rational control methods to be applied (Table 5.1). The potential impact of control methods is seen in Table 5.2.

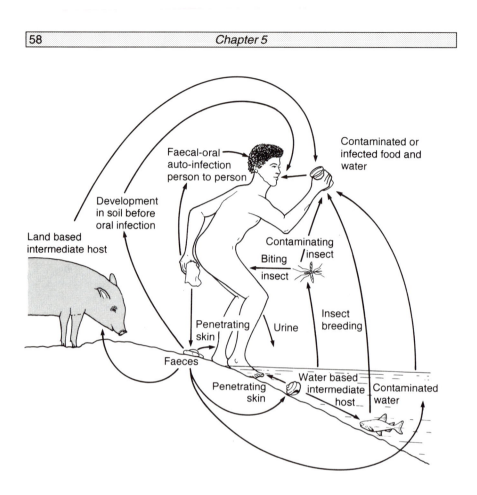

Fig. 5.3. Routes of transmission of the water- and sanitation-related diseases.

5.2.1 Personal Hygiene

Personal hygiene is the understanding by the individual of how infections can be transmitted to them or others by unclean habits and using appropriate methods to avoid them. Infection can be avoided by preventing bad habits, e.g. failing to use a latrine, or introducing good habits, e.g. hand washing before eating. Infections that can be reduced by personal hygiene are shown on p. 61.

Category 1 diseases are reduced by washing of the body and clothes, using copious quantities of water, which is best heated, with the addition of soap if available. Categories 2 and 3 diseases are reduced by rigorous hand washing after defecation and before eating.

Personal hygiene is closely related to the availability of water in sufficient quantity. Water quality is of less importance. Washing is improved by using warm water and soap solutions, which reduce surface

Table 5.1. A classification of water- and excreta-related diseases.

Category	Characteristics	Examples	Transmission	Control measures
1. Water-washed disease	Diseases of poor hygiene	Skin diseases, eye diseases, louse-borne typhus	Person to person (and autoinfection)	Personal hygiene Increase water quantity
2. Faecal–oral diseases	a. Low infective dose	*Enterobius*, amoebiasis, enteric viruses	Person to person (and autoinfection)	Increase water quantity Personal hygiene
	b. High infective dose. Able to multiply outside host	Diarrhoeal diseases, cholera, typhoid, hepatitis A	Contamination of food or water	Excreta disposal Cook food Improve water quality
3. Soil-mediated diseases (helminths)	a. Development in soil	*Ascaris*, Hookworm, *Strongyloides*	Larvae penetrate skin or swallowed	Personal hygiene Excreta disposal
	b. Development in animal (cow or pig) intermediate host	*Taenia* spp.	Cysts in meat	Meat inspection Cooked food
4. Water-based diseases	Helminths requiring intermediate hosts			
	a. Copepods	Guinea worm	Ingested in water	Improve water quality
	b. Snails only	Schistosomiasis	Penetrates skin	Reduce water contact
	c. Two intermediate hosts	*Fasciolopsis, Opisthorchis, Paragonimus, Diphyllobothrium*	Eating uncooked specific foods	Excreta disposal Cook food
5. Water- and excreta-related insect vectors	a. Breeding in water or sewage	Malaria, filariasis, arboviruses	Mosquitoes	Drain breeding sites Maintain water supplies and sanitation
	b. Breeding or biting near water	Onchocerciasis Trypanosomiasis	*Simulium* Tsetse fly	Water supply at site of use
	c. Breeding in excreta	Diarrhoeal diseases	Housefly	Excreta disposal

(Modified from Bradley, D.J. (1978), in Feachem, R.G. *et al.* (eds) *Water, Wastes and Health in Hot Climates.* Reprinted by permission of John Wiley & Sons Ltd, Chichester.)

Table 5.2. The potential impact of environmental control methods (compare with Table 5.1).

Disease category	Personal hygiene	Cooking of foods	Water supplies	Sanitation	Miscellaneous
1. Water-washed diseases	+++	–	++	+	–
2. Faecal–oral diseases	+++	+	++	+	–
3. Soil-mediated diseases	++	+++	–	+++	Meat inspection
4. Water-based diseases	–	+++	++	+	Reduce water contact
5. Water- and excreta-related insect vectors	–	–	±±	±±	Protection from insects

+++, Very effective; ++, moderately effective; +, effective; –, not effective; ±, can be either effective or not effective.

tension and emulsify oils, allowing bacteria to be more easily removed. However, large quantities of water can still be effective in the absence of soap.

Infections that can be reduced by personal hygiene

Category	Infection
1	Skin sepsis and ulcers
1	Conjunctivitis
1	Trachoma
1	Scabies
1	Yaws
1	Leprosy
1	*Tinea*
1	Louse-borne fevers
1	Flea-borne infections (including plague)
2	Enteric viruses (including hepatitis A and polio)
2	*Enterobius*
2	Amoebiasis
2	*Trichuris*
2	*Giardia*
2	*Shigella*
2	Typhoid
2	Other salmonellae
2	*Campylobacter*
2	Non-specific diarrhoeal diseases
2	Cholera
2	Leptospirosis
3a	*Ascaris*

5.2.2 Protection of Foods

Food-transmitted infections can spread through either contamination or the specific intermediate host. Flies indirectly contaminate food.

Protection of the food we eat can be by the following.

- Inspection of raw produce.
- Packaging and avoiding contamination.
- Suitable storage conditions and time–limits.
- Washing and correct preparation.
- Adequate and even cooking.
- Preventing contamination of cooked foods.
- Eating cooked foods immediately.

Reduction of Infection by food protection

Category	Infection	Type of food	Possible reduction by cooking and storage
2	Enteric viruses (including hepatitis A and polio)	All	+
2	*Hymenolepis*	All	+
2	Amoebiasis	All	+
2	*Trichuris*	All	+
2	*Giardia*	All	+
2	*Shigella*	All, especially dairy produce	++
2	Typhoid	All, especially dairy produce	++
2	Salmonellae	All, espeically dairy produce	++
2	*Campylobacter*	All, especially dairy produce	++
2	Non-specific diarrhoeal diseases	All, plus fly contamination	++
2	Cholera	Marine animals, salad	++
2	Leptospirosis	Rat-contaminated foods	++
2	Brucellosis	Milk produce	++
3a	*Ascaris*	All	+
3b	*Taenia*	Cow or pig meat	+++
4b	*Trichinella*	Pig	+++
4c	*Fasciolopsis*	Salad	+++
4c	*Opisthorchis*	Fish (freshwater)	+++
4c	*Paragonimus*	Crustacea (freshwater)	+++
4c	*Diphyllobothrium*	Fish (freshwater)	+++

Category 2 infections contaminate food before or after cooking. Flies are often involved. Even if contamination has occurred, correct storage and the disposal of cooked foods after a limited time can prevent sufficient multiplication of bacteria to reach an infective dose.

Categories 3b and 4c require specific intermediate hosts in their transmission, so their destruction or proper cooking is an effective means of control. Meat inspection is effective in *Taenia* infections (3b). Cooking needs to be at a sufficiently high temperature to kill off the intermediate stages, and procedures such as roasting on a spit or cooking meat 'underdone' do not provide high enough temperatures inside the meat.

5.2.3 Water Supplies

Contaminated water can be the vehicle of transmission of a number of disease-producing organisms. Water is also important in diseases of poor hygiene, as a medium for intermediate hosts and as a breeding place for vectors of disease.

The infections and possible improvements that may occur from installing a water supply are as follows.

Category	Infection	Water improvement required	Possible reduction produced (%)
1	Skin sepsis and ulcers	Increase water quantity	50
1	Conjunctivitis	Increase water quantity	70
1	Trachoma	Increase water quantity	60
1	Scabies	Increase water quantity	80
1	Yaws	Increase water quantity	70
1	Leprosy	Increase water quantity	50
1	*Tinea*	Increase water quantity	50
1	Louse-borne fevers	Increase water quantity	40
1	Flea-borne diseases (including plague)	Increase water quantity	40
2	Enteric viruses (including hepatitis A and polio)	Increase water quantity	10?
2	*Enterobius*	Increase water quantity	20
2	*Hymenolepis*	Increase water quantity	20
2	Amoebiasis	Increase water quantity	50
2	*Trichuris*	Increase water quantity	20
2	*Giardia*	Increase water quantity	30
2	*Shigella*	Improve water quality	50
2	Typhoid	Improve water quality	80
2	Other salmonellae	Improve water quality	50
2	*Campylobacter*	Improve water quality	50
2	Non-specific diarrhoeal diseases	Improve water quality	50
2	Cholera	Improve water quality	90
2	Leptospirosis	Improve water quality	80
3a	*Ascaris*	Increase water quantity	40
3a	Hydatid	Increase water quantity	40
3a	*Toxocara*	Increase water quantity	40
3a	Toxoplasmosis	Increase water quantity	40
4a	Guinea worm	Reduce water contact	100
4b	Schistosomiasis	Reduce water contact	60
5a	Malaria	Water piped to site of use and maintenance of water supplies	10
5a	Filariasis		10
5a	Arboviruses		10?
5b	Onchocerciasis	Water piped to site of use	20?
5b	Gambian trypanosomiasis		80

From Bradley, D.J. (1978) in Feachem, R.G. *et al.* (eds) *Water, Wastes and Health in Hot Climates*. Reprinted by permission of John Wiley & Sons Ltd.

The Provision of water

There are four aspects of water supply improvements which can help to control disease transmission. These are as follows.

- Increase water quantity.
- Improve water quality.
- Reduce water contact by bringing water to site of use.
- Prevent spillage by proper maintenance of supplies and drainage.

It will be noticed how this is the normal process in the supply of water. The first objective is to provide water in sufficient quantity. This is followed by improving its quality and finally piped systems are used. These will require maintenance if they are to function properly. If this is the pattern followed, it can be anticipated that the first group of diseases to be reduced will be the water-washed and faecal–oral, then the water-borne, etc.

In rural water supplies, where chlorine treatment of the water is costly, difficult to maintain or inappropriate, a different standard from that in large centralized supplies may be acceptable. This should not be considered to be unsatisfactory, as the provision of a properly constructed water supply is an improvement on what was used before. Also quality is closely related to quantity. By providing a greater volume of water at a more accessible site, quality will usually be improved.

Health aspects are the concern of the medical worker, whereas the villager looks upon water as a basic necessity. His or, rather, her (as women are nearly always the carriers of water) major concerns will be quite different. These are the following.

- Availability of water at a more convenient place (preferably in the village).
- A continuous and reliable supply.
- Additional water for crops and domestic animals.

It is a combination of these health and social factors that needs to be used in deciding the appropriateness and benefits of water supplies.

Economic and planning criteria

Everybody wants the best possible water supply he/she can get, but resources are limited so it will be many years before everyone has a supply. Decisions have to be made as to which sections of the community should be served, when they should receive their supply and the level of availability. There are many alternative strategies that may be, or inadvertently will be, used. They might include the following.

- Priority of an area on health grounds.
- Priority to an area of water scarcity.

- Encouragement of development to an area of high potential.
- Priority to communities that can contribute in money and labour.
- First come, first served.
- Political favouritism.

Other alternatives in the nature of the supply can also be considered.

- Supplying a large number of people with the simplest of supplies.
- Restricting supplies to certain demonstration areas with a high standard.
- Start with the most available natural water sources.
- Plan a major project, such as a dam, followed by extension of supply in subsequent years.

This will depend on how much the country, region, district or village is prepared to pay for the price of water. Savings can be made by the following.

- Economies of scale.
- Standardizing the equipment.
- Self-help labour.

The initial water master plan is best formulated by skilled engineers, but its execution can be carried out by a purpose-trained technician utilizing community effort. The plan needs to take account of health, engineering, political and community demands.

Water capacity and use

In selecting a suitable source, the amount of water it produces and its regularity need to be known. If a spring or stream does not flow all the year round, it is not suitable unless a dam is also built. Measurements of water flow should be made at the end of the dry season and the people asked if the source has ever dried up. A temporary dam can be made and the rate of filling a measured bucket estimates the flow. Wells can be mechanically pumped out and the fall noted for a given flow of water. Rainwater catchment is derived from the simple formula:

1 mm of rainfall on 1 m^2 of the roof in plan will give 0.8 litres of water

As an example, if the roof area in plan is 10 m × 5 m and the average annual rainfall is 650 mm, then 10 × 5 × 650 × 0.8 = 26,000 litres per year or 71 litres per day, on average.

The demand for water will be determined by the availability, the number of people and the use to which it is put. The availability is the most crucial factor, as water that has to be carried some distance will be used much more sparingly than when there is a tap inside the house. Average figures taken from a number of studies are as follows.

	Litres per person per day
Rural supply	20
Standpipe	40
Single tap in the home	80
Multiple taps with bath, WC, etc.	200–300

At least 50% extra capacity is allowed for future growth of the community and expansion of the supply. A water source is chosen where the expected demand on the supply will never be exceeded, even in the driest time of the year. If this is not possible, some form of storage will be required. Water use during the night is far less than during the day, so a poor supply can be boosted by providing a storage tank that fills at night. In areas of wide seasonal variation, more extensive storage facilities may be required to save the rain that falls in the few wet months, such as a dam.

Choice of water supply

Choosing a water source will depend on the following.

- Proximity to user.
- Reliability.
- Quantity of water.
- Quality of water.
- Technical feasibility.
- Resources available.
- Social desirability or taboo.
- Maintenance.

The alternative choices are illustrated in Figs 5.4 and 5.5. Rainwater naturally seeps through the earth until it finds an impervious layer (such as clay), on which it collects. Where this impervious layer comes to the surface the water runs out of the ground as a spring. It can also form the bed of a river or, in an enclosed area, a lake. This groundwater can be tapped by a shallow well. At a much deeper level, a second impervious layer can trap a large quantity of water. A deep well or borehole is required to reach this source of water. Island populations (Fig. 5.5) have particular problems in obtaining water and are generally left with only two alternatives. Providing they have suitable roofing material (e.g. corrugated iron), rainwater can be collected and stored in a tank. The alternative is to sink a well to tap the freshwater lens. Due to a fortunate quality of coral rock, it acts like a large sponge holding fresh water that has percolated through, floating on the denser sea water. Providing the

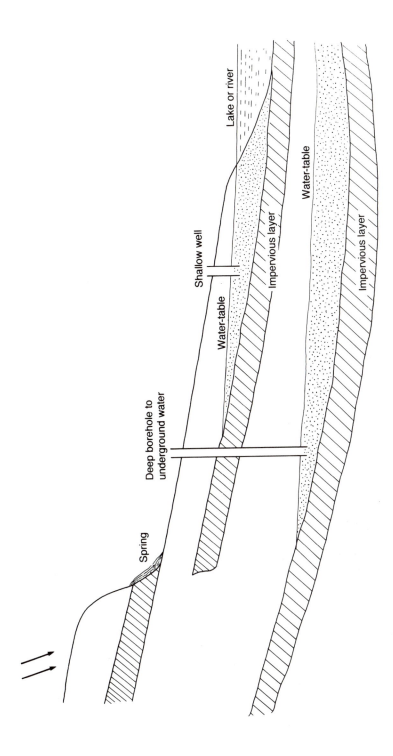

Fig. 5.4. Sources of water.

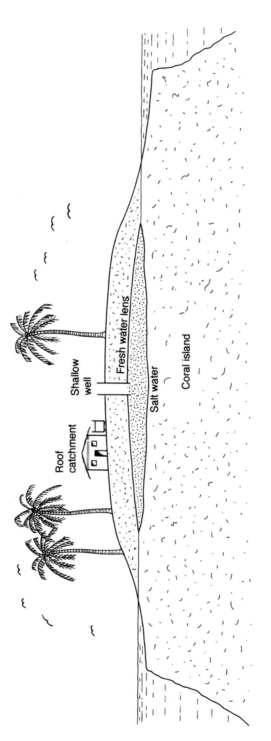

Fig. 5.5. Water catchment and the freshwater lens of coral islands.

well is sunk just far enough and not pumped out too hard, fresh water can be obtained. The advantages and disadvantages of different water sources are summarized in Table 5.3.

Wells are often a good supply, as long as contamination can be prevented. If they are sealed and a pump is provided, this will require maintenance. They have the advantage of being sited close to houses. Deep wells and boreholes need special equipment for their construction and complex pumps to lift water from these depths. They are mainly applicable in areas of severe water shortage, such as deserts.

Lakes and rivers provide convenient but poor-quality water. Other sources should be used if possible, but, if there is no alternative, then some form of water treatment, such as filtration and storage, should be incorporated.

Rainwater catchment is an underutilized source of pure water, either as a main method or as a subsidiary (for drinking water). So much good water runs to waste off large expanses of roof that have already been paid for in the construction of the building. For the additional cost of guttering and a tank, a family can have a good, safe source of water, inside or very close to the house. Storage tanks can either be close to the roof or large concrete structures built underground.

A constant spring that never dries up is a very suitable source, because it is comparatively free from contamination and can normally be led to an outlet without requiring pumping. This means that its maintenance costs will be very low, so greater capital expenditure can be allowed for protecting the spring and piping its water to the village.

The ideal is to find a source that has both constant quantity and good quality, but, where the latter is not achieved, quality can be improved by

Table 5.3. Sources of water, their advantages and disadvantages.

	Spring	Shallow well	Borehole	River	Lake	Catchment
Proximity	Distant	Near	Intermediate	Near	Near	Near
Reliability	Good	Variable	Good	Unreliable	Good	Unreliable
Quantity	Good	Moderate	Good	Variable	Good	Poor
Quality	Good	Moderate	Good	Poor	Poor	Good
Technology	Easy	Moderate	Difficult	Easy*	Easy*	Moderate
Cost	Low	Moderate	High	Low*	Low*	Moderate to high
Community preference	High	Moderate	Moderate	Low	Low	Moderate
Maintenance	Low	Moderate	High	Low	Low	Moderate

*These assessments are for taking water by hand from the river or lake. If a pump and supply system are used, the technology is difficult and the cost high.

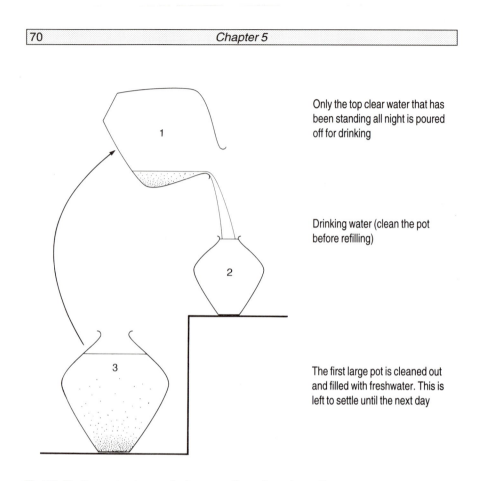

Only the top clear water that has
been standing all night is poured
off for drinking

Drinking water (clean the pot
before refilling)

The first large pot is cleaned out
and filled with freshwater. This is
left to settle until the next day

Fig. 5.6. The three pot system – a simple means of improving water quality.

simple methods, such as the three pot system (Fig. 5.6). This uses three
pots, the last to store clean water and the other two to store it overnight
in sequence, as shown in the illustration.

5.2.4 Sanitation

With food and water supplies, the emphasis is on the prevention of
contamination, but with sanitation it is reducing the source of contamination. Social habits concerned with excreta disposal are often strongly
held and, unless these are approached in a sensible manner, any system
will fail. Sanitation is not just the provision of latrines, but a complex and
interrelated subject involving the people, the water supplies and all the
other aspects of environmental health.

Health factors

As shown in Table 5.1, the main impact of sanitation is on groups 2, 3a, 4c and 5c. The installation of sanitation may produce a reduction in the following infections.

Category	Infection	Mode of action	Possible reduction from sanitation improvements
1	Trachoma	Through reduction of flies (group 5c)	+
2	Enteric viruses (including hepatitis A)	Reduces contamination of vegetables	+
2	Hymenolepis	Reduces contamination of food and water	+
2	Amoebiasis	Reduces contamination of vegetables	++
2	Trichuris	Reduces contamination of food and water	+
2	Giardia	Reduces contamination of food and water	+
2	Shigella	Reduces contamination of food and water	++
2	Typhoid	Reduces contamination of food and water	++
2	Other salmonellae	Reduces contamination of food and water	++
2	Campylobacter	Reduces contamination of food and water	++
2	Non-specific diarrhoeal diseases	Reduces contamination of food and water	++
2	Cholera	Reduces contamination of food and water	++
3a	Ascaris	Reduces soil contamination	+++
3a	Hookworm	Reduces soil contamination	+++
3a	Strongyloides	Reduces soil contamination	+++
3b	Taenia	Reduces soil contamination	+++
4b	Schistosomiasis	Reduces water contamination	+
4c	Fasciolopsis	Reduces water contamination	+
4c	Opisthorchis	Reduces water contamination	+
4c	Paragonimus	Reduces water contamination	+
4c	Diphyllobothrium	Reduces water contamination	+
5	Housefly-transmitted diseases	Controls flies	±±*
5	Filariasis	Reduces Culex quinquefasciatus breeding	+

*Sanitation facilities can be as responsible for increasing the fly nuisance as for decreasing it.

The provision of sanitation

When providing sanitation, there is a sharp contrast with water supplies; everybody wants a water supply, but nobody wants to change their defecation practice. This is quite simple to explain in that substances taken into the body can be understood as a direct cause of illness, whereas excreting something from the body cannot. Defecation is a necessary but private business, not a matter for discussion. There are also social reasons that are set by religious, racial or cultural rules. These may dictate where defecation can take place and where it cannot and, will probably separate the sexes and define particular anal cleansing practices. With all these patterns and customs that have been taught since childhood, any change becomes a long and difficult process. If a family can see the benefits of a latrine, they will install and look after it; the health authority can then assist in technical specifications and subsidize costs. Any attempt to impose systems or even build them free of charge will cause resentment or non-use.

Like water, sanitation has to be paid for, but here costs are even less accepted by the population. People are only prepared to pay for the minimum possible in getting rid of their excreta. Only in urban areas will it be considered necessary to pay for the removal of excrement; in rural areas there is sufficient space. A subsidizing scheme then becomes the main way in which sanitation can be improved. For instance, in pit-latrine construction, the villagers will need to dig their family's own hole, but might be sold a bag of cement at a reduced price or be provided with a squatting slab free of charge.

Cost is related to convenience, which is why people are prepared to pay for improved systems, their willingness to pay usually having nothing to do with health. A good pit latrine can be as effective in disease control as a conventional water-carried sewage system, the only difference being that the former is outside the house, while the latter carries excreta from within the house. The cost of this convenience is typically ten times that of a pit latrine.

In choosing the most appropriate excreta disposal system, the emphasis should be on simplicity. Only when a simpler method becomes outmoded because of rising standards and expectations will a more sophisticated system become appropriate. A simple incremental process, as illustrated in Fig. 5.7, can be planned. The first stage is to bury excreta, which will lead on to using a pit latrine. If pit latrines are already accepted by the community, demonstrating the advantages of improved pit latrines will be the next step. The type of facility will also be determined by the availability of water. As mentioned in Section 5.2.3, the provision of water should precede any sanitation programme, as personal hygiene can only be taught if there is water at hand to wash with. The quantity and nearness of this water will then determine the type of

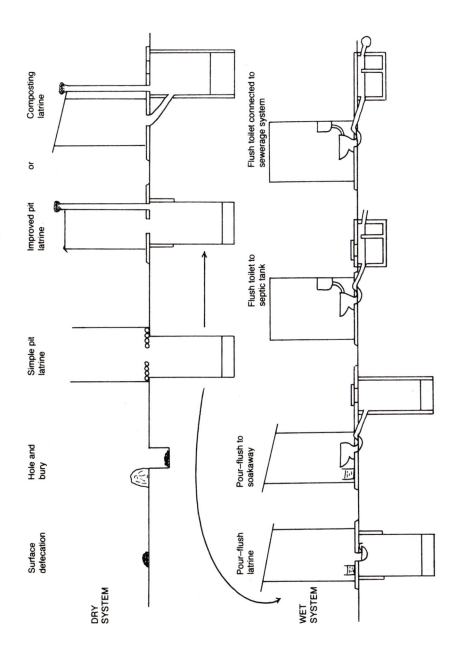

Fig. 5.7. Types of excreta disposal systems – incremental sanitation.

sanitary system that can be used. In the lower part of Fig. 5.7, the incremental progression of a water–utilizing sanitary system is shown. A pour–flush latrine can be installed where water is obtained from a village standpipe, but, with a septic tank or sewerage, a water flushing system requires in–house water connections.

Siting and contamination

The unit must be sited so that it does not contaminate the environment in such a way as to threaten the health of others. With a pit latrine, bacterial pollution can travel downwards for a distance of up to 2 m. If the contamination reaches the water-table, it will flow horizontally for up to 10 m. This means that any latrine should be sited at least this distance from a water supply, such as a well. The latrine should also be placed downhill from the well, although excessive pumping will draw water into the well from all directions, including possibly from a latrine. If a latrine is built less than 10 m from a river or stream, it can pollute it, as the water-table will be flowing towards the stream. Latrines in this situation can be potent sources of pollution if the river is used for drinking water. Pollution of the soil is a complex subject and the rough rule of 10 m distance between a latrine and source of drinking water is given as a guide. Contamination is dependent upon the following.

- The velocity of groundwater flow (should be less than 10 m in 10 days).
- The composition of the soil (not fissured, e.g. as in limestone).

Expert advice should be obtained before embarking on a latrine programme.

In a sealed system such as a septic tank or an aquaprivy, contamination of the soil will not take place unless there is a crack in the structure. However, the effluent is highly charged with pathogens and must be disposed of properly. Running it into a storm drain, as often happens, is a bad practice and a considerable danger. The easiest solution is to lead it into a soakaway, but precautions similar to a latrine need to be taken.

5.3 VECTOR CONTROL

Parasites are transmitted by vectors from one host to another, often utilizing the stage to undergo multiplication or development. In some parasites, e.g. malaria, the vector is the definitive host, whereas in others, such as *Wuchereria bancrofti*, it is the intermediate host. Whichever part the vector plays, it is a vital one for the parasite and it cannot continue if the vector is destroyed.

The time of changing from one host to another is a precarious time for the parasite and considerable loss may occur. Malaria gametocyte development must coincide with a mosquito taking a blood meal, and both male and female gametocytes are required for fertilization and maturation to take place in the insect's stomach. *W. bancrofti* suffers considerable parasite loss during the vector stage. However, the vector does not have to be completely destroyed, but has to be kept at levels too low for transmission to take place. So vector control means vector reduction, not vector eradication.

5.3.1 Mosquito Control

The various ways in which mosquitoes can be controlled are as follows.

- Adulticides.
- Repellents.
- Personal protection.
- Larvicides.
- Biological control.
- Environmental modification.

These are all illustrated in Fig. 5.8.

Adulticides

Killing the adult mosquito can either be done while it is flying, using a knock-down spray, or when it is resting, with a residual insecticide. Knock-down insecticides will kill adult mosquitoes at the time of application only, whereas residual insecticides continue to have a lethal effect for a considerable period of time.

Knock-down insecticides

Knock-down insecticides are used to control epidemics of vector-transmitted disease where an explosive increase in the number of flying adults is responsible. They have been used in malaria epidemics, but have perhaps their greatest value in dengue and the control of arbovirus infections. They are used as space sprays (aerosols), in the house, for mosquito survey counts and for disinfecting aircraft. Knock-down sprays commonly contain pyrethrum, derived from a species of chrysanthemum grown in highland areas of East Africa. They can be dispersed in aerosols, smoke generators (fogging) or ultra-low-volume (ULV) aerial sprays.

Residual spraying

Residual spraying is the main method for control of mosquito-transmitted disease. Residual insecticides continue to remain active for 6

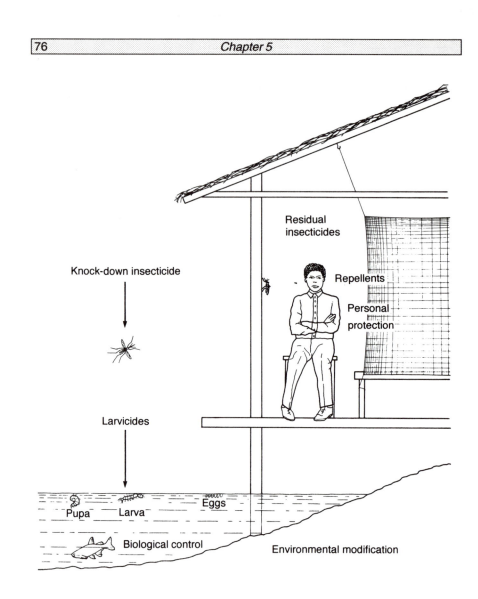

Fig. 5.8. Mosquito control methods.

months or more. By careful organization, repeated applications made at regular intervals can maintain a killing effect. Ideally they should be sprayed just before the start of the main transmission season, especially in areas where malaria is seasonal.

Residual insecticides act on the resting mosquito. Mosquitoes need to rest after they have taken a blood meal and generally choose the nearest place, which is the wall of the victim's house. If the wall is sprayed with residual insecticide, the mosquito will absorb a lethal dose through its legs.

Residual insecticides can be sprayed on surfaces either as solutions or as wettable powders. Few of the insecticides commonly used go into solution with a cheap and easily obtainable medium such as water, so emulsions and wettable powders are more commonly used. Emulsions are required on non-absorbent surfaces, while wettable powders are suitable for mud, leaf or other poor-quality walls. The wettable medium (generally water) soaks into the wall and leaves the powder on the surface. Some of the insecticide is taken into the porous surface, but this gradually comes out, maintaining a steady concentration. Once residual insecticide has been sprayed on a wall, it must not be washed or painted. Residual insecticide sprayed on a surface depends upon a number of factors.

- The proportion of active insecticide in the preparation.
- The amount of insecticide mixed with the fluid medium.
- Mixing, before and during application.
- The distance from the surface that it is sprayed.
- The speed of application.

These are all specified for a particular insecticide and spraypersons must be trained to ensure that the right concentration is delivered. To test this a measured area of plaster can be scraped and the insecticide content analysed.

Residual spraying is carried out by a team of spraypersons with manually operated sprayers, covering a village at a time. Houses are emptied and pets and domestic animals restrained in a suitable place some distance away (as they are sensitive to insecticides). Any insects, beetles and lizards that are killed should be swept up and disposed of before the domestic animals are allowed back into the houses. This takes a considerable amount of organization with a strict schedule of notification followed by spraying. The supervisor answers any questions, ensures that the work is done and arranges logistic support. If residual spraying is not adequately explained to people, organizational resistance will develop. The target is to spray every dwelling-house, whether permanently or temporarily occupied.

Deterrents and repellents

Deterrents and repellents can be either smokes or applications to the body in the form of creams and solutions. They do not kill the mosquito but deter it from biting.

Mosquito coils or heated pads have a combined deterrent and repellent action. They are made with small quantities of pyrethroids in a slow-burning base, but other insecticides can be added to enhance the activity. Used in a still atmosphere they can be most effective. If they do not prevent all the bites, they reduce the number, which is important in filariasis transmission. They reduce the probability of being bitten by an infective mosquito carrying any disease.

The most commonly used repellent is diethyltoluamide (DEET), which can be applied to the person, clothing, tents and mosquito nets. The solutions can either be dissolved in methylated spirit or emulsified with water and applied to the surface. It is not absorbed by synthetic fabrics and a cotton or wool base is essential if it is to remain for some time. Four weeks of activity are given if continuously exposed, but if the garments, such as a shawl or leg bands, are kept in a polythene bag, repellent action can continue for 3–6 months. Precaution should be taken in applying DEET to the skin, as some individuals are sensitive, while neurological toxicity can be produced in children. Natural repellents made from eucalyptus oil are preferable for application to the person.

Personal protection

Personal protection is a valuable precaution in reducing the number of mosquito bites. Clothing that covers the arms and legs, especially if combined with a repellent, can protect an individual most effectively. With the appearance of widespread insecticide resistance, greater reliance must now be placed on personal protection.

The use of *mosquito nets* for beds is a well-tried method of personal protection. Mosquito nets must have no tears and can be tucked under the mattress. A knock-down spray applied prior to retiring will prevent any mosquitoes entering the net when the occupant goes to bed. Young children should be placed under them before it gets dark. The sale of subsidized mosquito nets can be an effective method of malaria control, if they are subsequently impregnated with an insecticide.

Mosquito nets are *impregnated* with synthetic pyrethroids, such as permethrin, deltamethrin or lambda-cyhalothrin. Impregnated nets deter mosquitoes from entering should the net be torn or kill them if they touch the net. Nylon nets are better than cotton because they absorb less solution and are stronger, but this has to be offset by their greater cost. Additional advantages of impregnated bed nets are that they provide some protection for other people sleeping in the same room. They also kill fleas, lice, bedbugs and cockroaches and even if rolled up will still provide some protection. A modification of this method is to impregnate curtains that are used to cover the door, windows or any opening. These methods are used in community malaria control programmes.

Nets are impregnated by soaking them in a solution of the insecticide. Nets should first be washed and when dry dipped into a bowl or container of the solution. Unfortunately, cotton nets (or the cotton bases of synthetic nets) absorb more water than nylon/polyester nets so it is necessary to calculate this by soaking the net in a known volume of water, wringing out and measuring the amount absorbed. Some impregnated bed-net programmes are overcoming this problem by using standard-sized nets all made of the same material, but where this is not done weighing nets may allow the amount of water to be estimated for different kinds of nets. The area of the net is then measured to calculate the amount of insecticide, 200 mg m^{-2} permethrin, 25 mg m^{-2} deltamethrin or 10 mg m^{-2} lambda-cyhalothrin, which is mixed with the calculated volume of water. The net is then thoroughly mixed with the diluted insecticide, taking care to make sure that all parts of the netting are treated. It is then dried horizontally on a plastic sheet or a bed, as insecticide draining out will kill any bedbugs. Some people suffer from nasal congestion when sleeping under a net that has recently been impregnated with deltamethrin or lambda-cyhalothrin and it is probably better to not use the net for the first 2 days if either of these insecticides have been used. Otherwise they are perfectly safe and no long-term effects have been recorded.

Nets can either be impregnated individually, as villagers can easily be taught how to dip their own nets, or the solution can be made up in bulk according to the number of nets to be treated. Rubber gloves must be worn by anyone doing the impregnation. Once nets have been impregnated they should not be washed again until reimpregnation as this decreases the effectivness of the insecticide.

A less satisfactory alternative is to screen the whole house, but this is expensive and a torn area will destroy the whole effect. An intact ceiling is also required. Air-conditioning, by providing a sealed room, generally prevents mosquitoes from entering. Even so, it is preferable to use a knock-down spray in the evening to get rid of any mosquitoes that may have entered. However, the cost of whole-house screening, air-conditioning and knock-down sprays is considerably greater than using impregnated mosquito nets.

Larvicides

Larvicides act on mosquito larvae by blocking their breathing apparatus, destroying surface tension (so they sink to the bottom) or poisoning them. Paraffin (Kerosene) spread on water covers the syphon of the larvae and it dies from asphyxiation. High-spreading oils have been developed which inactivate the force of surface tension that larvae use to float on the surface. Insecticides kill off many other organisms (including fish), are expensive and are generally objected to by the public, and therefore are rarely used as larvicides, such preparations as temephos (Abate), with its very low toxicity, being a notable exception.

Larvicides are not efficient methods of mosquito control, their main use being in urban and periurban areas, especially against culicine vectors. Drains and gutters can be sprayed and temephos added to water containers and septic tanks. Surface sprays must be renewed at regular intervals.

In the control of *Culex quinquefasciatus*, the main vector of urban filariasis, which breeds in latrines, expanded polystyrene beads can be placed in the pit. Larvae are dislodged and prevented from breathing, while the functioning of the latrine is not disrupted. The polystyrene is manufactured as fine granules and when placed in boiling water it expands.

Biological control

Biological control is the use of natural methods to bring about a reduction in vectors. They can be predators, such as larvivorous fish, microbial organisms, e.g. *Bacillus thuringiensis* and *B. sphaericus*, or modifications to the insect. Male insects can be sterilized by radiation or chemosterilants and then released into the environment. If these sterile males compete successfully with the unsterilized males, the females will not be fertilized. Unfortunately, this technique requires the preparation and release of a sufficient number of males to outnumber those in the natural habitat, which is generally impractical. An alternative technique is to breed mosquitoes that are refractory to the target disease. This can either be through genetic manipulation or an introduced closely related natural species. Species replacement, as the method is called, offers some promise because similar but competitive species can be obtained from different parts of the world.

The problem with any biological method is that nature continues in a balance. If a predator destroys all its food supply, it will die, so an equilibrium is reached whereby the number of predators and those they prey on remain in sufficient numbers for both to exist. Biological control is therefore more an aid rather than the definitive method.

Environmental modification

Environmental modification implies a change of habitat, making it no longer suitable for the existence of the vector. It can include simple methods, such as burying all tin cans or cutting holes in old tires to drain water, to clearing vast tracks of forest for tsetse fly control. Any method of environmental modification on a large scale must carefully consider other systems that may be damaged. Clearing large areas of forest can affect the water retention of the soil; deforesting river banks can lead to severe erosion. On the other hand, filling in or draining a swamp can provide extra land. Eucalyptus trees, which take out large amounts of water from the soil, can be planted and subsequently used for firewood.

Specific methods of environmental modification, such as for trypanosomiasis, will be found under the particular disease, while the emphasis here will be on mosquito control. One of the most successful methods for reducing surface water and getting rid of breeding places is the construction of subsurface drains. This should be within the

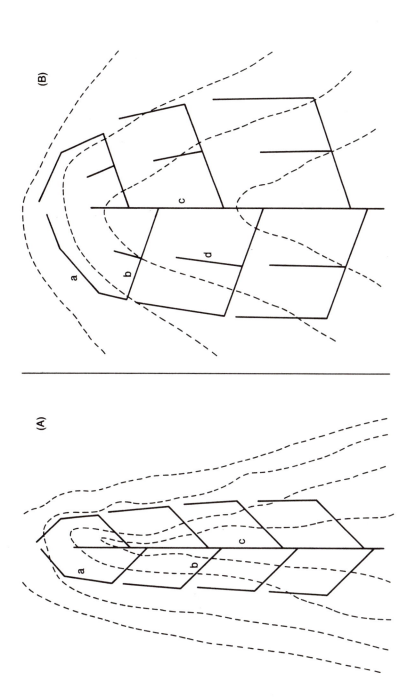

Fig. 5.9. Contour drains in a narrow ravine (A) and in a wide ravine (B). ----, Contours; ———, drains; a, contour or intercepting drain; b, collecting drain; c, main drain; d, intermediate drain. (From Stevenson, D. (1987) *Davey and Lightbody's The Control of Diseases in the Tropics*, H.K. Lewis, London. Reprinted by permission of Chapman & Hall.)

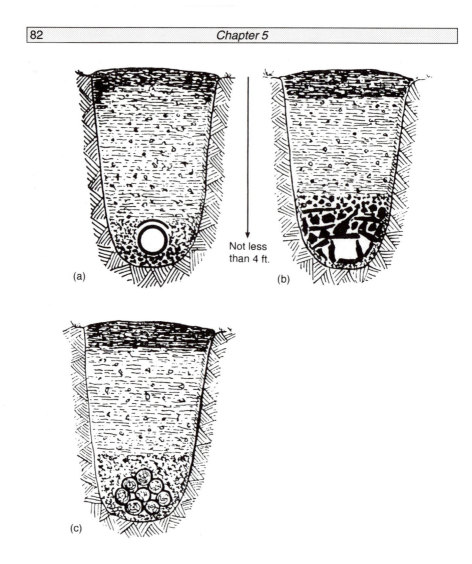

Not less
than 4 ft.

(a)

(b)

(c)

Fig. 5.10. Subsoil drain construction. (a) Tile–pipe drain. (b) Stone-packed drain. (c) Pole drain. (From Stevenson, D. (1987) *Davey and Lightbody's The Control of Diseases in the Tropics*, H.K. Lewis, London. Reprinted by permission of Chapman & Hall.)

ability of most health personnel. The system of drains should follow the contours (Fig. 5.9) and be at least 1.5 m below the surface. The gradient needs to be between 1 in 400 and 1 in 30. Three different methods of construction are illustrated in Fig. 5.10. The best is to use unjointed clay pipes on a bed of gravel. The upper surface of the pipes is covered with pieces of broken tile or other impervious material so as to make the water flow into the pipe from the sides and base. This forces the water to lose its sediment around the sides and not block the pipe. An

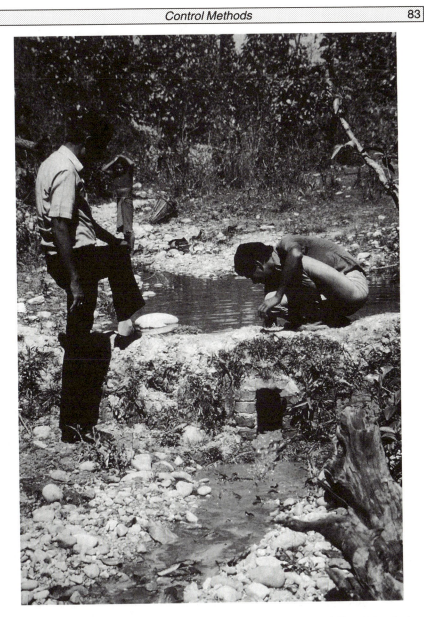

Fig. 5.11. A locally constructed dam for the control of *Anopheles fluviatilis* in Nepal. Every 3 days the bung is removed and the head of water rushing down the stream is sufficient to dislodge developing mosquitoes.

alternative design is to use stones, either loosely laid or in the form of a tunnel, covered with palm fronds or banana leaves. This allows the earth to compact down without clogging the stones. Another method is to use poles, particularly bamboos, which when drilled form an almost perfect pipe. These rot in time, but the channel made should still continue for some while after. Another method of environmental control is to use a siphon which flushes out mosquito larvae, or a simple dam as shown in Fig. 5.11.

5.3.2 Insecticides

Insecticides for vector control include the following.

- *Poisons*, e.g. Paris green, which was used extensively as a larvicide. *Anopheles gambiae* was eradicated from upper Egypt by this preparation. In view of the resistance to insecticides, it could be reconsidered.
- *Fumigants*, e.g. hydrogen cyanide, methyl bromide and ethyl formate, can be used on grain or clothing to destroy infestations.
- *Knock-down*, e.g. pyrethrum, bioresmethrin and bioallethrin.
- *Residual*, which are subdivided into organochlorines, organophosphates, carbonates and pyrethroids.

Organochlorines

Examples of organochlorines are dichlorodiphenyltrichloroethane (DDT), benzene hexachloride (BHC) and dieldrin. These were widely used in the early days of eradication programmes. DDT exhibits deterrence and irritancy, which may cause the mosquito to leave the surface before it has absorbed a lethal dose. BHC is a volatile substance, the vapours alone being sufficient to kill mosquitoes. This means it does not remain active for long and frequent applications are required. Dieldrin is non-volatile and kills by contact, but it is also toxic to humans and so considerable caution must be used.

Organophosphates

Organophosphates such as malathion and fenthion are volatile substances that require frequent application. They act by inhibiting cholinesterase at the nerve junctions, and can therefore produce temporary paralysis (and respiratory failure) in humans as well as insects. They do not have a long residual action, and so are not persistent in the environment. Chlorpyrifos (Dursban) and temephos (Abate) are low-toxic compounds widely used as larvicide.

Carbamates

Carbamates act in a similar manner to the organosphosphates except that they compete with the acetylcholinesterase rather than combining with it. This means that the action is more easily reversed, conferring an advantage to humans. Examples are propoxur and carbaryl.

Pyrethroids

Pyrethroids are synthetic substances derived originally from pyrethrum, but now modified so extensively that forms with a residual action have been developed. These are stable substances, with a low mammalian toxicity, but they are expensive to produce. However, only very small quantities are required. Examples are permethrin and deltamethrin.

5.3.3 Resistance

When an insecticide is being chosen for a control programme, the vector must be tested against various strengths of the insecticide to determine the discriminatory dose (this is when 99.9% mortality of the sample occurs). These tests need to be repeated from time to time during the course of the programme to determine whether the vector remains sensitive. If there are technical reasons why this cannot be done, resistance will probably only be noticed by an increase in number of insects or cases of the disease. This might, however, indicate deficiencies in the spraying programme and these should be ruled out first. Correct application of insecticide can be measured as mentioned above, while a simple field test for suspected resistance can be performed by placing a few of the insects in a glass jar held against the sprayed surface for a minute. If they are not all killed, resistance should be suspected and entomological assistance obtained.

Resistance may be partial or complete. If partial, then increasing the concentration of insecticide may be sufficient to control the vector. Unfortunately, complete resistance is likely to develop soon. Resistance is a genetic character and resistant strains are selected out under pressure of insecticides. Initially resistance to one insecticide was found, but subsequently cross-resistance has developed, making several insecticides ineffective. Some species now have multiple resistance. Biological control or trying a completely different strategy may be effective.

5.3.4 Ectoparasite Control

Ectoparasites live on the outside of the body; examples are fleas, lice, bedbugs, mites and ticks. They are responsible for transmitting a number of diseases. There are various control methods.

- Personal hygiene.

- Reduction of interpersonal contact from overcrowding and clothes sharing.
- Regular and effective washing of clothes and bedding.
- Repellents.
- Improved house construction.
- Insecticides.

Ectoparasites favour dirty dark places, whether they are searching for a suitable habitat on a person or a vantage place in housing from which to mount an attack. Fleas and lice are not removed by washing, but the regular use of warm water and soap considerably deters them. If this is combined with clothes washing, fleas can rapidly be controlled. Where possible, clothes and bedding should be boiled or at least subjected to very hot water, as fleas are not affected by cold water. Some communities practice head shaving to control lice. Although this is rather a drastic measure, short hair certainly makes them easier to control.

Fleas and lice favour overcrowded conditions such as occur during wars, during famines or in refugee camps. Efforts should be made to reduce overcrowding but, where this is impossible, at least washing and laundry facilities should be provided. Wearing of other people's clothes and sharing combs are common methods of transferring ectoparasites in tropical areas.

Repellents have been used successfully in areas where infection is likely. Impregnated socks and trousers are effective when passing through microhabitats of scrub typhus or sylvatic plague. Ticks, bedbugs and reduviids are kept off by repellents.

Bedbugs, ticks and reduviid bugs live in cracks in the walls of poorly constructed houses. They come out at night and attack sleeping persons, some transmitting disease (relapsing fever, typhus and Chagas' disease). Improving house construction or applying a layer of unbroken plaster to a wall discourages these arthropods permanently. Bed nets can protect the individual from being bitten.

Insecticides are especially useful in epidemic conditions. Dusting clothing, using a puffer to supply the insecticide up trouser legs and skirts and down collars and sleeves can quickly reduce the number of ectoparasites in concentrations of people. Insecticide solutions can be applied to the hair to kill off head lice or to clothing if repellents are not available. Rat burrows and runs should be dusted with insecticides to kill off plague-carrying fleas before rat catching. Benzyl benzoate or benzene hexachloride are effective against scabies mites. Further details on ectoparasites will be found in Chapter 17.

6

Notification and Health Regulations

6.1 INTERNATIONAL HEALTH REGULATIONS

International health regulations require that certain diseases are notified. The purpose is to warn other countries and intended travellers to the country of the health risks involved. Assistance can also be requested, once the disease has been notified.

Diseases subject to the International Health Regulations (1969, 1974) are as follows.

- Plague.
- Cholera.
- Yellow fever.

Diseases under surveillance by the World Health Organization (WHO) are as follows.

- Louse-borne typhus.
- Relapsing fever.
- Paralytic poliomyelitis.
- Malaria.
- Influenza.
- Acquired immune deficiency syndrome (AIDS).
- Smallpox.

Initial case is notified by telex or fax to:

- EPIDNATIONS, Geneva.

Subsequent weekly summaries are sent.

In addition, a region, e.g. the South Pacific Commission or Association of Caribbean States, may initiate its own regulations, for example for the following.

- Dengue.
- Diphtheria.
- Typhoid.
- Whooping cough.
- Scrub typhus.

6.2 NATIONAL HEALTH REGULATIONS

Countries have their own system of national notification for some diseases, including the following.

- Tuberculosis.
- Leprosy.
- Sleeping sickness.

6.3 SURVEILLANCE

The principles of surveillance were mentioned in Section 3.25. A country at particular risk may be advised to set up a surveillance system of international or national importance. Some suggestions are as follows.

- In plague areas any case of fever, glandular enlargement and death.
- Any person dying from diarrhoea.
- Any person dying of jaundice in the yellow fever zone (Fig. 6.1).
- *Aedes aegypti* index.
- Severe case of chickenpox or other unusual pox rashes.
- Any case of acute flaccid paralysis following a feverish illness.

Any case coming within one of these categories is reported immediately to the responsible medical officer or doctor in charge, who is required to investigate the report.

WHO have set up an international surveillance team to investigate any case of suspected smallpox reported. The suspected case must be isolated and WHO informed immediately. There is also concern about emergent diseases, and the strengthening of surveillance systems and the linking of one reporting country with another will assist in detecting new diseases before they become a serious problem.

6.4 VACCINATION REQUIREMENTS

The only vaccination now required for international travel is

- yellow fever

for persons who come from or are liable to pass through the yellow fever

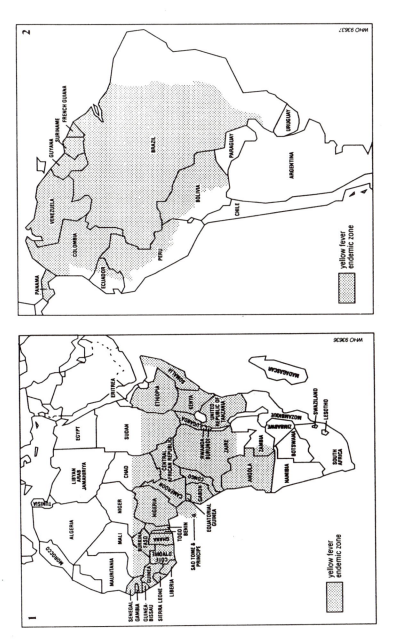

Fig. 6.1. The yellow fever endemic zones in Africa (Map 1) and Central and South America (Map 2). Yellow fever endemic zones are areas where there is a potential risk of infection on account of the presence of vectors and animal reservoirs. Some countries consider these zones are infected areas, and require an international certificate of vaccination against yellow fever from travellers arriving from these areas. (Reproduced, by permission, from WHO (1995) *International Travel and Health, Vaccination Requirements and Health Advice*, World Health Organization, Geneva.)

zone (Fig. 6.1). Cholera vaccination is no longer required by international regulations. A yellow fever vaccination must be recorded on the prescribed form with the signature of the doctor, the batch number and the official stamp of the vaccination centre. WHO publishes lists of officially recognized yellow fever vaccination centres. The vaccination is valid for 10 years, 10 days after the date of the vaccination or revaccination.

Part II

Communicable Diseases

Transmission is the key to the epidemiology and control of communicable diseases. Normally diseases are classified by agent (e.g. bacterial or viral) or symptom complexes (e.g. hepatitis), which are useful to the clinician needing to make a diagnosis and treat individual cases, but for the community physician and epidemiologist it is the method of transmission that determines the method of control to be used. So in this section an epidemiology classification is used, grouping together diseases that have a similar transmission and means of control. The divisions are as follows.

	Chapter
Water-washed diseases	7
Faecal–oral diseases	8
Soil-mediated infections	9
Diseases of water contact	10
Food-borne diseases	11
Infectious skin rashes	12
Respiratory infections	13
Leprosy (unknown means of transmission)	14
Diseases transmitted via body fluids	15
Insect-borne diseases	16
Ectoparasite zoonoses	17
Domestic zoonoses	18

No classification system is perfect and not every disease fits neatly into the 12 categories. For many diseases there are more than one means of transmission and these can also be important in developing control methods. However, the categories are sufficiently broad to encompass minor differences. Bringing diseases together into such a system demonstrates similarities and associations, making it easier to understand the complexities of the many communicable diseases.

Not every communicable disease is covered – only those that are of worldwide importance, are major problems in certain parts of the world or illustrate a particular disease pattern. An attempt is made to list all diseases and their means of transmission in Section 19.1 (which is arranged in alphabetical order) and readers may find it easier to refer to this first before turning to the fuller description in the following pages.

Note: In keeping with accepted scientific notation the negative indices style has been used instead of 'per' or '/', e.g.

20 mg kg^{-1} instead of 20 mg per kg or 20 mg/kg.

100 mg m^{-2} instead of 100 mg per m^2 or 100 mg/m^2.

7

Water-washed Diseases

The simplest disease transmission is by person-to-person contact (see Fig. 1.3). The diseases of poor hygiene arise from direct contact of the skin, conjunctiva or mucous membrane. Alternatively organisms from the skin or in conjunctival secretions can be transported by an intermediate vehicle. The essential mechanism is contamination from lack of hygiene.

There are two groups of diseases in this category, skin diseases and eye diseases and it is convenient to describe them in this order. The skin diseases include infections of scabies and lice and the superficial fungal diseases. Tropical ulcers, for which a means of transmission has still not been defined, are conveniently included here. The eye diseases of public-health significance are trachoma, epidemic haemorrhagic conjunctivitis and ophthalmia neonatorum.

The main method of control of the diseases of poor hygiene is to increase water *quantity*. They are the first category in Table 5.2, called the water-washed diseases. Personal hygiene is encouraged by providing an adequate volume of water for washing.

7.1 SCABIES

Infection of the skin by a mite, *Sarcoptes scabiei*, causes a skin rash and intense itching. The mite burrows into the superficial layers of the skin, favouring the wrists and hands, although in heavy infections it may be found in almost any area of the body, but not the head or face. Due to scratching, the affected skin can become thickened and discoloured leading to a mistaken diagnosis of eczema. Secondary infection is common and glomerulonephritis can occur.

Scabies is due to close personal contact permitting the mite to pass from one person to another. It can be transmitted by shared clothing and is potentiated by poor hygiene. It mainly occurs in children, but anyone who comes in contact with infected individuals, e.g. mothers and school-teachers, can catch scabies. Scabies is a community problem and treatment of an individual is insufficient unless the whole family, school or village is similarly treated. In communities with poor hygiene the provision of adequate water is the most effective method of controlling the disease. People should be encouraged to wash themselves with soap and water and to wash their clothes and bedding.

Specific treatment is by benzyl benzoate, but this may need to be accompanied by an antibiotic if there is secondary infection. The patient is first given a warm bath and then a 10% emulsion of benzyl benzoate liberally applied to the whole body. This is left for 24 hours before being washed off. Treatment is repeated after 4–7 days to kill off larvae that have hatched from eggs. The whole family is treated at the same time, ensuring that only clean clothes and bedding are used. Alternatively 1% gamma-benzene hexachloride (Lindane) or tetraethylthiuram mono-sulphide (Tetmasol) is applied twice daily. If none of the special preparations are available, repeated applications of oil to the skin can be effective. Any oil usually used by people to rub on the skin, such as coconut oil, is effective. As the mite lives in a small burrow through which it respires, to seal the opening off with a film of oil asphyxiates it. This requires careful and repeated application to the whole body after washing.

Where possible, infected individuals should be prevented from infecting others, e.g. by keeping children away from school until they are clear. A careful search should be made for unreported or unrecognized cases in the community.

7.2 LICE

Lice are potential vectors of typhus (see Section 17.2.3) and relapsing fever (see Section 17.9) but the main worry of people is personal infection. Washing with warm water and soap at frequent intervals is the main method of prevention. Specific treatment is with a 10% dichlorodiphenyl-trichloroethane (DDT) dusting powder, repeated after a week, or in resistant cases with 1% gamma-benzene hexachloride (Lindane) or 2% temephos (Abate). Shaving of heads is a rigorous but effective method of control of head lice, but not of body lice.

7.3 SUPERFICIAL FUNGAL INFECTIONS (DERMATOMYCOSIS)

Just as viruses, bacteria and parasites attack the skin, fungi also find it a suitable medium on which to grow. Fungi either attack specific sites, such as moist skin in the feet or groin – *Tinea pedis*, the nails – *T. unguium* or the scalp – *T. capitis*, or are generalized on the body – *T. corporis, T. versicolor* or *T. imbricata. T. corporis* (often called ringworm) produces well-defined circular lesions that spread out from the centre, causing slight depigmentation as they proceed, whereas *T. versicolor* produces a blotchy hypopigmentation that can sometimes be misdiagnosed as leprosy. *T. imbricata* is particularly common in Western Pacific islands, producing serpiginous scaly designs that can cover the whole body. Children are most commonly affected.

Prevention is by body washing with soap and water and by not sharing clothes, towels, combs, etc. Local applications, such as acetylsalicylic acid ointment or benzoic acid compound (Whitfield's ointment), are effective if applied regularly for some 3 weeks. In resistant cases griseofulvin can be used, but it is expensive.

7.4 TROPICAL ULCERS

Tropical ulcers are a common debilitating condition, but the method of transmission is still not understood. They cause tissue loss and pain, which temporarily invalid the person, making daily work an agonizing undertaking. The condition can last for several months and, even when it heals, the victim is left with a scar that may lead to contracture. All ages and both sexes are susceptible.

There are two types of tropical ulcer, a non–specific variety and one due to *Mycobacterium ulcerans*, often called Buruli ulcer. These should both be differentiated from yaws, (see Section 15.1).

7.4.1 Non-specific Tropical Ulcers

Tropical ulcers are found in the warm moist areas of the world where the temperature and humidity are fairly constant. The ulcer follows a minute scratch or cut that becomes contaminated from the surroundings, especially by flies. Scratching of the wound by the host can be a potent method of instilling organisms into the skin.

No specific organism is isolated from the ulcer and treatment is empirical. During the invasive stage, antibiotics should be given, both systemically and locally, and the limb rested. Once the ulcer has formed, antibiotics have no effect and a cleaning solution, such as Eusol, should be applied. In coastal areas, soaking the affected limb in sea water is a cost-free method of cleaning out the ulcer. Skin grafting may be necessary.

Tropical ulcers can be prevented by taking scrupulous care over minor cuts and abrasions. As soon as any break in the skin surface occurs, it should be cleaned, an antiseptic applied and the ulcer covered with a dressing. Where dressings are in short supply, certain kinds of leaves can be used.

7.4.2 Buruli Ulcer (Mycobacterium ulcerans)

A more severe form of tropical ulcer, Buruli ulcer, is found in central Africa, Central and South America, South-East Asia and New Guinea. When the exudate is examined it is found to contain *Mycobacterium ulcerans*. Children and young adults are afflicted.

The method of transmission is not known, but it has been hypothesized that the mycobacterium enters the skin through either an abrasion or an inoculation by an insect. There is at first just a small papule surrounded by shiny skin, but this soon breaks down to reveal a large necrotic ulcer with undermined edges. Tissue damage may be extensive, involving bone and other structures.

Antimycobacterial drugs such as streptomycin, dapsone or thiambutosine have been found helpful, but essentially treatment is surgical – excision of the early ulcer and skin grafting of the large areas of tissue loss.

Several trials have been made with bacillus Calmette–Guérin (BCG) vaccination and, although this showed some early protection, it was not sustained. Health education in areas of high endemicity, with the provision of facilities for treating lesions as soon as they occur, has reduced the period of debility and the severity of the deformities.

7.5 TRACHOMA

A common infectious disease, trachoma is the major cause of blindness in the world.

Commencing as a keratoconjunctivitis, the first sign is red eye. There may be irritation and discharge but it is passed off as a self-limiting infection. A follicular infiltration of the conjunctiva then takes place particularly in the upper lid. Blood vessels grow into the periphery of the eye, forming pannus. Trachoma is often complicated by secondary infection. It is at the late stages of the disease, when it is non-infectious, that scarring, particularly of the upper eyelid, turns the eyelashes inwards to rub on the eye, a condition called entropion. This constant rubbing of the eyeball, aided by the dryness of the conjunctiva, damages the cornea, leading to scarring and finally blindness.

Diagnosis is usually made on clinical grounds, but can be confirmed by finding the characteristic inclusion bodies (containing the causative organism *Chlamydia trachomatis*) in scrapings taken from the

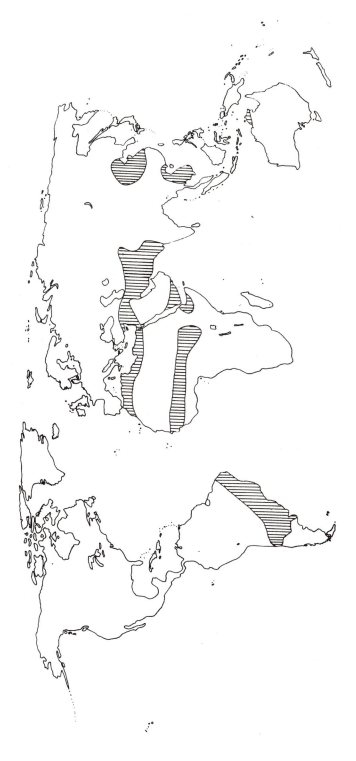

Fig. 7.1. The distribution of trachoma.

conjunctiva. The incubation period is 5–12 days and the period of communicability as long as there are active lesions.

Trachoma is found mainly in dry regions of the world (Fig. 7.1). It is a disease of poor sanitary conditions where a combination of close contact and dirty conditions encourages transmission. Within the family unit transmission is from child to child or by flies, which are attracted to the discharges around the eyes. In endemic areas 80–90% of children are infected by the age of 3 years. Cycles of reinfection and recrudescence continue to damage the eye and lead to blindness at school age. In conditions of improved sanitation there is a natural cycle lasting until the age of 11, with little residual damage. Females develop trachoma and blindness as adults more commonly than males, because they are directly concerned with looking after children. The usual method of wiping away secretions with hands, towels or clothing, which is then used by the adult, on themselves or other children, is a typical pattern of transmission. The chance of acquiring infection is increased by large families with short birth intervals, as there are more children of a young age living in close proximity.

Flies proliferate in rubbish and excrement, reaching their maximum numbers during the dry sunny period of the year. The damp, moist conditions in open pit latrines may be more important in encouraging fly breeding than non-use of latrines. Any flushing mechanism or improved latrine will discourage flies.

Long-term preventive measures are to improve sanitation and provide water supplies. The use of water to wash away secretions and to clean clothes and the surroundings is perhaps the single most effective method. Face washing has been shown to reduce the risk of developing trachoma. Regular daily face washing should be encouraged.

A strategy for a control programme is as follows.

- Conduct a survey to find the worst-affected areas.
- Give mass treatment.
- Conduct health education through schools, stressing regular face washing.
- Provide backup services.

Mass treatment is given more easily in schools, but it is preferable to treat in the home, where the main transmission takes place. A single dose of azithromycin ($20 \, \mathrm{mg \, kg^{-1}}$) is better than topical tetracycline plus oral erythromycin, although more expensive.

Preventing blindness once scarring and entropion have developed is very easily done by a simple operation that a medical assistant can be trained to do.

7.6 EPIDEMIC HAEMORRHAGIC CONJUNCTIVITIS

First recognized in Ghana in 1969, epidemic acute haemorrhagic conjunctivitis has caused epidemics in a number of parts of the world which have given their name to the disease, e.g. Nairobi eye.

Enterovirus 70 is the most important aetiological agent and has been responsible for tens of millions of cases. The infection starts suddenly with pain and subconjunctival haemorrhages. There is often much swelling and discomfort. It is self-limiting within 1–2 weeks. In a few cases there are systemic effects involving the upper respiratory tract or central nervous system (CNS). CNS effects are identical to those of poliomyelitis and residual paralysis can occur.

The incubation period is short, 1–3 days, transmission occurring from the discharges of infected eyes. Where there are systemic infections, transmission may be by the respiratory route. As with trachoma, intrafamilial transmission is common and, in situations of poor hygiene and overcrowding, large epidemics can occur.

There is no treatment, so mass administration of eye ointment is not applicable, but methods to improve hygiene and reduce overcrowding will prevent major epidemics. Careful hand washing, use of separate towels and sterilization of ophthalmological instruments are important in preventing transmission.

Similar in its epidemic presentation is *epidemic keratoconjunctivitis*, but as well as conjunctivitis a keratitis develops 7 days after onset in some 50% of cases. This normally resolves in about 2 weeks, but a minority are left with conjunctival scarring. The causative organism is adenovirus 8, but bacterial superinfection is common and this responds to topical antibiotics. Mode of spread and prevention are similar to epidemic haemorrhagic conjunctivitis.

7.7 OPHTHALMIA NEONATORUM

Infection of the eye of the newborn infant with *Neisseria gonorrhoea* or *Chlamydia trachomatis* can occur as a result of infection in the mother. As the infant passes through the birth canal, its eyes become contaminated with infectious dicharges. This leads to conjunctivitis in 5–14 days and in gonococcal infection is an important cause of blindness, especially in developing countries.

The *incubation period* is 1–5 days in gonococcal infection and 5–12 with *Chlamydia*.

Prevention of initial infection in the mother (see Sections 15.5 and 15.6) is the best strategy and any vaginal discharge occurring during pregnancy should be examined, cultured and treated. At delivery all babies' eyes should be routinely wiped and a 1% aqueous solution of silver nitrate instilled. Wiping both eyes at delivery alone can reduce the incidence of infection if silver nitrate is not available and should always be practised.

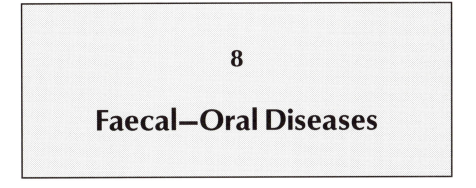

8

Faecal–Oral Diseases

The faecal–oral group of diseases are transmitted by person-to-person contact, through water or food via the oral route. Breaking the faecal–oral cycle is the basis of control by personal hygiene, increase in water quantity, improvement in water quality, food hygiene and the provision of sanitation.

Many of the diseases in this group cause diarrhoea (Table 8.1).

8.1 AMOEBIASIS

Amoebiasis is caused by the protozoan, *Entamoeba histolytica*, which exists in an amoeboid form in the human large intestine. The pathogenic amoeba enters a mucosal fold and feeds on red blood cells. Penetrating through the muscularis mucosae, an abscess forms which results in vascular necrosis. This leads to tissue disintegration and the development of an ulcer (the so-called flask-shaped ulcer). Active amoebae can be found in the base of an ulcer. In a chronic infection an amoeboma can be formed which may be confused with carcinoma.

If the amoebic ulcer penetrates a blood vessel, fresh blood is passed in the stool, which is a characteristic feature in the diagnosis. Amoebae are also carried in the breached circulatory system to various parts of the body, the liver being the commonest, forming a liver abscess. The right lobe is the commonest site and liver damage a predisposing cause. The expanding abscess can track outwards through the peritoneum, abdominal wall and on to the skin, or upwards to form a subphrenic abscess or enter the pleural cavity. The most serious site of amoebic abscess development is in the brain. All these features are illustrated in Fig. 8.1.

Cysts are formed in the large intestines and passed into the environment in the faeces. They survive in faeces for only a few days but if they

Table 8.1. Diarrhoeas.

Presentation	Disease	Organism	Characteristics
Acute watery diarrhoea	Salmonellosis Food poisoning	*Salmonella, Staphylococci B. cereus C. perfringens V. parahaemolytica*	Sudden onset with vomiting in group of people associated by food
	Gastroenteritis (bacterial)	*E. coli* or non-specific	Common, mainly in children, epidemic
	Gastroenteritis (viral)	Rotavirus and other enteroviruses	Occurs in children, often in institutions (hospitals,
	Cryptosporidiosis	*Cryptosporidium*	schools, etc.)
	Cholera	*V. cholerae*	Severe, dehydration, rice-water stools, epidemic
Acute diarrhoea with *blood*	Bacillary dysentery	*Shigella* sp.	Severe, seasonal, all ages
	Campylobacter	*C. jejuni*	Sporadic, from contaminated food, animal reservoir
Chronic diarrhoea	Giardiasis	*G. lamblia*	Mainly children, can cause malabsorption
	(Sprue or malabsorption syndromes)		Adults, mostly males, nutritional deficiencies especially of folic acid
Chronic diarrhoea with *blood*	Amoebiasis	*E. histolytica*	Cooler climates, mainly adults
	Balantidiasis	*B. coli*	Similar to amoebiasis, associated with pigs
	Schistosomiasis	*S. mansoni*	Endemic areas, characteristic eggs in stools

B.(cereus), Bacillus; C.(perfringens), Clostridium; V.(parahaemolytica), Vibrio; E.(coli), Escherichia; V.(cholerae), Vibrio; C.(jejuni), Campylobacter; G.(lamblia), Giardia; E.(histolytica), Entamoeba; B.(coli), Balantidium; S.(mansoni), Schistosoma.
Many other diseases cause diarrhoea, e.g. measles, malaria, tonsillitis.

enter water they remain viable for considerably longer periods. Infection occurs through drinking contaminated water or eating irrigated salad vegetables. Flies can carry cysts for some 5 hours. In circumstances of poor hygiene, direct faecal–oral transfer via food or by utensils can take place.

Amoebiasis is a disease of poor hygiene, more commonly found in cooler areas than hot. In the tropics it predominantly occurs in highland areas or where there is a large temperature fluctuation. Cysts can survive

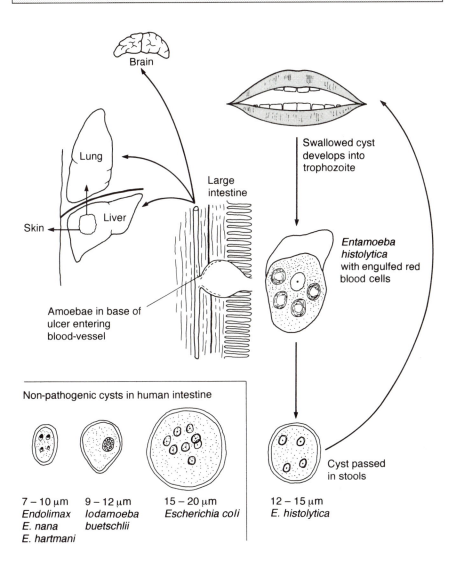

Fig 8.1. Amoebiasis.

in the cold for considerable periods, but they are killed by a temperature over 43°C, which must be obtained in any composting system where human faeces are used. Survival of amoebic cysts is a useful indicator of ineffective decomposition (see Fig. 1.2).

Amoebiasis is an infection of adult life and the longer the period of residence in an endemic area, the greater the chance of becoming infected. The *Incubation period* is 2–4 weeks, illness presenting as an acute diarrhoea with frank blood, as chronic diarrhoea or as an abscess with no apparent transitional period of diarrhoea. Liver abscess is more common in males than females. Symptoms of an abscess are fever, weight loss and localized tenderness. Amoebic pus is characteristically a pale reddish brown colour (without odour) and can be discharged on to the skin from a penetrating ulcer or coughed up from the lung.

Diagnosis is made by examining fresh stool specimens within half an hour for motile amoebae with ingested red blood cells. Amoebae are occasionally found in amoebic pus, which similarly must be examined as soon as possible as the active forms rapidly die off. The finding of cysts indicates infection, but a search must be made of fresh stool or pus for motile amoebae. Liver abscess is diagnosed by X-ray (raised diaphragm) or by ultrasound. The abscess is usually not tapped, unless in differential diagnosis from a bacterial abscess or it is about to burst.

Treatment of all stages of the disease is by metronidazole, 2.4 g single dose for 3 days or 2 g daily for 5 days, or by other derivatives of the 5-nitroimidazole group of compounds (tinidazole, ornidazole and nimorazole). Cyst passers can be given diloxanide furoate (Furomate), 500 mg 8-hourly for 10 days.

Control is by personal hygiene, food hygiene and the proper provision of water and sanitation. Sand filtration, especially if it is combined with alum flocculation, removes cysts from water supplies. A high concentration of chlorine is required to kill cysts (3.5 parts per million (ppm) residual), although they are more sensitive to iodine.

8.2 *GIARDIA*

The small flagellate *Giardia intestinalis* (*lamblia*) is a common commensal of the human small intestine. Heavy infections in children, especially those in institutions or debilitated by other conditions, can produce a persistent diarrhoea. Faeces are loose and greasy with an unpleasant odour. Bloating and abdominal distension can occur. Chronic infections can produce partial villous atrophy with a resulting malabsorption syndrome. *Giardia* is one of the causes of travellers' diarrhoea. The *incubation period* is 5–20 days.

The characteristic 'face'-shaped flagellate is occasionally seen in the faeces, easily detected by its high motility. The small cysts are more commonly found. Jejunal biopsy or the duodenal string test may be performed in the differential diagnosis of the malabsorption syndrome.

Treatment is with tinidazole, either as a single dose of 2 g or 300 mg a day for 7 days. Metronidazole can also be used.

The cysts can survive for several weeks in fresh water and are not killed by normal levels of chlorine. Transmission is by person-to-person transfer of cysts from the faeces of an infected individual or by contamination of food or water. An animal reservoir might also be responsible.

Control is through the following.

- Personal hygiene.
- Proper sewage disposal.
- Protection of water supplies.
- Water treatment (iodine five to ten drops per litre of water).
- Hygienic food preparation and handling.

8.3 CRYPTOSPORIDIOSIS

Cryptosporidiosis presents as an acute watery diarrhoea associated with abdominal pain. Fever, anorexia, nausea and vomiting can occur, especially in children. There may be repeat attacks, but these do not normally continue for more than a month. In the immunodeficient, especially acquired immune deficiency syndrome (AIDS) patients, the disease enters a chronic and progressive course.

Cryptosporidium is a protozoan parasite found in poultry, fish, reptiles and mammals, especially cattle, sheep, dogs and cats, from which the infection can be acquired. Transmission is from person to person via the faecal–oral route or from faecally contaminated water. The oocyst can survive in nature for a considerable period of time. The infecting dose is very low.

Diagnosis is by finding the oocyst in faecal samples. Alternatively, the intestinal stages can be looked for in intestinal biopsy specimens. Supportive treatment is with oral rehydration to replace fluid loss.

Cryptosporidiosis has a worldwide distribution, being found particularly in conditions of poor hygiene. It is endemic in many developing countries, where infection is acquired at an early age. Massive epidemics have occurred in developed countries where the water purification system has failed (such as the Milwaukee epidemic, where there were 0.5 million cases). In other areas it is a disease of animal handlers, homosexuals and institutions.

The incubation period is about a week (range 1–12 days) and the period of communicability continues for up to 6 months in faecal material. Prevention is through personal hygiene, the provision and use of sanitation, safe water supplies and hygiene precautions with domestic animals and pets.

8.4 GASTROENTERITIS

Gastroenteritis is a common form of diarrhoea that predominantly attacks children. It is endemic in developing countries, but seasonal epidemics occur. Attempts to find a specific organism are often unsuccessful and not essential as management and control are the same. Strains of toxigenic *Escherichia coli* and enteric viruses, particularly rotavirus, are the main organisms.

The *incubation period* is some 12–72 hours (generally 48), after which a profuse, watery diarrhoea commences with occasional vomiting. Despite the fluid nature of the stools, faecal material is always present and never the rice-water stool characteristic of cholera.

Water and electrolytes are lost, which in the young child may be sufficient to cause dehydration and ionic imbalance, leading to death. Normally, it is a self-limiting condition but, in unhygienic surroundings or where babies' bottles are used, repeated infections occur. These lead to chronic loss of nutrients and subsequent malnutrition. A serious infection in neonates, mortality decreases with age until in adults it is just a passing inconvenience (travellers' diarrhoea).

Management is by replacement of fluid and electrolytes using an oral rehydration solution (ORS) in the moderately dehydrated and following intravenous replacement in the severely dehydrated.

The following, dissolved in 1 litre of water, is a suitable ORS.

Sodium chloride (salt)	3.5 g (Na^+ 90 mmol)
Sodium citrate	2.9 g (citrate 10 mmol)
Potassium chloride	1.5 g (K^+ 20 mmol, Cl^- 88 mmol)
Glucose (dextrose)	20.0 g (glucose 111 mmol)

These ingredients can be obtained separately or in packets of ready-prepared ingredients. In the absence of prepared packets a simpler formulation can be prepared, as shown in Fig. 8.2. This consists of mixing salt, sugar and water; potassium is not an essential constituent, but if the juice of one orange can be added this is useful. Tea-leaves also contain potassium, so the mixture can be prepared as tea, with salt and sugar added. Teaspoons vary in size and it is dangerous to give too much salt, so a useful check is for the mother to taste the solution before administering it to her child. If it tastes salty, more water is added.

A naturally available rehydration solution is the fluid from a green coconut. A 7-month coconut has been found to be most suitable. Rice water made from a handful of rice boiled in a saucepan of water until it disappears, plus the appropriate amount of salt for the volume of water, makes a simple rehydration solution. Carrot water can also be used. If

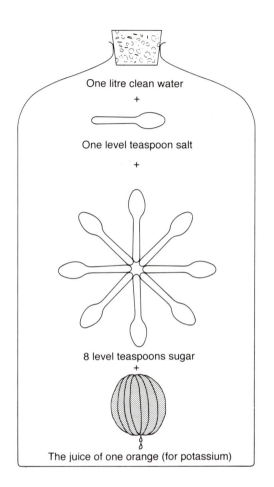

One litre clean water

+

One level teaspoon salt

+

8 level teaspoons sugar

+

The juice of one orange (for potassium)

Fig 8.2. Preparing a simple oral rehydration solution.

mothers are taught how to make up these solutions, they can treat their own children as soon as they start to get diarrhoea. The mother should use a cup and a spoon and sit with her child, giving it small quantities of fluid at frequent intervals. Severe dehydration can usually be prevented from developing by primary care from the mother.

There is no need to use an antibiotic or an antispasmodic, both of which are contraindicated. Lactobacilli, which inhibit *E. coli*, colonize the gut in the breast-fed infant. In some countries lactobacilli are administered in yoghurt (curd).

Epidemics occur in families or groups of children sharing similar surroundings. Infection is often seasonal, with the beginning of the rains often heralding an outbreak. This would suggest transmission by water, and simple control measures such as the boiling of water can stop the epidemic.

Control is by:

- promotion of breast-feeding;
- promoting the use of ORS in the community;
- improvement in water supply and sanitation;
- promoting personal and domestic hygiene;
- rotavirus vaccination (and other vaccines, e.g. measles).

Breast-feeding not only provides a sterile milk formula in the correct proportions (in contrast to the often contaminated bottle) but also promotes lactobacilli and contains lactoferrins and lysozymes. Promoting breast-feeding and the administration of ORS solution in the community are the main control strategies. Improvement in water supplies and sanitation, with promotion of personal hygiene, are long-term measures. A rotavirus vaccine is being developed which could reduce some 6% of diarrhoeal episodes and up to 20% of deaths.

8.5 BACILLARY DYSENTERY (SHIGELLOSIS)

Bacillary dysentery presents as an acute diarrhoeal illness with blood in the stools, more acute and severe than amoebic dysentery. In mild infections, blood may be absent and the presentation may be similar to that of gastroenteritis. In severe cases, the stools are a mixture of pus and blood and tenesmus is common. Fever accompanies the illness and nausea or frank vomiting can occur. *The incubation period* is 1–7 days.

Bacillary dysentery is due to *Shigella* invading the bowel. The species and strains of *Shigella* are numerous. There are four main groups.

- A. *S. dysenteriae* and 10 serotypes.
- B. *S. flexneri* and 6 serotypes.
- C. *S. boydi* and 15 serotypes.
- D. *S. sonnei.*

The most severe are group A organisms and the least group D (*S. sonnei*), but severity is also determined by age and general level of health. A moderate mortality can occur in the very young and very old.

Management is the same as for other diarrhoeas, to replace fluid and electrolytes lost. ORS is adequate and effective in all but the severely dehydrated. There is, however, a place for antibiotics, although sensitivity must be determined, as many organisms are resistant to a wide range of preparations. Ampicillin, tetracyclines, chloramphenicol, co-trimoxazole, nalidixic acid and the quinolones (Ciprofloxacin, Ofloxacin, Norfloxacin) can be used.

Transmission is by the faecal–oral route and only ten to 100 organisms are required to produce the disease. Bacillary dysentery can occur in small outbreaks among families, suggesting food as the mode of transfer. Seasonal epidemics coinciding with the arrival of the rains indicates water-borne spread. Flies can be important in the hot dry months, when garbage accumulates and massive fly breeding takes place. The carrier state is found, and sporadic epidemics in institutions might indicate a food handler with insanitary habits. The development of antibiotic resistance makes control more difficult and the disease can relentlessly spread through a country.

If bacteriological facilities permit, the organism should be identified, typed and sensitivity determined. A suitable transport medium is Carey Blair. Where this is not possible, a simple epidemiological investigation may provide sufficient information to indicate the mode of transmission. Appropriate control measures, as covered in Chapter 5 can be implemented. A search for carriers is generally unsatisfactory and investigation should be restricted to food handlers. Management of an epidemic is similar to that of cholera (see Section 8.6).

8.6 CHOLERA

A profound diarrhoea of rapid onset that leads to dehydration and death should be considered as a case of cholera until proved otherwise. The diarrhoea contains no faecal particles but is watery and flecked with mucus (not cells), the so-called rice-water stools. The passage of large quantities of fluid leads to rapid and extreme dehydration, which can be fatal. Vomiting can also be present in the early stages.

The causative organism, *Vibrio cholerae*, can be identified from the diarrhoeal discharge, from the vomitus or by rectal swab. The characteristic vibrio mobility can be seen by dark-ground or phase-contrast microscopy and is inhibited by specific antiserum. Confirmation of the diagnosis is made by culture on TCBS sucrose agar. A suitable transport medium is Carey Blair, or alternatively 1% alkaline (pH 8.5) peptone water, which can also be used for water samples.

Classical cholera is restricted to south Asia, caused by *V. cholerae* 01, but recently *V. cholerae* non-01 (vibrio 0139) has been responsible for epidemics in India, Bangladesh, Myanmar, Thailand and Malaysia. The El Tor biotype has infected Asia, Africa, Europe, the Western Pacific and South America. First isolated from pilgrims to Mecca in the quarantine station of El Tor in West Sinai (now Egypt) in 1906, it differs from the classical variety by producing a soluble haemolysin.

The El Tor biotype is classified as either Ogawa or Inaba of the classical serotypes. The importance of the El Tor biotype is that it can survive longer in water, is more infectious, can cause mild infections and more frequently produces the carrier state. These characteristics have all

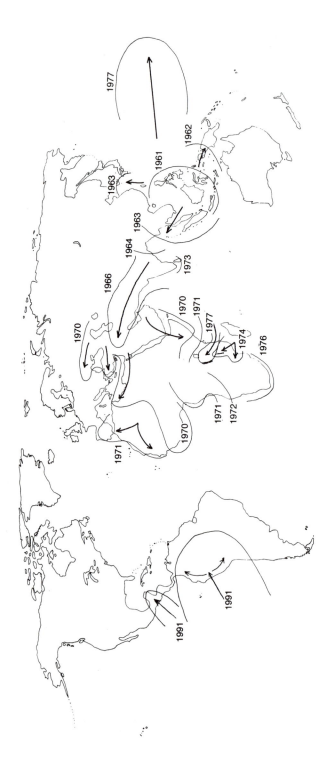

Fig. 8.3. The spread of El Tor cholera 1961–1991

assisted in the extensive spread of this organism from a focus in Sulawesi (Indonesia) since 1961 (Fig. 8.3).

The vibrio binds to the cells and produces an enterotoxin, which activates adenyl cyclase, an intracellular enzyme that initiates a system of fluid and ion transport from the plasma to the intestinal lumen. There is no mucosal damage and increased permeability is unlikely, which explains why glucose and electrolytes can still be absorbed by the mucosa. This allows large quantities of low-protein fluid, bicarbonate and potassium to escape through an essentially undamaged intestine. Management is to correct dehydration in this otherwise self-limiting disease.

Fluid replacement must be rapid and adequate, the most easily available being the first choice. If rehydration can be started as soon as cholera symptoms begin, oral rehydration will be all that is required. ORS can either be prepared from ready-mixed packets of salts (see Section 8.4) or by making a sugar–salt solution (see Fig. 8.2). Unfortunately, most cases have already lost considerable body fluid on presentation, which means that they will require intravenous infusion. If available, Ringer–lactate solution (Hartmann's) contains the nearest approximation of electrolytes to that being passed in the diarrhoeal fluid. As a second best a mixture of two units of normal saline and one of sodium bicarbonate can be used. The patient should be rehydrated intravenously as rapidly as possible, and then ORS substituted once the patient can swallow. This allows the body mechanisms to regulate electrolytes, as ionic imbalance can rapidly occur with intravenous infusion, from which many patients succumb. The body fluid deficit should be restored, followed by a maintenance of the equivalent amount of bowel loss. Fluid loss can be measured into a bucket under the bed. A bed or cholera cot is not essential and the patient can be nursed on a plastic sheet laid on the ground with the earth hollowed out under the pelvis to take a receptacle to collect the fluid outpouring.

Tetracycline is not essential in treatment, but shortens the duration of the illness and reduces the quantity of fluid replacement required. Tetracycline is given in a dose of 500 mg 6-hourly for 3 days, or Doxycycline in a single dose of 300 mg. Sensitivity must be monitored, as the development of tetracycline resistance will necessitate a change of treatment.

The management of a cholera epidemic requires speed and good organization. Essentially treatment is taken to the people by setting up treatment centres at strategic places in the vicinity of the epidemic. These can be dispensaries, schools, church halls or even tents, supplied with staff and fluids. Cholera patients do not need to be treated in hospital.

Classical cholera is a disease of water transmission, whereas El Tor is by both water and food. Generally, epidemic cholera is transmitted by water and endemic cholera by food. It is the endemic nature of El Tor and its persistence in the environment that has been responsible for its prodigious spread. Carriers are of short duration, 70% of cholera cases are free of vibrios at the end of the first week and 98% by the end of the third. Long-term carriers are rare and of no epidemiological importance.

For every clinical case of El Tor cholera, there can be as many as 100 asymptomatic cases. This would explain how epidemics spread from one region to another, but not how infection persists. It may appear in a seasonal pattern (Fig. 8.4) with no cases in between.

It is possible that vibrios may be able to persist in an aquatic environment, such as the mucilaginous covering of water plants, fish or even amoebae. Another explanation of persistence of the vibrio is that person-to-person transmission takes place, maintaining the organism in an asymptomatic cycle. When a susceptible person enters the cycle, or there is an environmental or climatic change, it breaks out and multiplies again.

A case of cholera can excrete between 10^7 and 10^9 V. cholerae ml^{-1} of diarrhoeal discharge and since the volume of this discharge may be in excess of 20 litres per day the potential for contamination of the environment is enormous. Clearly, though, since the severe case is unlikely to be anything but a transitory source, it is the asymptomatic case passing 10^2–10^5 organisms g^{-1} of stool in a spasmodic manner that poses the greatest hazard.

V. cholerae in water are easily destroyed by sunlight, chemical action or competing bacteria. However, where these elements are not present, it can survive in fresh water for some time and in saline for at least a week. The level of salinity needs to be between 0.01 and 0.1%, as is found in estuarine or lagoon water. V. cholerae in this saline environment can be taken up by shellfish or fish, which then form an alternative method of infection when eaten uncooked. The isolation of V. cholerae from river water has been an enigma, because epidemiological investigations show this source of infection to be important, but bacteriologists have not isolated organisms in sufficient numbers. One possible explanation is the presence of non-agglutinable vibrios (NAG, alternatively known as non-cholera vibrios), which are closely related to V. cholerae except that they do not agglutinate antisera. These are known to be mutations, and shifts between typical vibrios and non-agglutinable forms may occur. If this is a regular feature in nature, it could help to explain where cholera goes to (especially the classical form) during interepidemic periods. The recent appearance of non-O1 cholera (vibrio 0139) supports this view.

V. cholerae has been found to remain viable in crude sewage for over a month and in sewage-contaminated soil for up to 10 days, a possible source of infection of rivers or wells. It has been isolated from a number of foodstuffs, especially those with a pH of between 6 and 8 such as milk produce (e.g. ice-cream), sugar solutions, meat extracts or articles of food preserved by salt. Uncooked fish have been responsible for outbreaks, as

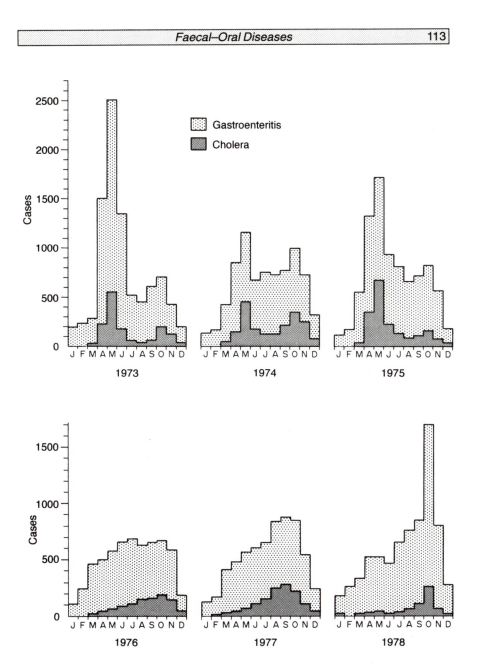

Fig. 8.4. Similar pattern of gastroenteritis and cholera in Calcutta, India (1973–1978). (Reproduced, with permission, from the Indian Council of Medical Research (1978) *National Institute of Cholera and Enteric Diseases, Annual Report*, Indian Council of Medical Research, Calcutta.)

have vegetables that have been washed or irrigated by sewage effluent.

Direct person-to-person spread or via fomites, such as utensils or drinking straws (in home-brewed alcohol parties), do not appear to be as important as expected. Even for persons attending the death of a cholera case, it is more likely that infection will result from drinking water or consuming food that has been prepared for the mourning ceremony, rather than from the dead person or his/her shrouds.

A high dose of V. cholerae is required to infect the healthy subject. Some 10^6–10^8 organisms are needed, but, if they have a decreased gastric acidity, 10^3 organisms may be sufficient. Lowered gastric acidity is found more commonly than expected and may be related to malnutrition or diet. Cannabis smoking is known to depress gastric acidity.

The incubation period is between 1 and 5 days. Humans are the only known reservoir, but the persistence of the organism in the environment, possibly in a changing form, as discussed above, may be another source. In endemic areas cholera is a disease of children (adults having developed immunity in childhood), whereas in its epidemic form adults are the more usual victims. The disease is associated with poverty and poor hygienic practices.

Control is aimed at the cause. All too often a panic situation develops, foods are banned, vaccination is given and quarantine is instigated. If cholera is epidemic and preliminary investigations indicate that water is the vehicle of transmission, the supply should be sterilized by super-chlorination (adding two to three times the calculated amount of chlorine required for the volume of water) or everybody told to boil the water. Boiling water is unpopular as it uses vital firewood, it monopolizes scarce cooking pots and the water has a flat taste. However, there is no reason why water cannot be boiled at the same time as the meal is cooked and simple clay pots used instead of metal ones. Boiled water can be re-aerated by shaking it up. A not so safe, but easier, method is to leave water to stand and then decant off the supernatant. A simple way of doing this is the three pot system (see Fig. 5.6). Chlorine can be added to a well or communal water supply, but any vegetable matter in the water will inactivate chlorine and several times that calculated may be required.

The banning or restriction of food should only be made on good epidemiological evidence. If fish are properly cooked before being eaten, they are unlikely to be a source. Disruption of a fish-eating practice may have dire consequences on other aspects of people's health. It is more often the fisherman rather than the fish or the farmers rather than their produce that are the purveyors of cholera.

Quarantine is rarely effective, as bribery or evasion of the barricades by the few who might be carrying the infection negates the hardships borne by the many who are not. Giving tetracycline to immediate contacts of cases will reduce the number of asymptomatic carriers, but the widespread distribution of the drug will encourage tetracycline resistance.

Cholera vaccination gives about 50% protection and only lasts for 6 months; it does not prevent the asymptomatic disease state and so can actively encourage the spread of infection. Vaccination is therefore not recommended as a method of control. However, newer vaccines are in the development stage and may well be valuable in the control of epidemics.

Persons dying from cholera should be buried promptly and the ceremony kept to a minimum. Disinfectants and hand-washing facilities should be provided at treatment centres and when bodies are prepared for burial. Flies should be controlled by disposing of or covering all faecal discharges, although they have not been shown to play a significant role in transmission.

Surveillance for cholera is both national and international. An outbreak of cholera must be reported to the World Health Organization (WHO). This provides an advance warning system to neighbouring countries. Nationally a warning system can be implemented for diarrhoeal diseases where an increase in number of cases or of persons dying from diarrhoea may indicate an underlying outbreak of cholera (Fig. 8.4). Where cholera exhibits a seasonal pattern, the population and health staff can be placed on the alert when the next season starts.

8.7 TYPHOID

Although transmitted by the faecal–oral route, typhoid manifests mainly as a systemic infection, generally presenting as a fever. The fever starts gradually, increasing in a stepwise fashion over the first 1–2 weeks, with a progressive malaise, disorientation and drowsiness. At the end of the first week a rash of characteristic rose spots may appear (not seen in black skins). The *Incubation period* is 7–21 days, with a mean of 14. The incubation period depends upon the infecting dose.

The stools are normally constipated at first, but may later change to diarrhoea. The organism, *Salmonella typhi*, can localize in the Peyer's patches of the small intestine, resulting in ulceration, haemorrhage and perforation.

Diagnosis is difficult and depends upon finding the organism in blood, stool or urine. A blood culture (3–5 ml) taken in the first week is the most satisfactory. Culture from the stools can be achieved if repeated examinations are made from the start of the illness, with a greater likelihood of becoming positive as the illness progresses, provided antibiotics have not been used. Finding the organism from the urine, in which it is excreted spasmodically, is more difficult. Where the diagnosis has still not been made and the investigation is considered necessary, *S. typhi* can be cultured from the bone marrow or bile (by the duodenal string test). Bone-marrow culture has the advantage of being positive occasionally, even if the patient has received antibiotics. Sewage culture can be used in the investigation of epidemics.

The Widal test on the patient's serum can indicate infection, but a search for S. *typhi* must also be made to confirm the diagnosis. The Widal test has three components, the H (flagellar), the O (somatic) and the Vi antigens. The H antibody titre can be raised by any *Salmonella* infection and remain raised (giving an estimate of previous exposure), whereas the O antibody indicates recent infection. However, both H and O levels will be raised by recent typhoid immunization, thus negating any value of the test. A titre of 1/40 or higher is required. Added weight is given to the diagnosis by making a series of tests and demonstrating a rising titre. The Vi antibody is produced during the acute stage of the disease and persists while the organism is present, and so has a value in detecting the carrier state.

Treatment is with chloramphenicol 2 g daily for 14 days. Co-trimoxazole is also effective. Over the last few years, multiply resistant organisms have been reported from all over the world. Some of the newer agents which can be used include the quinalones, e.g. Ciprofloxacin, Ofloxacin, etc. Prolonged treatment of the carrier with ampicillin, 1 g three times a day for 11 weeks, has been successful. Relapse occurs in about 5% of treated acute cases.

The *carrier* state is the most important epidemiological feature, with persistence of the organism in some individuals for periods in excess of 50 years. About 3% of typhoid cases are found to be still excreting organisms after 1 year. People become more prone to act as carriers if they have a chronic irritational process, such as cholecystitis and especially the presence of stones (in which S. *typhi* are able to survive). *Opisthorchis sinensis* has also been associated with the development of faecal carriers. Urinary carriers often suffer from an abnormality of the urinary tract, such as calculus, and *Schistosoma haematobium* is a predisposing cause.

S. *typhi* has been found to survive periods of 4 weeks in fresh water, but if the water is stored in bright sunlight (as in a reservoir) the number of organisms rapidly dies off. S. *typhi* survives in aerobic conditions with organic nutrient, as found in contaminated streams. If the stream is polluted with raw sewage, the organism can survive for over 5 weeks and within solid faecal material for considerable periods of time. Sea water is bactericidal to S. *typhi*, but, where a sewage outfall is near a shellfish bed, the organism is filtered and concentrated, providing a potent source of infection if the shellfish is eaten raw.

Milk and dairy produce provide ideal culture media and can become infected during handling by a carrier or rinsing of containers with polluted water. Contaminated ice-cream has been responsible for several outbreaks. Pasteurization of milk at 60°C is effective in killing S. *typhi*. Infection of meat products and canned foods is less common, but can occur in the cooling process (if carried out in polluted water).

Flies can transmit the organism from faeces to food, whereas person-to-person infection is uncommon. Secondary cases form a very small proportion of an epidemic, so serial transmission in an unhygienic environment is not a feature.

The main method of transmission is water, contaminated by faecal material from a carrier. These water-borne outbreaks may not always be explosive, and where low–grade infection of the water source is taking place, groups of cases, spread over time, may occur.

In most tropical areas the disease is *endemic*, with seasonal outbreaks. Water is probably the main vehicle of transmission, but may be more related to collections of people gathering at scarce water sources (as occurs in the dry season), rather than epidemics occurring with the early rains. Endemic typhoid is maintained by subclinical infections, especially in undiagnosed children, which produce a degree of immunity. It has been suggested that these subclinical infections result from persons swallowing lower bacterial doses than the critical threshold.

An *infecting dose* of at least 10^3 organisms is required (except in persons suffering from achlorhydria), but it may need to be as high as 10^9. The main effect of vaccination appears to be to offer protection against lower-dose infecting inocula (less than 10^5 organisms).

Control relies on the protection of water supplies and the sanitary disposal of faeces. Placing latrines too close to wells, fractures in water mains and accidental contamination by sewage are ways in which outbreaks occur. Drinking water taken from polluted streams can be boiled, chlorinated or left to stand (the three pot system in Fig. 5.6). Reservoirs and settling tanks can reduce the level of organisms below the infecting dose.

Where the outbreak can be traced to a food source, a search for carriers can be made. Stool specimens should be obtained from persons involved in the preparation of the food. If a carrier is discovered, he/she should be prohibited from preparing food. This cannot always be applied to domestic catering, so careful instruction in personal hygiene should be tried. The organism can persist under the nails, so these should be kept short. Food must be protected from flies and stored only for limited periods. All shellfish must be properly cooked.

Typhoid vaccine has a variable effect, offering protection to persons who receive a low infecting dose, but none to those who ingest a high dose of organisms. It may therefore be useful for individual protection, but not on a mass immunization basis. The live oral vaccine (Ty 21a) gives protection for at least 3 years and may also give cross-immunity against *S. paratyphi* B. It is administered in three capsules taken orally on days 1, 3 and 5. A vaccine containing the polysaccharide Vi antigen is also available, administered parenterally in a single dose. These both produce fewer reactions than the whole-bacteria vaccine.

8.7.1 Paratyphoid

Paratyphoid is similar to typhoid, but with fewer systemic effects, diarrhoea being a more important feature. The paratyphoid group is more commonly food-borne (see under food poisoning, Section 11.1).

8.8 HEPATITIS A (HAV)

Infectious hepatitis is a viral infection (picornavirus) producing inflammation, infiltration and necrosis of the liver, resulting in biliary stasis and jaundice. The *incubation period* is 15–50 days, generally about 28, during which time the person feels lethargic, anorexic and depressed and has fever, vomiting, diarrhoea and abdominal discomfort. The appearance of jaundice reveals the diagnosis, and the person begins to feel better.

The period of infectivity is the latter half of the incubation period until about 1 week after jaundice appears, so that most cases have already transmitted the virus to family and contacts before they report for medical attention. A large number of asymptomatic cases occur. There is an increase in symptomatic and severe cases with a rise in age. HAV is a mild disease, leading to spontaneous cure in the large majority, with only a few cases developing acute fulminant hepatitis and even, rarely, severe chronic liver damage.

Hepatitis is endemic in most tropical countries, children coming into contact early in life and developing a degree of immunity. Non-immune persons, such as those from an area of good sanitation, coming into this environment are likely to develop the disease. It is mainly a disease of poor sanitation, with water and food as the principal vehicles of transmission, but it can also occur when sanitation is good. The carrier state is not important. Epidemics occur when sewage contaminates water supplies, producing infection in people who have previously acquired some immunity, suggesting that the disease may be dose-dependent. Where there is a large infecting inoculum, infection can occur despite previous experience of the disease.

HAV vaccine protects the individual at risk, but is unfortunately too expensive to be used on a community scale. Long-term prevention is by sanitary methods. Good personal hygiene prevents contamination by infected food handlers during the prodromal stage of the disease. Salads, cold meats and raw seafood are common vehicles of transmission.

8.9 HEPATITIS E (HEV)

An enteric (E) virus bearing many similarities to HAV has been identified. It has been responsible for large epidemics and appears to be endemic in south and South-East Asia, especially Myanmar and Vietnam.

The main difference from HAV is that HEV results in a high mortality in pregnant women (up to 40%). It is thought to be water-borne and mainly occurs in epidemics, when extra precautions must be taken to protect pregnant women. Incubation period, means of transmission and control are very similar to those of HAV.

8.10 POLIOMYELITIS (POLIO)

A widespread and common disease in developing countries (Fig. 8.5) the serious sequelae of polio are found in a comparatively small number of children (three to ten per 1000). Commencing with fever, general malaise and headache, the majority of cases resolve after these mild symptoms, but approximately 1% proceeds to paralytic disease. The virus has a predilection for nerve cells, especially those with a motor function (the anterior horn cells of the spinal cord and the motor nuclei of the cranial nerves). These cells are destroyed and a flaccid paralysis results. As a generalization, the paralysis is more common in the lower part of the body, becoming less common the higher up it affects. Unilateral is more common than bilateral lameness. The severe form of bulbar poliomyelitis is generally fatal in poor countries where respirators and intensive nursing care are not available. Site of paralysis is associated with injections or operations and these should be avoided if there is any suggestion of poliomyelitis.

Diagnosis of the disabled case is made on clinical grounds, differentiating it from the spastic paralysis of birth injury, with which it is commonly confused. In polio there will be a history of normal birth with commencement of walking, followed by a feverish illness and the development of flaccid paralysis. The paralysis is limited to well demarcated muscle groups and there is no sensory loss. A similar history may be given for meningitis, but the damage will be central with accompanying mental deficiency. These features are important to the epidemiologist conducting a lameness survey (see below). The *incubation period* is 5–30 days with a mean of 10.

Transmission is generally from faecal contamination, although the virus initially multiplies in the oropharynx, from which it can also be transmitted. It then goes to the gastrointestinal tract, where it is excreted for several weeks. A disease of low hygiene, young children (4–5 months) meet the virus with only a small proportion showing overt disease: 80–90% have an unapparent subclinical disease, 5–10% suffer from fever, headache and minor clinical signs and only 1% go on to paralysis. Paralysis is more common at an older age, so a non-immune person coming into an endemic environment is at far greater

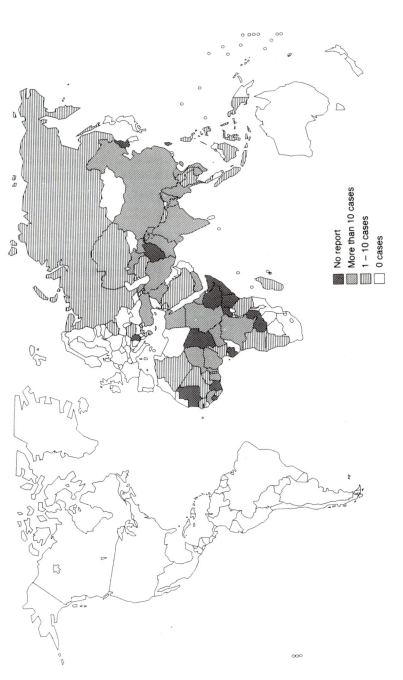

Fig. 8.5. Global incidence of indigenous poliomyelitis, 1994. (Reproduced with permission from WHO (1995) *Weekly Epidemiological Record* 14, World Health Organization, Geneva.)

No report
More than 10 cases
1 – 10 cases
0 cases

danger of developing paralytic poliomyelitis. Raising standards of hygiene will also have the same effect because it spares people from meeting the virus as young children and allows a pool of susceptibles to develop. In time, the number of non-immunes will be sufficient for an epidemic to take place. There will also be a higher proportion of paralysed cases (peak age 5–9 years) and many deaths. So sadly the raising of living standards will change polio from an endemic disease with a few paralysed cases to an epidemic disease of increased severity. In epidemic poliomyelitis where sanitation is good, pharyngeal spread becomes a more important method of transmission. Poliovirus strains vary in their neurovirulence, with the more virulent strains having a greater tendency to spread. This could be due to a lower infective dose of the virulent virus being required to produce disease.

Two types of vaccine, the killed (Salk) and the attenuated living (Sabin), are available. The Salk vaccine is given by intramuscular injection and is expensive to produce because it contains many organisms. But it induces a high level of immunity, which is not antagonized by inhibitory factors in the gut. The Sabin vaccine is easily administered orally, is cheaper and produces an intestinal immunity in addition to systemic immunity, which can block infection with wild strains of poliovirus. Multiplication of the virus in the intestine makes it very useful in preventing epidemics and allows it to spread to non-vaccinated persons in conditions of poor hygiene, so protecting them as well. Unfortunately, the inhibiting action of antibodies in breast milk and colonization of the gut by other enteroviruses can reduce its effectiveness. Increasing the dosage and telling mothers not to breast-feed for at least an hour after administration can help.

There are three strains of the poliovirus (1, 2 and 3), and the vaccine should be given on three separate occasions, separated by periods of at least 1 month, to ensure that immunity develops to each of the strains. Polio vaccine is conveniently administered at the same time as diphtheria, pertussis and tetanus (DPT). A preliminary dose can be given soon after birth in areas where wild poliovirus is circulating.

There is a slight risk of a live attenuated virus becoming more virulent, so it is preferable to vaccinate the majority of the population all at one time. Also, in a situation of rising sanitary standards, epidemic poliomyelitis will only be prevented if there are sufficient people immunized to produce 'herd immunity'. For these reasons, mass campaigns can be effective, as preferred in countries of South America. These should always be followed up by static clinics vaccinating newborns and missed persons. The WHO in its bid to eradicate polio from the world recommends national immunization days (NID), in which all children under 5 are vaccinated, irrespective of previous immunization status, followed by mop-up operations in areas of low coverage or where continuing transmission has been identified.

To assess the extent of poliomyelitis and determine the effectiveness of a vaccination campaign, a *lameness survey* can be conducted. The standard method is to demarcate areas within the country by random selection and then examine children in consecutive households until 2000 under-15-year-olds have been seen. The head of the household is asked to give details of all his/her children and they are then examined for signs of polio disability. (Other forms of disability must be excluded.) If children who come within the survey are at school they should be examined at school. In tropical countries there is a higher incidence of polio cases in urban than in rural areas, so these two categories must be included in the survey in proportion to the population distribution. There may also be other features which may suggest a difference in endemicity, such as highland and lowland areas. This means that a multistage random sample, rather than a simple random-sample technique, should be used.

If the lameness survey only examines lameness of the lower limbs, the results should be multiplied by 1.25 to allow for cases with deformity of the upper part of the body. In order to compensate for those who died with severe disease or recovered from their temporary deformity, a correction factor of 1.33 is used.

An alternative technique is to use a school postal survey. With this method forms are sent to all schools and the schoolteacher is asked to fill in the proportion of disabled in the school. This is a less sensitive method as many physically disabled children do not attend school.

Surveillance developed for poliomyelitis eradication looks for cases of acute flaccid paralysis (AFP) in children. These are investigated by stool examination, enquiry and search for other cases and by conducting remedial measures around the case, vaccinating all contacts.

If it is proposed to set up a disability service, all ages of polio deformity need to be included. For assessment of disease level and vaccine coverage, age-specific disability rates should be calculated, using the local or national population distribution. As disability rates should be greater in young children in a normally distributed population, an alteration to this pattern may indicate an improvement in vaccine coverage.

8.11 *ENTEROBIUS* (PINWORM)

Enterobius vermicularis, a nematode worm, has a unique history in that the gravid female leaves the intestines to lay her eggs. She migrates out of the anus at night and lays them on the perianal skin before dying. This activity of the female causes the patient to scratch so that eggs are transferred to the fingers where they may subsequently produce reinfection or be passed on to someone else. Masses of eggs are liberated on each occasion, so that infection of family groups, dormitories of schoolchildren or other groups of people occurs at the same time. Eggs can be collected from the perianal skin by using an adhesive-tape slide.

The main symptom is intense pruritus ani, and rarely there is appendicitis. Treatment is with piperazine or mebendazole, but it is preferable to treat everyone in the group at the same time to break the transmission cycle.

Good personal hygiene, particularly cutting of fingernails and hand washing, is the means of control. Bedding also gets contaminated and eggs are scattered during bed making. So frequent washing of bed linen and underclothes needs to be carried out at the same time as treatment.

9

Soil-mediated Infections

The soil can be a source of infection for a group of helminth diseases and the bacterial infection, tetanus. Transmission can either be direct from the soil, as with tetanus bacilli, by swallowing helminth eggs or by the larvae penetrating the skin. Developmental stages often take place in the soil. Prevention of soil contamination through personal hygiene and prevention of contamination through sanitation are the main methods of control.

9.1 *TRICHURIS* (WHIPWORM)

Trichuris trichiura has a characteristic egg, which is commonly seen when faecal specimens are examined (Fig. 9.1). The egg develops in the soil and, when swallowed directly or as a contaminant of food, changes into an adult in the caecum.

It is a very common parasite (perhaps 540 million people are infected) but produces hardly any pathology unless the infection is very heavy. When there are over 16,000 eggs g^{-1} of faeces, a chronic bloody diarrhoea, anaemia, rectal prolapse and occasionally appendicitis can result. These infections tend to occur where the child eats earth (pica), which can be a result of iron deficiency. Heavy infections are probably potentiated by nutritional deficiencies, especially of zinc. Treatment with mebendazole or albendazole is effective.

Hand washing and the careful preparation of vegetables are the main methods of control. Parents should discourage their children from eating earth.

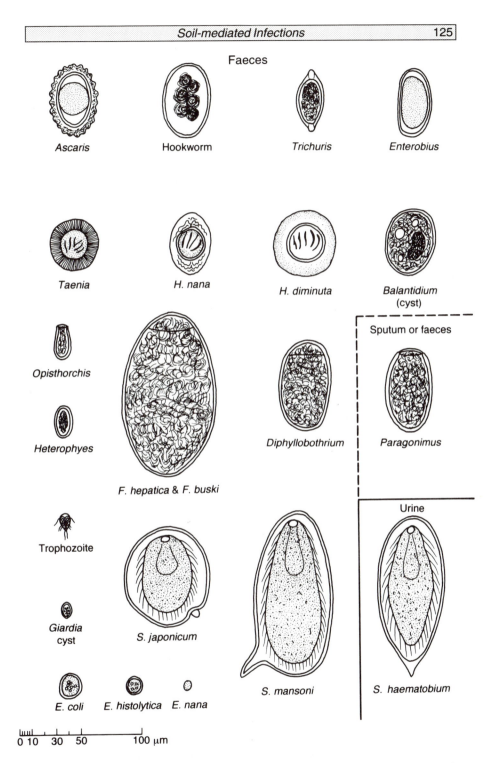

Fig. 9.1. Parasite eggs found in faeces, urine and sputum. *E.* (*coli*), *Escherichia*; *H.* (*nana*), *H.* (*diminuta*), *Hymenolepis*; *F.* (*hepatica*), *Fasciola*; *F.* (*buski*), *Fasciolopsis*; *S.* (*japonicum*), *S.* (*mansoni*), *S.* (*haematobium*), *Schistosoma*; *E.* (*histolytica*), *Entamoeba*; *E.* (*nana*), *Endolimax*.

9.2 ASCARIS

Ascaris lumbricoides is a very common nematode infection, found in all parts of the world and all strata of society. When swallowed, the fertile egg hatches in the stomach and the larva penetrates the intestinal mucosa to enter the bloodstream, passing through the venous and pulmonary circulations to the lungs, where it breaks through the alveolar wall to emerge in the bronchiole. Migrating up to a main bronchus, it ascends the trachea and is swallowed back into the gastrointestinal tract. By the time it reaches the intestines, it has developed into an adult, the fertilized female laying eggs into the excrement (Fig. 9.2). Direct smear examination of the stool is sufficient for diagnosis (see Fig. 9.1).

This common intestinal parasite (1000 million people estimated infected) can occur in considerable numbers without causing any symptoms. When the larvae pass through the lungs, pneumonitis and possible haemoptysis can occur. Otherwise the sheer number of worms can cause intestinal obstruction or blocking of vital structures, such as the common bile duct. Where nutrition is marginal, the loss of nutrient can be sufficient to tip a child into malnutrition. It has been calculated that 25 worms can produce a loss of 4 g protein daily from a diet containing 40–50 g protein. Vitamin A and C deficiency can also occur. Performance in school is reduced with heavy *Ascaris* infections.

Personal hygiene, food hygiene and proper sanitary facilities can break the transmission cycle. The egg is extremely resistant, being unaffected by cold, drying and disinfectants. A temperature of 45°C is required to kill them. Personal treatment is by pyrantel pamoate or mebendazole, 100 mg twice daily for 3 days.

9.3 HOOKWORMS

The two common hookworm infections of man are *Ancylostoma duodenale* and *Necator americanus*. The eggs are passed in the faeces and hatch within 24–48 hours to liberate an intermediate (rhabditiform) larva. After some days it moults to produce the infective filariform larva. In suitable conditions of moist warm soil this larva can live for several months awaiting the opportunity to penetrate through the skin of a new host. (The ingested third-stage larvae of *Ancylostoma* can also produce infection.) The larvae migrate to a blood or lymphatic vessel and are then carried in the circulation to the lungs. Here they break out of the alveoli, find their way up the trachea and enter the gastrointestinal tract. The adult stage is finally reached in the duodenum or jejunum, the fertilized female producing characteristic oval eggs (Fig. 9.3).

Despite its extensive journey through the human body, like *Ascaris* it is very well adapted to its host and only produces symptoms when heavy

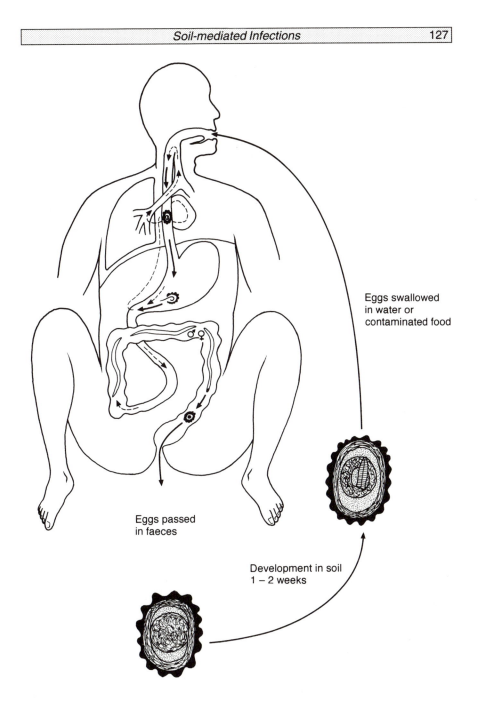

Eggs swallowed
in water or
contaminated food

Eggs passed
in faeces

Development in soil
1 – 2 weeks

Fig. 9.2. *Ascaris lumbricoides.*

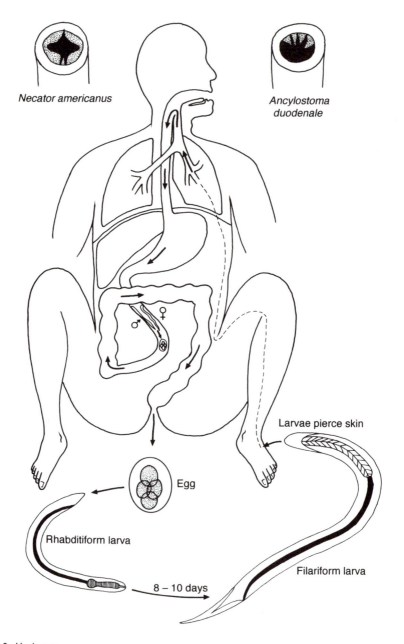

Necator americanus

Ancylostoma
duodenale

Larvae pierce skin

Egg

Rhabditiform larva

Filariform larva

8 – 10 days

Fig. 9.3. Hookworm.

infections occur. The passage through the skin can result in a transient urticaria (ground itch), while that through the lungs can cause pneumonitis and haemoptysis. Occasionally the haemoptysis can be sufficient to suggest a possible diagnosis of tuberculosis. The main effects result from the adult worms attached to the intestine, where they invaginate a piece of mucosa, from which they extract blood and nutrients. The degree of anaemia produced depends upon the worm load, and one estimate calculates that 60–120 worms (measured by 30 worms excreting 1000 eggs g^{-1} faeces) will result in slight anaemia, whereas over 300 worms (10,000 eggs g^{-1} faeces) will cause severe anaemia. Anaemia results from frank blood loss and depletion of iron reserves. The newly established worm may produce several bleeding points and, if the sexes are unbalanced, the search for a mate can result in increased activity. These effects will naturally be most profound in the growing child and the pregnant woman. Malaria, malnutrition and other intercurrent infections, in combination with hookworms, accentuate the seriousness of this infection.

N. *americanus*, despite its name, is the more widely distributed, being found extensively throughout the tropical belt and well north of the tropic of Cancer in America and East Asia. A. *duodenale* is found in East Asia and the Mediterranean (Fig. 9.4). It has been suggested, that N. *americanus* was taken from Africa to the Americas as a result of the slave trade. Altogether, some 720 million of the world population have hookworms.

Ideal conditions for development are moist, shaded, humus-type soil at 30°C for N. *americanus* and 25°C for A. *duodenale*. The two worms are identified by the characteristic mouthparts of the adult worms, illustrated in Fig. 9.3. Non-human hookworms can produce cutaneous larva migrans (see Section 18.4)

Diagnosis is made by finding the eggs in faeces (Fig. 9.1). A number of drugs are effective in treatment: albendazole, pyrantel pamoate, mebendazole and bephenium. In the debilitated child, supporting therapy will need to accompany deworming.

Control is by use of pit latrines or other methods of sanitation. The wearing of footwear effectively prevents penetration by the larvae. The open-sandal type of footwear often worn (thongs, flip-flops) is not effective and infection can readily occur. Mass treatment can be given to reduce the parasite load, but without health education and the proper use of latrines it will only produce a temporary improvement.

9.4 *STRONGYLOIDES*

Strongyloides stercoralis has several alternative cycles of development and it is the type of cycle which determines the nature and degree of pathological change.

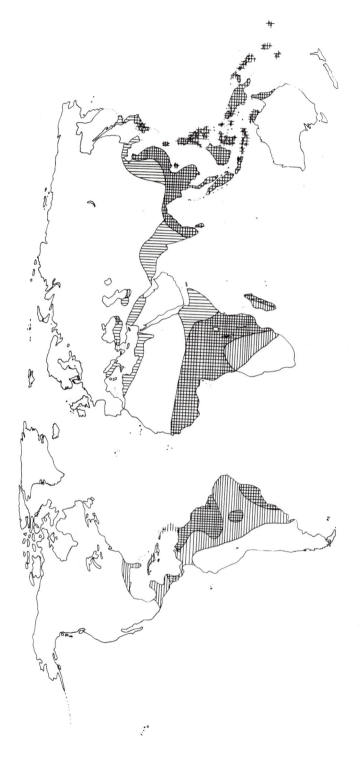

Fig. 9.4. Distribution of the hookworms. ▤, *Necator americanus*; ▦, *Ancylostoma duodenale*.

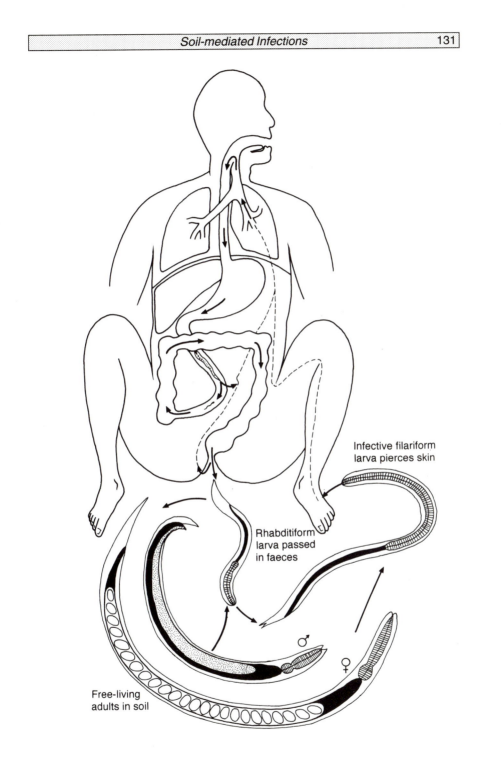

Infective filariform
larva pierces skin

Rhabditiform
larva passed
in faeces

♂

♀

Free-living
adults in soil

Fig. 9.5. *Strongyloides stercoralis.*

S. stercoralis is very similar to the hookworms: an infective filariform larva develops in warm moist soil, penetrates the skin and follows the same internal route to the final resting site in the small intestine. But it differs markedly in that no eggs are passed to the outside; only rhabditiform larvae are found in the faeces. If environmental conditions are favourable, a free-living cycle takes place. The rhabditiform larvae develop into adults in the soil and this cycle can be repeated, increasing the number of potential parasites. If conditions change, filariform larvae are produced, or, if the conditions are unsuitable for the free-living cycle, the rhabditiform larvae passed in the faeces change directly into filariform larvae. Direct autoinfection can also occur, the rhabditiform larvae penetrating the intestinal mucosa to enter the bloodstream, without ever leaving the body. Swallowed larvae can also complete their development by entering the body through the intestinal mucosa (Fig. 9.5). (Achlorhydria, as occurs in malnutrition, makes infection easier by the oral route.) It is the abnormal cycle of autoinfection that can lead to wandering larvae producing linear urticaria (larva currens) or 'eosinophilic lung'. Larva currens can persist for periods in excess of 40 years.

Diagnosis is made by finding the rhabditiform larvae in the faeces or in the aspirate of the duodenal string test. Treatment is by thiabendazole, albendazole or mebendazole. Control is the same as for hookworm.

9.5 TETANUS

Tetanus occurs worldwide, with higher rates in Africa and the Western Pacific, as seen in Figure 9.6. Infection results from the organism entering an abraded surface, favouring anaerobic conditions. Liberated toxin produces severe muscle spasms. It is a serious infection in the neonate due to contamination of the umbilical cord. As well as good hygiene, immunization is the main method of control.

Clostridium tetani is a Gram-positive rod with spherical, terminal spores that give it a characteristic drumstick appearance. It is found naturally in the soil, where it survives in anaerobic conditions. Many types of soils have been found to harbour C. tetani but it is more common in cultivated soils, especially those manured with animal faeces. The organism is found in horse and cattle dung and, less commonly, in pig, sheep and dog faeces. It is occasionally found in human excreta, particularly in people associated with animals.

The vegetative form of the organism is sensitive to antibiotics, disinfectants and heat, but as a spore it is resistant to all but the superheated steam of an autoclave. Indeed, the spores of C. tetani are used to test the effectiveness of the sterilizing process because, if it cannot survive, then no other organism can (apart from anthrax).

Spores can survive for considerable periods of time, but when they

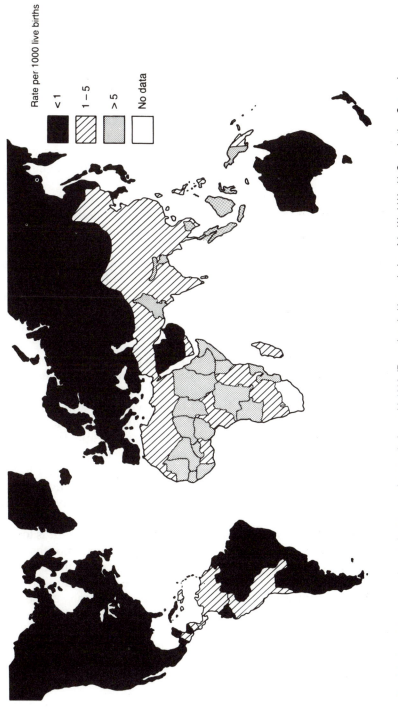

Fig. 9.6. Estimated number of deaths from neonatal tetanus in the world, 1992. (Reproduced with permission of the World Health Organization, Geneva.)

Rate per 1000 live births

- < 1
- 1 – 5
- > 5
- No data

enter a wound or umbilical stump, in which a low oxygen reduction potential permits them to grow anaerobically, infection takes place. It is the moist, contaminated umbilical stump or the traumatized wound that provides suitable conditions. It is not the replication of the organism that is important, but the toxin that is produced. The exotoxin has a high affinity for nervous tissue and as little as 0.1 mg is sufficient to kill a man. Toxin is absorbed along the nerves, reaching the spinal cord, where the generalized features of the disease are produced.

The *incubation period* is variable, from 4 to 21 days, but most cases occur within 14 days. There is a relationship between incubation period and severity, with an incubation period of less than 9 days having a mortality of 60% and more than 9 days 25%. This is due to a higher dose of toxin.

The adult presents with muscle spasm and rigidity. There may be trismus, in which the muscle of the jaw and later the back become rigid, leading to lockjaw and opisthotonos. Muscle spasms can produce the characteristic half smile, half snarl of risus sardonicus or generalized opisthotonos. These spasms are initiated by external stimuli such as touch or attempts at intubation and every care must be taken to protect the patient from such stimuli. Neonatal tetanus generally presents as a difficulty in sucking; then the rigidity of muscles and generalized convulsions develop. It usually commences within 5 to 10 days of birth.

Tetanus is a self-limiting disease and if the patient can be kept alive for 3 weeks, complete recovery will take place. But keeping the patient alive for this period of time is the problem. It is the toxin that is causing the symptoms and, once this is fixed in the nerves, only support can be given to the patient to maintain respiration, urinary output and nutrient intake. The patient is sedated to reduce the spasms and in all ways expertly nursed. The contaminated wound must be cleaned and excised, antitoxin or immunoglobulin administered and penicillin given to kill any remaining organisms. Sadly, the mortality of tetanus is high, 40% in adults and 90% in neonates, so the objective should always be to try and prevent it.

Tetanus immunization is given in two doses of adsorbed tetanus toxoid (0.5 ml), separated by 4 weeks, and a third dose of 1 ml six months later. This is preferably given as part of the routine childhood immunizations, but where this was missed it can be given at any age in life. Immunization will provide immunity for at least 10 years and sometimes 20. Booster doses every 10 years will maintain a high level of immunity. The benefits of alternative strategies are shown in Fig. 9.7.

In the event of a person being injured and presenting with a contaminated wound that could produce tetanus, the following action should be taken.

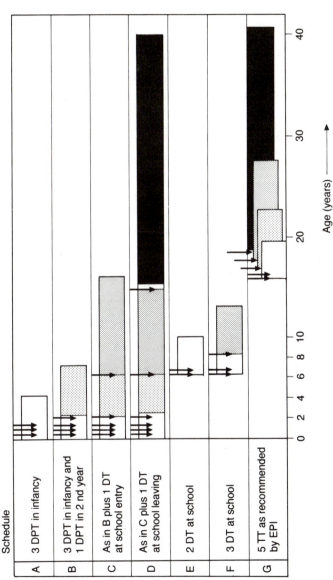

Fig. 9.7. Expected duration of tetanus immunity after different immunization schedules. DPT, diphtheria, pertussis and tetanus; DT, diphtheria and tetanus; TT, tetanus toxoid; EPI, Expanded Programme of Immunization. (Reproduced with permission of the World Health Organization, Geneva.)

- Clean out the wound.
- Give penicillin.
- If the person has been immunized within the last 10 years, give a booster dose of toxoid only.
- If there is no record of tetanus immunization or protection is in doubt, give the first dose of tetanus toxoid, plus 250 units of human tetanus immunoglobulin or 1500 units of equine tetanus antitoxin, following a test dose. Instruct the person to return at 4 weeks and then 6 months to complete the course of immunization.

In developing countries the most serious problem is neonatal tetanus. It is mainly due to the customary practices of treating the umbilical cord

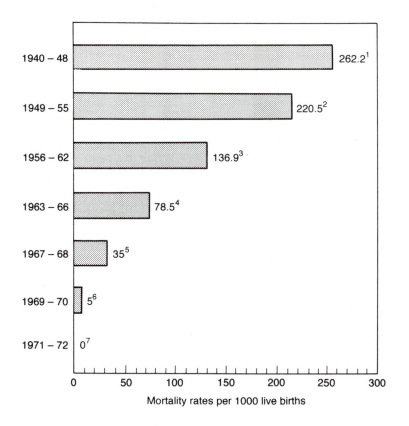

Mortality rates per 1000 live births

Fig. 9.8. Neonatal mortality per 1000 live births in rural Haiti, 1940–1972, from a retrospective study of 2574 mothers. 1, Before national programme for training tradition birth attendants (TBAs); 2, national programme for training TBAs; 3, hospital treatment for tetanus, training of TBAs by hospital nurse; 4, immunization of pregnant women in hospital clinics; 5, immunization of women in market-places by hospital team; 6, immunization after door-to-door invitation by community workers. (Reproduced with permission of the World Health Organization, Geneva.)

in the newborn. These can involve covering the stump with an unsterile dressing or even traditional methods of placing cow dung on it. Such practices should be outlawed and traditional midwives taught how to clean the cord and apply iodine, spirit or a similar antiseptic. The objective is to dry out the cord stump.

The most effective way of preventing neonatal tetanus is the immunization of all women of childbearing age. The policy is to give all women a lifetime total of five doses of tetanus toxoid. This is preferable to waiting until the woman becomes pregnant because many women do not attend antenatal clinic, especially those likely to use traditional applications to the umbilical cord stump. The effectiveness of various strategies for controlling neonatal tetanus in Haiti are shown in Fig. 9.8.

People who live close to their animals place themselves and their newborn children at greatest risk of developing tetanus. Animal manure is used for fertilizing the soil, as a fuel or as a plaster on the walls of houses. Domestic animals either share the same house as their owners or live in such close proximity that the surrounding soil is contaminated by their faeces. These are the conditions in which *C. tetani* abound, posing an ever-present threat to the family. Health education about these dangers, stressing personal hygiene, can in time produce an improvement in the situation. While this must be an ideal, the long-term objective must be to produce a level of immunity in the community by vaccination.

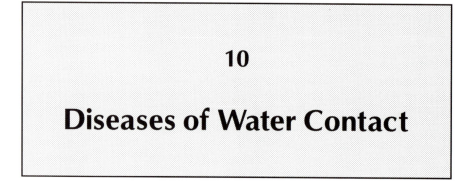

10

Diseases of Water Contact

Schistosomiasis and dracunculiasis are transmitted by contact with water. Minimizing water contact is the main method of control.

10.1 SCHISTOSOMIASIS

The main parasites are *Schistosoma haematobium*, *S. mansoni* and *S. japonicum*. Other species, such as *S. intercalatum* and *S. mekongi* do occur, but their epidemiology and control are similar to one of the three main types. (As well as species differences, there are also strain variations.)

10.1.1 Distribution

S. haematobium and *S. mansoni* were originally diseases of Africa, where they are widely distributed, but with the massive exodus of slaves that took place in the seventeenth and eighteenth centuries this legacy was carried with them. The East African slave trade carried *S. mansoni* to the Arabian peninsula and *S. haematobium* to the Yemen and Iraq. The Western trade carried only *S. mansoni*, which found a suitable snail host in South America and the West Indies. *S. japonicum* probably originated in China, but is also found in Japan, the Philippines and Indonesia (Fig. 10.1). Domestic and wild animals, especially the water buffalo, are reservoirs of *S. japonicum* in these countries. A separate species, *S. intercalatum*, pathogenically similar to *S. mansoni*, with which it was previously included, is found in Zaire, Congo and Cameroon. *S. mekongi* is restricted to the lower part of the Mekong River in Cambodia and Vietnam.

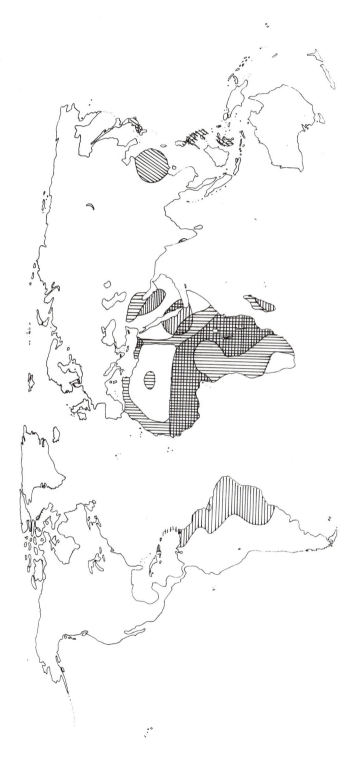

Fig. 10.1. Schistosomiasis distribution. ▤, *Schistosoma mansoni*; Ⅲ, *S. haematobium*; ▨, *S. japonicum*.

10.1.2 Parasite

S. haematobium is unique in the human parasite world in using urine as a route of transmission. The eggs of S. mansoni and S. japonicum are passed in the stools. With the passage of the eggs through the bladder or intestinal wall, many are trapped and less than 50% leave the body and develop further. On reaching water, a temperature of 10 to 30°C and the presence of light are required for hatching.

The eggs hatch to produce miracidia which swim actively using geotactic and phototactic behaviour to search out a molluscan host. A chemical substance, 'miraxone', inadvertently liberated by snails, attracts miracidia to home in and penetrate them. Miracidia live for 8–12 hours, but their chance of penetration decreases with age. Some 40% of snails are infected at a distance of 5 m in still water, but, where the water is moving, similar infection rates can occur at a far greater distance. Normally, infection occurs in water flowing at 10 cm s^{-1} or less. Even after surviving the rigours of the journey, when miracidia have entered the correct species of snail, many are inactivated and only a small proportion develop into sporocysts. This is determined by the part of the snail entered and the immunity to reinfection developed by the snail (Fig. 10.2).

Cercariae are stimulated by light to emerge from the snail when the ambient temperature is between 10°C and 30°C. Cercarial emergence increases as daylight penetrates the watery environment, producing a peak for S. mansoni at 12 noon and for S. haematobium in the mid- to late afternoon. With S. japonicum the stimulus produced by light is delayed and maximal cercarial liberation occurs at 11 p.m. The number of cercariae issuing from a snail can be immense, in the order of 1000–3000 day^{-1}, but this depends upon the species and relative size of the snail. Where more than one miracidium has penetrated a snail, there is depression of cercarial production; this may also occur if the snail is host to other trematode infections. Cercarial output is greatest in S. mansoni, less in S. haematobium and least of all in S. japonicum. Cercariae survive for 24 hours, but their greatest chance of penetrating the host is when they are young. When cercariae enter the host within 2 hours of release only 30% die, but this rises to 50% at 8 hours and 85% at 24 hours.

On penetrating the subcutaneous layer of the host, the cercaria becomes a schistosomule, migrates to the lungs and finally develops into an adult in the portal vessels of the liver. Both male and female worms are required, so that pairing can take place prior to migration to the final destination in the mesenteric or vesical plexus. Adult worms can live for 20–30 years and are active egg producers for 3–8 years, although viable eggs have been produced for over 30 years. The egg output per day in S. haematobium is some 20–250, in S. mansoni 100–300 and in S. japonicum 1500–3500. It is this massive output of eggs in the Far Eastern form of

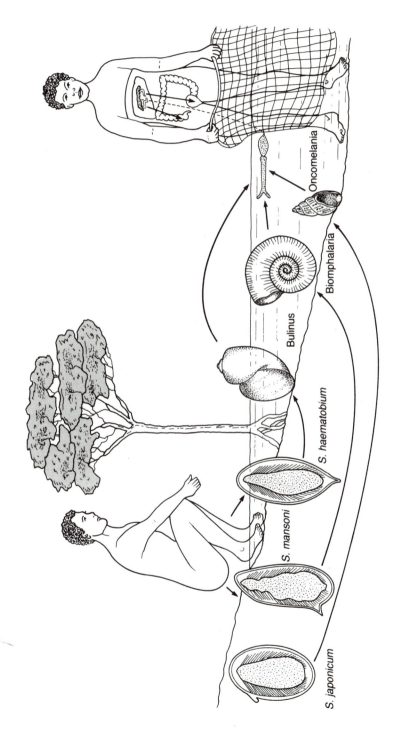

Fig. 10.2. Schistosomiasis.

schistosomiasis that leads to the more rapidly developing and severe pathology.

10.1.3 Snail

The snail intermediate hosts are species specific, *Bulinus* spp. for *S. haematobium*, *Biomphalaria* spp. for *S. mansoni* and *Oncomelania* spp. for *S. japonicum*. They are illustrated in Fig. 10.2. They can adapt to a wide range of habitats, from natural waterways to temporary ponds and cultivated rice fields. Whenever there is sufficient organic matter on which to feed, snails will be found. Within a body of water, distribution may be quite irregular, with dense colonies in some places and complete absence in others. These are various factors which may influence snail colonization.

- *Electrolyte concentration.* Snails demand a minimum calcium concentration and cannot tolerate a high salt content or a low pH.
- *Light* is not required by the snail, and they can often survive in near-total darkness.
- *Rainfall* may herald the end of the dry season and provide water in which snail populations can increase, but if the rainfall is too heavy it may flush out the snails, resulting in a subsequent decrease. Snail populations may therefore follow a seasonal pattern.
- *Temperature* rise encourages expansion of population up to a maximum of approximately 30°C.
- *Density* is a limiting factor and reduced growth results from a high density of snails.
- *Aestivation* or the ability of snails to survive out of the water for weeks or months allows populations of snails to continue from one season to another, possibly also transferring immature infections of *S. haematobium* and *S. mansoni*. The snail host of *S. japonicum* can survive conditions of desiccation best of all.

Snails are capable of self-fertilization, although cross-fertilization is more common. Their reproductive capacity is phenomenal and a single snail can produce a colony within 40 days and be infective in 60. When conditions are optimal, many species of snails will double their population in 2–3 weeks. In measuring the age of snail populations, size of snails is a useful indicator. A large number of small samples from several different areas is preferable to a few large samples in estimating the numbers and density in watercourses.

Infection rates in snails are generally low, only some 1–2% of the colony being infective, but even so this level is sufficient to account for high prevalence rates in the human population.

10.1.4 Person

The last performer in the trilogy, the person, acts both as the infector and the infected and these two different aspects of involvement need to be considered separately.

As an infector, persons contaminate water by either urinating or defecating into or near watercourses. Egg output is variable between individuals and at times in their life. There are a few individuals with heavy infections and egg outputs, while the majority have light infections. In areas of high endemicity, children between 5 and 14 are responsible for over 50% of the contamination. As the infection rate declines, older age-groups become more important.

People are infected by making contact with water. This can be from collecting water, from washing (both clothes and the person), occupational (such as fishing) or for recreation. Children are most commonly infected when they play in the water, while in adults it is when they carry out their domestic duties or occupation. Infection is generally due to repeated water contact over a long period of time, but can occur from a single immersion if it coincides with a large number of cercariae in the water.

10.1.5 Diagnosis

Diagnosis is made by finding the characteristic eggs (Fig. 9.1). In *S. haematobium* they are seen in the urine, best collected between 11 a.m. and 3 p.m., when egg output is at a maximum. Leaving the urine to stand, centrifuging it or passing it through a filter increases the chance of finding eggs. *S. mansoni, S. japonicum* and *S. intercalatum* are diagnosed by finding eggs in the faeces. A rectal snip can also be done. While the qualitative diagnosis is required in the individual case, quantitative estimates are more valuable in epidemiological investigations.

In *S. haematobium*, the simplest method is to pass 10 ml of urine through a membrane filter. The paper or membrane is taken out, dried and stained with ninhydrin and the eggs counted directly. Immunological methods have also come into their own and a complement fixation test or the immunofluorescence antibody technique (IFAT) are useful in surveys. The enzyme-linked immunosorbent assay (ELISA) test has now been developed for schistosomiasis.

Infection and egg output increase up to about the age of 15 years and then decline. Individuals vary in their response as some persons acquire heavy infections and are subject to severe pathological changes. These are related to the number of worms, which can be measured by the number of eggs produced. In *S. haematobium*, the production of 50 eggs ml^{-1} of urine or above, is regarded as the level of severe pathology, and much of present-day control strategy is aimed at reducing this level.

10.1.6 Control

There are two approaches to the control of schistosomiasis.

- Reduce the transmission of the parasite.
- Reduce the level of infection in individuals.

The first attempts to control the parasite while the second aims at minimizing the pathological effects.

There are various methods of control.

- Reduce contamination of the environment.
- Reduce the snail intermediate host.
- Reduce water contact by the human host.
- Reduce the human reservoir by mass chemotherapy.
- Reduce the animal reservoir in S. *japonicum*.
- Vaccination.

Or a combination of methods may be used.

Reduce contamination of the environment

Humans pollute their environment by urinating or defecating into bodies of water. This can be minimized by encouraging the use of latrines. Unfortunately, it is very difficult to get everybody in a family or community always to use a latrine and the few non-users will be sufficient to maintain a level of pollution (see Section 2.4.2). There is also the longevity of the adult worms, meaning that prevalence rates will remain static in the community for a considerable period of time.

Reduction of the snail intermediate host

The snail is a vulnerable link in the life cycle of the parasite and can be attacked in an effort to break transmission. There are various methods that can be used.

- Predators.
- Biological control.
- Water management and engineering.
- Molluscicides.

Various kinds of fish are natural predators, but they will only reduce snails to a certain level unless they have an alternative source of food. Such species as *Tilapia* and *Gambusia* are effective.

Snails, especially of the *Marisa* and *Helisoma* genera, compete for food supplies and *Marisa* will even prey on the eggs and juveniles of *Biomphalaria*. Another approach to biological control is the sterile–male technique but, since many snails are hermaphrodite, it is only suitable with *Oncomelania*.

Where small and temporary ponds are foci of infection, they can be filled or drained. Filling can best be done by controlled tipping of household refuse. Where canals and irrigation systems are responsible, lining with concrete, increasing the rate of flow and any method to reduce vegetation can discourage snail habitation. Unfortunately, these methods are rarely effective on their own and need to be combined with molluscicides.

A commonly used molluscicide is niclosamide (Bayluscide), which can be administered as a liquid, suitable for treating moving water, or as granules, in lakes and ponds. Continuous application is required to have a sustained effect on the snail population. It has the disadvantage of killing fish and is expensive. Cheaper preparations, such as copper sulphate, are still in limited use and naturally occurring plant preparations such as endod (*Phytolacca dodecandra*) have shown promise.

The remarkable recovery of snail populations, once control methods are removed, and the cost of molluscicides make snail reduction a less effective approach to schistosomiasis control.

Reduction of water contact

Preventing water contact can be highly effective in the individual. There are various ways of encouraging this.

- Health education, especially to schoolchildren, but this is often ineffective unless an alternative, e.g. a swimming-pool, is provided.
- Providing places to wash has been disappointingly ineffective for the cost involved.
- Where areas of absent or minimal transmission occur in occupational or recreational bodies of water, people can be encouraged to use these, rather than the heavily infected parts.

Reduction of human infection by mass chemotherapy

With the discovery of effective preparations, such as praziquantel, single-dose mass drug administration is now a good method of control. A suitable target population is schoolchildren between 5 and 15 years of age, where mass therapy is used. Alternatively, only the positive cases or those with heavy infections are treated, following a simple diagnostic procedure. Individual treatment, based on worm-load estimation, aims at disease control, by reducing morbidity. It permits limited resources to be more widely spread and attempts the less ambitious target of disease rather than transmission reduction.

Chapter 10

Reduction of the animal reservoir

Animal reservoirs are responsible for maintaining S. *japonicum*. In order of importance, they are dogs, cows, pigs, rats and water buffaloes. As most of these are domestic animals, proper animal management can reduce contamination of the environment. Vaccination of domestic animals can be used.

Baboons and monkeys have been shown to be reservoirs of S. *mansoni* and could play a part in maintaining infection. There is little prospect of controlling these animals.

Vaccination

There are difficulties in preparing a vaccine because the schistosome is able to absorb host antigen and mask its presence, but one has been shown to be reasonably effective in cattle.

10.1.7 Strategies of Schistosomiasis Control

Various different approaches to the control of schistosomiasis have been tried depending on the resources and nature of the disease.

Raising of economic standards by the provision of water supplies and sanitation, environmental engineering and water management have been shown to be effective on a long-term basis in countries such as Japan and China.

In well-controlled irrigation schemes, the use of molluscicides on its own may be effective. Where discipline and motivation of the population are less certain, a double approach of mass chemotherapy and reduction of water contact is more effective.

When resources are meagre and greatest benefit for limited finance is required, treatment of high worm-load cases is the method of choice.

Effectiveness of control strategies can be measured by the following.

- Change in incidence rate.
- A shift in peak prevalence to an older age-group.
- Reduction in the geometric mean egg output.
- Greater awareness of socio-economic values, e.g. the use of water supplies and sanitation facilities.

10.2 GUINEA WORM

Dracunculus medinensis is the largest of all human nematode worms, with the adult female exceeding 100 cm on occasions. She migrates to lie in one

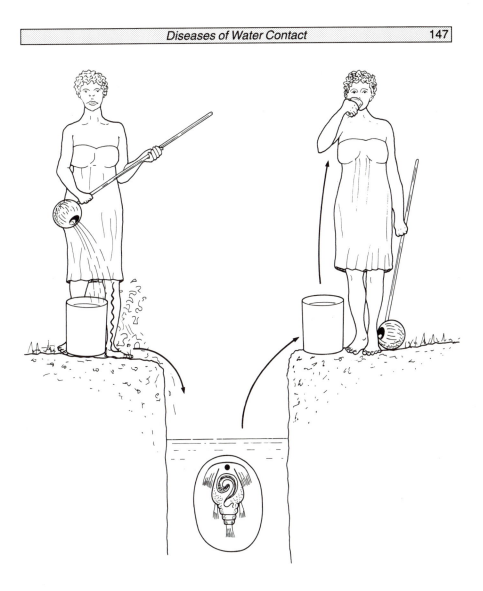

Fig. 10.3. *Dracunculus medinensis.*

of the lower limbs, forming a blister in the skin near her vulval opening. When the blister comes into contact with water it bursts, discharging large numbers of larvae. These larvae are ingested by a copepod in the water and after a period of some 2 weeks develop into the infective form. When the copepod is swallowed with the water, the larvae are liberated. The larvae penetrate the gut mucosa and wander in the subcutaneous tissues until they become adults. Some 9 months after the larvae were swallowed, the fertilized adult female has migrated to the lower extremity to repeat the cycle.

The presence of this large worm in the tissues can result in a number of unpleasant sequelae. Once the blister has burst, the nematode can be removed by gradually winding it out. A broken worm can lead to secondary infection. By keeping the sore clean and using niridazole, mebendazole or metronidazole, the extraction is made easier (probably more from their anti-inflammatory action than from any specific effect). The track produced by the worm is a ready passage for secondary infection and there is an increased incidence of tetanus. The worms have a predilection for wandering into the joints, causing disability.

Diagnosis is normally clinical, but the characteristic larvae can be obtained from an erupted blister by placing a few drops of water to encourage the worm to discharge.

The parasite is found in India, Pakistan, southern Iran, West Africa, S.W. Asia and the Sudan in some 80 million people. It is characteristically spread by spilt water washing back into unprotected wells (as shown in Fig. 10.3), or else through the use of shallow walk-in wells. It has perhaps one of the easiest and most effective control methods, by simply protecting a well with a wall that rises a few metres above ground level and a surrounding apron to drain any spilt water away. A piped water supply is a more expensive alternative, while any system of filtration will remove the copepods.

The World Health Organization (WHO) has launched a programme of eradication of dracunculiasis, with a target of the end of the century. Very good progress is being made and the infection is disappearing from a number of areas. It is likely that some affected countries will soon be able to declare the disease eradicated.

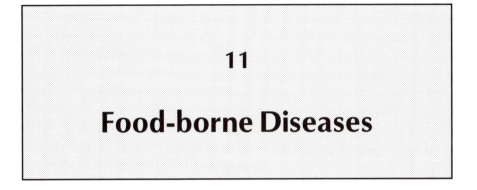

11

Food-borne Diseases

The ingestion of food provides a self-made mechanism for the transfer of disease organisms. This is another method of direct person-to-person transfer. Control is by personal hygiene and cooking of food.

11.1 FOOD POISONING

Food poisoning can be due either to bacteria, viruses or contamination from an organic or inorganic poison (Table 11.1). The most common is that produced by bacteria. The main types of bacterial food poisoning are due to:

- salmonellae;
- staphylococci;
- clostridia.

Due to the similarity of presentation, it is more convenient to consider them as a group, rather than individually. Onset is sudden, with fever and generally vomiting and/or diarrhoea in a family or group of persons who have shared the same meal. The *incubation period* is very short: for staphylococci between 1 and 6 hours, longer for salmonellae – 6–72 hours (usually 12 to 36) – and for clostridia 12–24 hours or several days. Less commonly, food poisoning can be due to *Bacillus cereus* (1–12 hours) or *Vibrio parahaemolyticus* (12–48 hours).

Salmonellae generally infect the food in the living state, such as in cattle, poultry or eggs, but unhygienic practice in the slaughtering of animals or preparation of foodstuffs can also be responsible. They are killed by proper cooking and no toxin is produced, so examination of the meal should reveal an improperly cooked source. In contrast, staphylococcal food poisoning results from the toxin, so the food may be adequately cooked and no bacteria isolated. *V. parahaemolyticus* is

Table 11.1. Food poisoning.

Agent	Period of onset (hours)	Symptoms	Types of food
Bacterial food poisoning			
Staphylococcal	1–6	Sudden, vomiting more	Stored food
Bacillus cereus	1–12	than diarrhoea	
Salmonella	12–36	Vomiting, diarrhoea and fever	Improperly cooked meat, eggs and milk produce
Clostridium perfringens	9–24	Abdominal cramps, diarrhoea, shock	Cooked meat, especially pig
Clostridium botulinum	9–24	Ptosis, dry mouth, paralysis	Preserved foods
Vibrio parahaemolyticus	12–48	Abdominal pain, diarrhoea and fever	Undercooked or raw fish
Fish poisoning			
Ciguatera	1–30	Paraesthesiae, malaise, sweating, diarrhoea and vomiting	Barracudas, snappers, sea bass, groupers
Tetraodontoxins	½–3	Hypersalivation, vomiting, paraesthesiae, vertigo, pains	Puffer fish
Shellfish	½–3	Paraethesiae and paralysis	Clams and mussels
Plant foods			
Akee (*Blighia sapida*)	2–3	Vomiting, convulsions, death	Unripe akee fruit
Cassava (cyanide)		Vomiting, diarrhoea, abdominal pain, headache, coma	Improperly processed root
Contaminants			
Triorthocresyl phosphate	Days	Neuropathy	Cooking oil

particularly associated with seafood or food that has been washed with contaminated sea water.

Clostridial food poisoning can be caused by several types of organisms. *Clostridium botulinum* infection results in a severe disease, botulism, which is characteristic of home-preserved foods and is found worldwide. In New Guinea and the Western Pacific islands *C. perfringens* (*welchii*) is responsible for enteritis necroticans or *pigbel*. This is associated with feasting, generally with pig meat but also meat from other animals such as cattle. It affects children, particularly males, and leads to an acute necrosis of the small and large intestine, with a high fatality rate. The disease is probably accentuated by a protease inhibitor contained in sweet potato, which prevents breakdown of the toxin. *C. perfringens* produces a mild disease of short duration in other parts of the world.

Clostridia have resistant spores, which can remain in the soil for long periods, and their contamination of partly cooked and reheated food allows multiplication and production of the toxin. *Staphylococcal* food poisoning is transmitted by food handlers contaminating partly cooked foods, in which toxin production occurs.

The treatment of cases of food poisoning is supportive, with fluids and electrolytes (either orally or intravenous). In *pigbel*, gut resection or colostomy has been life-saving.

From the characteristics of the disease and the rapidity of onset, a diagnosis can be made. A search is required to discover a common food that has been eaten by all the persons that have succumbed to the illness. This foodstuff is likely to be one particular ingredient of the meal, rather than the whole meal, and samples should be taken for culture. If nothing is grown, this does not rule out staphylococcal or clostridial food poisoning and finer questioning on foodstuffs consumed might be the only way to discover the offending item (see Section 2.2.5).

There is often a seasonality in food poisoning, *Salmonella* and *Shigella* in the summer months and *C. jejuni* in spring and autumn. *C. perfringens* occurs throughout the year.

All suspect food must be destroyed and, if it is part of a common foodstuff, all must be traced and disposed of. The source of contamination, such as an abattoir, must be looked for and control measures implemented. Prevention is by proper cooking of food and personal hygiene. Where repeated attacks occur, a search for a carrier should be made among food handlers. Anyone with a septic or discharging sore should be banned from handling and preparing food.

Fish poisoning is commonly found among island communities or coastal people in which fish is a major item of diet. At certain times of the year and when hurricanes, seismic shocks or similar disturbances of the coral reef occur, an algal growth containing the dinoflagellate (*Gambierdiscus toxicus*) develops. Fish feed on this, which affects their flesh, producing *ciguatera poisoning*. Fish that are normally quite edible, such as barracuda, snappers, sea bass and groupers, become poisonous at these periods. Ciguatoxin is not destroyed by cooking. Symptoms are normally mild with paraesthesia, malaise, sweating, diarrhoea and vomiting, but in the young or those who have consumed a large quantity of poison the condition is more serious. Some fish are known to be poisonous, such as the puffer fish, and invariably produce severe symptoms, often with a fatal outcome. They are regarded as a delicacy in Japan.

Shellfish poisoning, especially clams and mussels, has a similar aetiology to ciguatera poisoning, except that the dinoflagellate *Gonyaulux tamarensis* is filtered and a toxin absorbed. Respiratory and motor paralysis can occur.

More generalized outbreaks involving large numbers of people, not necessarily associated with each other and presenting with bizarre symptoms, such as paralysis, may be caused by an organic or inorganic poison contaminating the food. Examples are cyanide poisoning from poorly processed bitter cassava, eating unripe akees (a fruit popular in the Caribbean) or contaminants in cooking oil.

11.2 *CAMPYLOBACTER*

An acute diarrhoeal disease with abdominal pain, malaise, fever and vomiting occurs with infection by *Campylobacter jejuni*. It is often self-limiting within 4 days to a week, but in severe cases pus and blood are found in the stools, similar to bacillary dysentery. The *incubation period* is 1–10 days.

Children are most commonly infected. In developing countries, it is predominantly found in children under 2. Domestic animals, including poultry, pigs, cattle and dogs, are reservoirs of the organism and their consumption as food or humans' close association with them potentiates transmission. Unpasteurized milk and unchlorinated water can also be responsible. Proper cooking of foodstuffs and control of pets are the main preventive methods.

11.3 THE INTESTINAL FLUKE (*FASCIOLOPSIS*)

The eggs of the large human fluke *Fasciolopsis buski* are passed in faeces. This may be directly into water or the eggs may be washed there following rains. In the water, they hatch and liberate a miracidium, which must find a snail of the genus *Segmentina*. Developing first into a sporocyst and then a redia, numerous cercaria are produced (Fig. 11.1). On leaving the snail, they encyst on water plants, which are subsequently eaten raw by humans. These plants include water caltrop (*Trapa* sp.), water chestnut (*Eliocharis tuberosa*) and water bamboo (*Zizania aquatica*). Beds of these water plants are often grown in ponds fertilized by human sewage, so there is considerable opportunity for transmission. Even if the foods are subsequently cooked, they are often first peeled with the teeth so that cercariae are still swallowed.

The adult worm lives in the intestines, causing direct damage, with an inflammatory reaction at the site of attachment, sometimes leading to an abscess and haemorrhage. As well as these local effects, the toxic action of the parasite can lead to oedema and weakness with prostration, ending fatally in the debilitated child.

A reservoir of infection is maintained in sheep, cattle, pigs and other domestic herbivores. Distribution is concentrated in East Asia especially China, Taiwan, Thailand, Borneo and Malaysia, in some 15 million people. Diagnosis is made by finding the large egg in the faeces, a giant

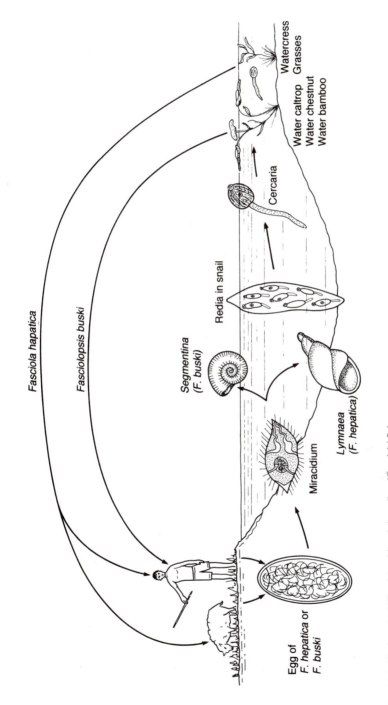

Fig. 11.1. The intestinal (*Fasciolopsis*) and sheep liver (*Fasciola*) flukes.

among parasites (see Fig. 9.1). This egg is indistinguishable from that of *Fasciola hepatica*. Treatment is with praziquantel 25 mg kg^{-1} three times a day for 1–2 days.

Control is by the proper preparation and cooking of water plants. Much can be done to reduce transmission by regulating the use of human faeces as a fertilizer. Domestic animals should be kept away from water-plant cultivation ponds.

11.4 THE SHEEP LIVER FLUKE (*FASCIOLA HEPATICA*)

Completing its normal life cycle in the sheep, humans are incidentally infected with *Fasciola hepatica*. Cattle and goats also act as reservoirs.

The life cycle is similar to *Fasciolopsis* in that eggs passed in the faeces, on contact with water, liberate a miracidium, which invades snails of the genus *Lymnaea* (Fig. 11.1). After passing through sporocyst and redia stages, the cercaria encyst on grass or water plants (e.g. watercress). When these are eaten by humans, they become infected; otherwise the cycle continues with the sheep grazing on the contaminated grass.

The adult worm has a predilection for the liver, piercing the gut wall and migrating through the liver substance to lie in the biliary passages. This migration and residence in the liver causes extensive damage, leading to fibrosis and cirrhosis.

Diagnosis is easily made by finding in the stool the very large egg, which is almost identical to that of *Fasciolopsis* (see Fig. 9.1). Treatment is with praziquantel, as for fasciolopsiasis.

In known endemic areas, careful control is required in the growing and consumption of water plants, such as cress. The close association of humans with sheep or their other domestic animals greatly increases the opportunity for infection.

11.5 THE FISH-TRANSMITTED LIVER FLUKES

Another group of smaller trematode flukes also has a predilection for the liver tissues. There are two intermediate hosts, a snail and fish. *Opisthorchis sinensis* (previously called *Clonorchis*) lives in the bile-ducts of humans, dogs, cats and pigs. The small operculated eggs passed in the faeces are eaten by the snail before the miracidium is liberated. The range of susceptible snails involves members of *Bulimus*, *Bithynia* and *Parafossarulus*. The sporocyst and redia stages are passed through in the snail, with the free-swimming cercaria seeking out a suitable fish and encysting in its flesh (Fig. 11.2). Humans acquire infection by eating the fish raw, pickled or smoked.

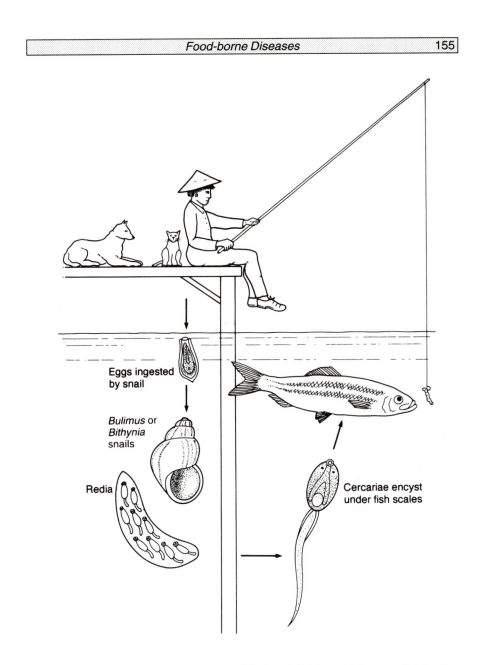

Fig. 11.2. The fish-transmitted liver flukes *Opisthorchis sinensis*, *Opisthorchis felineus* and *Opisthorchis viverrini*.

The adult fluke ascends the bile–duct and lodges in the bile–duct branches, resulting in trauma and inflammation. Dilatation of the biliary system causes a distortion of the liver architecture, which can lead to biliary stasis, hepatic engorgement, fatty infiltration and finally cirrhosis.

It is a risk factor for cholangiocarcinoma. Migration of the flukes up the pancreatic duct can damage the pancreas, leading to recurrent pancreatitis.

Distribution is very similar to that of *Fasciolopsis*, being found in China, Japan, Korea, Taiwan and Vietnam. Some 30 million suffer from the disease. Cats and dogs are also reservoirs of infection.

Diagnosis is made by finding the egg in the faeces (see Fig. 9.1). Treatment is with praziquantel 25 mg kg^{-1} three times a day for 1–2 days.

Control is by the proper cooking of fish. Members of the carp family (*Cyprinus*), the so-called 'milk fish', are a delicacy, being eaten raw. These are grown in fish farms as part of a system of aquaculture, fertilized by human faeces. Regulation of this practice is required to reduce this unpleasant infection.

There are a number of less common trematodes that share the same life cycle. *Opisthorchis viverrini* is found in Thailand and Laos, where raw fish paste is a favourite food additive. *Opisthorchis felineus* occurs in central and eastern Europe, similarly causing disease of the liver. *Heterophyes heterophyes* and *Metagonimus yokogawi*, found in Asia, do not attack the liver, but remain in the intestines. The eggs of all of these flukes are very similar (see Fig. 9.1).

11.6 THE LUNG FLUKE

Unique among all the parasites, *Paragonimus westermani* selectively inhabits the lung. This means that the egg is passed in the sputum, although if this is swallowed it will be found in the faeces. On reaching water, the miracidium frees itself from the egg capsule and searches for a snail of the genus *Semisulcospira* (Fig. 11.3). Passing through the sporocyst and redia stages, the cercaria encysts in the gills and muscles of freshwater crabs and crayfish. Humans are infected by eating uncooked crab or crayfish. The liberated metacercaria pass through the intestinal wall and penetrate the diaphragm to enter the lung. Occasionally they find their way to unusual sites, the brain being particularly serious.

Foreign-body reaction to the parasite in the lung results in fibrosis, compensatory dilatation and abscess formation. Haemoptysis is often an important feature, mimicking tuberculosis.

This is essentially an infection of East Asia, where an animal reservoir (mainly cats and dogs) helps to maintain the disease. Closely related species are *P. africanus* and *P. uterobilateralis* in West Africa, *P. pulmonalis* in Japan, Korea and Taiwan, *P. philippinensis* in the Philippines, *P. heterotremus* in Thailand and Laos and *P. kellicotti*, *P. caliensis* and *P. mexicanus* in Central and South America. In all, it has been calculated that some 5 million people suffer from the lung fluke.

Diagnosis is made by finding the egg in the sputum or faeces (see Fig.

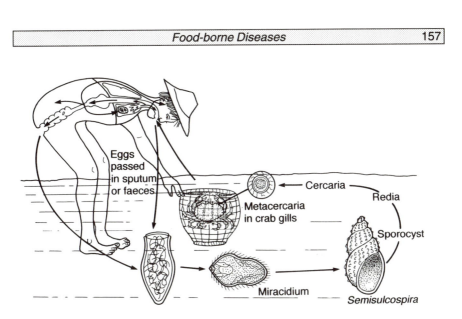

Fig. 13.3. The seasonal variation of meningococcal meningitis in relation to relative humidity.

9.1) and should always be considered in a case of haemoptysis. Treatment is by praziquantel 25 mg kg⁻¹ three times a day for 2 consecutive days.

Control is most effectively achieved by ensuring that all crab and crayfish meat is properly cooked. It is a focal disease, so that identifying foci and taking preventive action can reduce the danger.

11.7 THE FISH TAPEWORM

The large tapeworm *Diphyllobothrium latum* is found in the intestines of humans, dogs, cats, foxes and bears and a number of other mammalian hosts. Eggs are passed in the faeces and on contact with water, they liberate a *coracidium*, which is ingested by a copepod (Fig. 11.4). The coracidium develops in the copepod to a larval form, a *procercoid*, which, when eaten by a fish, burrows its way into the muscles of the fish and develops into a *plerocercoid*. When the raw or improperly cooked fish is eaten by humans, the liberated plerocercoid attaches itself to the intestinal wall and develops into an adult tapeworm.

Such a large worm (10 m or more) in the intestines can consume a considerable quantity of nutrients, but its main pathology is due to the specific absorption of vitamin B_{12}. This can result in megaloblastic anaemia in the host.

The parasite is found in the cooler parts of the world, around the great lakes of Europe and America and also in China and Japan. It is a disease of some 13 million people.

Diagnosis is made by finding the egg in the faeces (see Fig. 9.1).

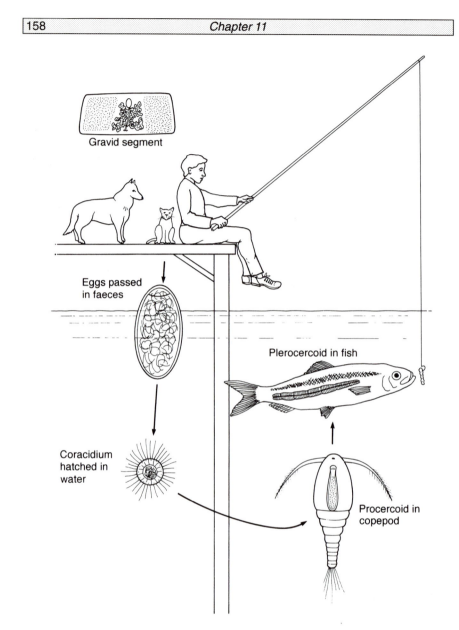

Fig. 11.4. The fish tapeworm – *Diphyllobothrium latum*.

Niclosamide, as a single dose of 2 g, or praziquantel, as a single dose of 5–10 mg kg^{-1}, is used for treatment.

Control is by ensuring that fish are properly cooked.

11.8 THE BEEF AND PORK TAPEWORMS

Perhaps the commonest (over 60 million infected) and most cosmopolitan of all the tapeworms, *Taenia saginata* is contracted by eating infected beef. The adult worm lives in the small intestine of humans. As the worm matures, gravid segments break off and are passed in the faeces. Cattle inadvertently eat the proglottids (mature segments) or the discharged eggs contaminate the pasture. An alternative method for cattle to become infected is to drink water polluted by sewage. The eggs develop into cysticerci in cattle, favouring the muscles of the jaw, heart, diaphragm, shoulder and oesophagus. Humans acquire the disease by eating improperly cooked beef containing the cysticercus.

The pork tapeworm *Taenia solium* follows essentially the same cycle, humans obtaining their infection from eating improperly cooked pork. The major difference is that the intermediate stage of the cysticercus can also occur in humans. This happens by swallowing eggs directly, either by autoinfection, from eggs in food or water or through sewage contamination. Also any gastric disturbance that might cause the regurgitation of proglottids into the stomach (including improper treatment) can lead to the liberation of vast quantities of eggs, with the result that cysticerci are produced anywhere in the body, including the brain, orbit and muscle.

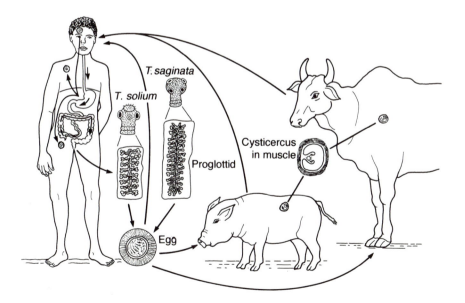

Fig. 11.5. The tapeworms – *Taenia solium* and *Taenia saginata*.

The adult worm of either species causes little pathology except that it shares the food supply of its host, which can result in debility when nutrition is poor. The serious problems are due to the cysticercus cellulosae (from *T. solium*). The cysts die and calcify, those in the brain being a common cause of epilepsy or even mental disorder.

Diagnosis is made by finding the proglottids in the faeces, the patient often diagnosing him/herself. It is very important to distinguish between *T. saginata* and *T. solium* in view of the danger of inducing cysticercosis. *T. saginata* has 18–30 compound branches of the uterus on each side, whereas *T. solium* has only eight to 12 (Fig. 11.5). Treatment for both worms is with niclosamide 2 g as a single dose. Alternatively praziquantel as a single dose of 5–10 mg kg^{-1} can be given. Praziquantel at a dose of 50 mg kg^{-1} for 15 days can be used for cerebral cysticercosis, in conjunction with corticosteroids, as an in-patient.

These two worms are found in areas of beef and pork eating where there is a ready transmission cycle in operation. Finding the worm in humans means that it is probably reasonably common in that area, whereas, in other places where beef and pork eating are just as much part of the usual diet, they are not found. *T. saginata* is increasing in Europe, probably because of human sewage contamination of animal drinking-water. It has also been found that birds feeding on sewage can carry eggs long distances and then deposit them on pasture land. Flies might have a place in transmission. *T. solium* is common in Mexico, Chile, Africa, India, Indonesia and Russia.

The main means of control is the proper cooking of meat. The underdone steak or joint of meat, where internal temperatures are not high enough to kill the cysticercus, are common ways in which transmission can still take place, despite cooking. Proper control of slaughtering in official abattoirs, with meat inspection, can prevent the dissemination of infected meat. Condemned carcasses must be burnt.

Where a localized cycle of infection is occurring, investigation may reveal a sewage leak or other source of contamination that can easily be rectified.

11.8 TRICHINOSIS

The nematode worms use every available means to disseminate themselves, from being swallowed directly as an egg, as a larva which pierces the skin, to being carried by vectors. *Trichinella spiralis*, *T. nelsoni* and *T. nativa* mimic the tapeworm and encyst in the flesh of animals. The cycle is a simple one, the encysted larvae in the muscles are eaten by another animal, and the liberated cyst develops into an adult to produce numerous new larvae, which are then carried to all parts of the body in the circulation. Only those larvae which reach striated muscle survive, the

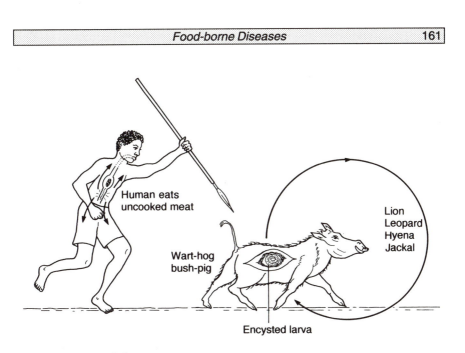

Human eats
uncooked meat

Lion
Leopard
Hyena
Jackal

Wart-hog
bush-pig

Encysted larva

Fig. 11.6. *Trichinella spiralis.*

diaphragm, tongue, throat, eye and thorax being the favoured sites.

In the different climatic zones of the world, where different groups of animals live off each other, several transmission cycles have evolved. In Africa the wart-hog and the bush-pig form the vital link in the cycle (Fig. 11.6). As they are the favoured prey of lions and leopards, these carnivores, with the hyenas and jackals that finish off the remains, all become infected. The general scavenging nature of the wart-hog and pig inadvertently eating the remains of dead animals allows the cycle to be completed. Humans come in as an intruder, a dead end to the cycle, when they feast upon a bush-pig they have recently killed.

The severity of the disease depends upon the dose of larvae that have encysted in the tissues. During the second week of the infection there is headache, insomnia, pain, dyspnoea and pyrexia, with oedema of the orbit and eosinophilia. If the symptoms are sufficiently severe, death can occur; otherwise, once the attack is over, the cysts cause no further trouble and gradually die.

Diagnosis is made by muscle biopsy of the deltoid or thigh muscles, where the encysted larvae are found. Treatment is symptomatic, with steroids. Mebendazole should also be given at a dose of 200 mg a day for 4 days.

Approximately 40 million of the world's population are affected, although trichinosis commonly occurs as a localized outbreak, with a group of people all contracting the disease at the same time. A classic example is for a wild pig to be killed and cooked over a fire by turning it on a spit. By this means, only the outside meat is well cooked; inside the temperature has not been sufficient to kill the larvae. The participants at the feast will all start having symptoms at much the same time. By counting back 2 weeks from these cases, the source of infection can be localized. Outbreaks in industrialized countries and the urban areas of developing countries are commonly caused by eating sausages, especially of the salami type. Where such a source is suspected, it should be investigated and food hygiene practices enforced.

12

Infectious Skin Rashes

This chapter covers a group of diseases in which a skin rash is a common feature and is generally involved in the infectious process. Transmission is by direct contact.

12.1 CHICKENPOX (VARICELLA)

A generally mild viral disease, chickenpox is a common infection of children. There is an acute febrile illness, followed by a characteristic skin rash of macules, papules, vesicles, pustules and dried crusts. The lesions occur in groups, appearing over several days, so pocks of different stages will be seen at the same time. In chickenpox the rash is distributed centrally, appearing on the chest and abdomen and sparsely on the feet and hands.

The majority of people contract the disease in childhood, when it is an inconvenience rather than a life-threatening condition, but if this has not occurred and they subsequently develop the illness as adults it can be very serious. This is a particular problem in island and isolated communities, where varicella can be a fatal disease in the elderly. Pregnant women who contract the disease in late pregnancy or shortly after delivery are at risk of severe generalized chickenpox, with a 30% mortality. Neonates who develop chickenpox within 10 days of birth are liable to a serious generalized infection. Chickenpox in early pregnancy may result in congenital malformations. Death results from generalized viraemia, cardiomyopathy or pneumonia.

The infection is transmitted by fluid from the vesicles. These can occur in the pharynx before the main rash, when transmission is by droplets. Otherwise spread is by direct skin contact, by airborne dispersion of vesicle fluid or through articles soiled by discharges. The *incubation period* is from 2 to 3 weeks and the period of communicability from

3 days before the onset of the rash to 6 days after its first appearance.

One attack of chickenpox confers lifelong immunity, so it is preferable for children to have the disease rather than be protected and run the risk of developing it as adults. The virus remains latent in the body, lodged in nerve bundles, and in later life, especially during a debilitating disease (such as human immunodeficiency virus (HIV) infection), the identical virus (varicella zoster) causes *shingles*. This presents as a vesicular rash with erythema, in a well-defined area of skin supplied by the affected dorsal-root ganglia. Pain and paraesthesia occur along the course of the affected nerve.

Control of the disease is not practised, as acquiring the infection as a child prevents more serious complications as an adult. Special groups such as neonates, pregnant women and the sick should be protected by preventing cases of chickenpox from coming into contact with them. In hospital, cases of chickenpox should be isolated.

The main concern in the diagnosis of chickenpox is to differentiate it from smallpox. Any case of a pox rash where the patient dies or where the pocks have an unusual distribution should be a smallpox suspect. The differential diagnosis of smallpox is given in the next section.

12.2 SMALLPOX

One of the major triumphs of international health cooperation has been the eradication of smallpox. This remarkable achievement was certified worldwide by the Global Commission on 9 October 1979, 2 years after the last case of naturally acquired disease was found.

Remote though it is, there is the possibility of a case being discovered, so the World Health Organization (WHO) has set up an international surveillance team to investigate any suspicious case. Any suspect must be strictly isolated and WHO informed.

The characteristics of smallpox are as follows.

- Clear-cut prodromal period of fever, headache and prostration, of sudden onset.
- Peripheral distribution of the rash (including soles and palms).
- Lesions pass through the same stages at the same time.
- Fever intensifies as the rash progresses to the pustular stage.
- Lesions are deeply seated, flat-topped and centrally depressed.

12.3 MONKEYPOX

Monkeypox is a rare zoonosis, significant because it produces a disease similar to smallpox. Localized to tropical rain-forest areas of West and

Central Africa. Most cases have been reported from Zaire. Although it is a disease of monkeys, it occasionally affects humans. It has a comparable case-fatality rate to smallpox, although the secondary attack rate is much lower (15%).

Smallpox vaccination (vaccinia virus) protects against monkeypox, so the waning level of vaccination poses the theoretical possibility of it spreading. However, the well-defined distribution and the low secondary attack rate in close contacts make it unlikely to develop into a similarly serious disease.

There are also other animal poxvirus diseases which have infected or could infect humans. Examples are cowpox, camelpox, tanapox, yabapox, buffalopox, sheeppox and goatpox. There is very little evidence to suggest that any of these diseases can cause an infection in humans that is likely to be spread from person to person to any marked extent. The importance of all these obscure pox infections is to recognize that they can occur and to differentiate them from smallpox.

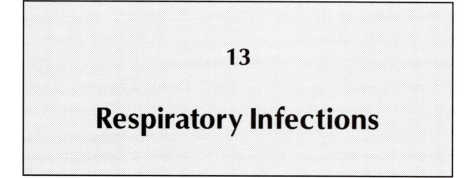

13

Respiratory Infections

The vulnerable respiratory apparatus is easily invaded by microorganisms. Breathing is continuous and, as respiratory gases are wafted in and out, infecting organisms find free passage deep inside the body.

The site of entry is commonly the nasopharynx, but entry can also occur through the oropharynx and the conjunctiva. The lacrimal glands drain into the nasopharynx and experimental studies have shown that this is often a more certain method of infection than directly through the nares. The respiratory system also includes connections to the middle ear, the sinuses and the gastrointestinal tract.

The ciliated lining and mucus-secreting cells of the respiratory tract can act as non-specific host defence mechanisms, entrapping microorganisms and passing them to the exterior. In attempting to expel these secretions from the body by coughing or spitting, organisms may be transmitted to another host. The lymphoid tissues, especially the tonsils and adenoids, guard the respiratory apparatus, but sometimes may themselves become foci of infection.

Respiratory diseases are usually transmitted by direct contact between individuals and generally the closer the contact the greater the chance of spread. As contact between human beings is a necessary part of life, control becomes more difficult and non-specific. Even so, the respiratory diseases are an enigma, because the voluminous quantities of expelled organisms are sufficient to infect entire populations, and yet only some individuals manifest the disease state.

Infective dose and host response determine whether infection will occur. Environmental factors which increase infective dose (e.g. overcrowding) or reduce the host's resistance (malnutrition) can have a marked effect.

13.1 ACUTE RESPIRATORY INFECTIONS

The acute respiratory infections (ARI) are the commonest causes of ill health in the world. The World Health Organization (WHO) has estimated that there are 14–15 million deaths a year in children under 5 and a third of these are due to ARI. Yet, despite their importance, they are a poorly defined group of diseases. They include the common cold, influenza, pneumonia, bronchitis and a number of other infections. They can be separated by clinical criteria, but it is the differing response of the individual to the organism that determines the clinical severity and management. A mild infection from an upper-respiratory-tract infection in one person may develop in another to a life-threatening attack of pneumonia. It is therefore not only the organism that determines the disease, but also the patient's response to the organism.

13.1.1. Organisms

A number of different organisms have been implicated, including rhinoviruses, adenoviruses, myxoviruses, *Mycoplasma* and bacteria such as the pneumococci, *Bordetella pertussis* and *Haemophilus influenzae*.

As well as there being a wide range of viruses, each species may have a number of serotypes, with new ones appearing from time to time. The host can respond by producing an appropriate immune response, but because of the large number of serotypes it is a continuous process. Infection will cause illness in some people, but not in others who have developed an immune response to the specific organism or an antigenically similar serotype. New antigenic mutation, as occurs in influenza, can cause epidemic or pandemic spread.

13.1.2 Host Factors

As already mentioned, response of the host is a major determinant of the disease process. Even with a well-defined organism such as A/Hong Kong/68(H3 N2), the cause of Hong Kong flu, infection was mild in some people, while it was fatal in others. Host factors are difficult to elucidate, but they include the following.

- Age. Young children develop obstructive diseases, such as croup (laryngotracheobronchitis) and bronchiolitis; tonsillitis is commonest in school-age children, whereas influenza and pneumonia are important causes of death in the elderly. In young children mortality is inversely related to age.
- *Portal of entry*. Volunteers have been more easily infected by some

organisms applied to the conjunctiva than through the nasopharynx.
- *Nutrition.* Low-birth-weight and malnourished children have a higher morbidity and mortality. Certain nutritional deficiencies, such as vitamin A and zinc, contribute to the development of a more severe disease and higher death rate. Breast-feeding appears to have a protective effect.
- *Socio-economic.* ARI is a disease of poverty, with a higher incidence in lower socio-economic groups and those that live in urban slums. Higher rates of lower-respiratory-tract disease have been found with increasing family size. Much of the reason for this increase appears to be due to increased contact and agglomeration, as shown by children attending day-care facilities or school, where infection occurs irrespective of social class.
- *Air pollution.* A correlation with domestic air pollution has been shown in South Africa and Nepal. Passive smoking may affect pulmonary function and make the child more susceptible to infection, as well as influencing the child to become a smoker.
- *Climate.* More respiratory infections are found in the cooler parts of the world or in the higher-altitude regions of the tropics. There is a distinct seasonal effect in many countries, with more respiratory infections in the winter. However, cold alone is not a causative factor. The 'cold' derives its name from the belief that becoming chilled or standing in a draught is responsible, but, when volunteers are subjected to these stresses and inoculated with rhinoviruses, they develop no more 'colds' than controls.
- *Other infections.* Any infection which causes damage to the respiratory mucosa will allow a mild infecting organism to progress to more serious consequences. The most important of these diseases is measles, post-measles pneumonia being particularly common.

13.1.3 Secondary Infection

Secondary infection by bacteria is responsible for pneumonia, bronchitis and pyogenic lung diseases. Many of these bacteria are already present as commensal organisms in the upper respiratory tract, but in hospital infections typed organisms can be shown to have been transmitted from one person to another.

13.1.4 Treatment

Treatment is supportive for mild infection and the active administration of antibiotics to the severe case. The mild infection is best treated at home and kept away from sources of other infection which may cause more serious disease, while the severe case requires early treatment to prevent complications and death. In children the *respiratory rate* and *chest indrawing* are used to decide management.

- *Mild cases*, with a respiratory rate of less than 50 min^{-1}, are treated at home with supportive therapy. The mother should be encouraged to nurse her child, giving it plenty of fluids (breast-feeding or from a cup), regular feeding, cleaning the nose, maintaining it at a comfortable temperature and avoiding contact with others.
- *Moderate case* (respiratory rate over 50 min^{-1} but *No chest indrawing*) should be given antibiotics (oral co-trimoxazole, oral ampicillin or intramuscular penicillin) and nursed at home.
- *Severe case* (with chest indrawing or cyanosis or too sick to feed) must be admitted as an in-patient and treated with an antibiotic and given active support. Benzyl penicillin or chloramphenicol are probably the most appropriate antibiotics.

13.1.5 Management

The first step in management of a child with ARI is to separate the mild from the moderate and to treat the moderate and severe. The essence is speed and active treatment. This can easily be taught at primary health-care level. The mother can be educated on the management of her child with a mild infection and when to refer. It is the delay in referral and treatment that will allow a moderate case to become severe and the severe to die.

The village health worker can identify and treat the mild or moderate case of ARI, using simple diagnostic criteria and a standard treatment protocol. Training and supervision of primary health-care workers is a priority in the management of ARI.

13.1.6 Prevention

With such an ill-defined disease complex, where a virus can cause a fatal obstructive illness in a young child and yet a mild transient infection in an attending adult, preventive action is varied.

Contact

Acute respiratory infections are just as common in industrialized countries as they are in developing countries, but infant deaths from respiratory infections in the former have declined. The reason would appear to be due to smaller families and greater birth intervals, permitting increased individual care of children and better nutrition. The child is reared at home and does not need to be carried round where it is exposed at a very young age to infecting organisms.

Health education

Important points are to teach people to cough away from people, to cover the mouth when coughing, not to spit or smoke and to provide proper ventilation for smoke and fumes.

Immunization

Against childhood infections

The danger of developing pneumonia after measles is a serious problem, so prevention of measles will reduce the severe forms of ARI. Indeed, measles immunization is perhaps the single most effective preventive method. Measles immunization is covered in Section 13.2. Pertussis, diphtheria and bacillus Calmette–Guérin (BCG) immunization should also be encouraged.

Influenza vaccine

The difficulty of developing vaccines against ARI is due to the large number of serotypes and their ability to undergo mutation. Fortunately, with influenza there are only three viruses and a limited number of serotypes. A is responsible for pandemics, B for smaller localized outbreaks and C produces mild infections, so a vaccine is only produced against influenza A. The virus contains haemagglutinin (H) and neuraminidase (N) subunits, which can both undergo antigenic shift and so evade the host response to the previous influenza A infection. These strains are classified by antigenic subunit types and the year and place that they were first identified. For example, the influenza pandemic that originated from Singapore in 1957 is called A/Singapore/1/57(H2N2). So far there have been three antigenic shifts of the H antigen and two of the N antigen. Each of these antigenic subunits is unique and a vaccine must contain the correct make-up of the invading virus. The difficulty is deciding what combination to include in the vaccine, as one containing many antigenic subunits has a low potency for any of them, whereas a specific one may not be correct for the prevalent disease strain. The WHO collaboration centre, with reference laboratories throughout the world, provides advance warning to assist countries producing vaccine, but new techniques, such as virus manipulation to anticipate natural change in the virus, could allow banks of virus to be kept in store.

Other vaccines

Recent trials have shown that a pneumococcal vaccine is effective in areas where ARI with a high mortality rate is common. A vaccine has also been developed against *H. influenzae* and it is hoped that this can be combined with diphtheria, pertussis and tetanus (DPT) in routine vaccination programmes. Viral vaccines against respiratory syncytial virus, parainfluenza and the adenoviruses are in preparation.

13.2 MEASLES

Measles presents as a skin rash, but is transmitted via the respiratory route, from nasal and pharyngeal secretions.

Measles is a severe disease in developing countries and accounts for a considerable amount of mortality and morbidity in the childhood population. It is not a new disease and there is evidence that it has been present in these countries for several hundred years. But the pattern of measles has changed from a sporadic epidemic, with all ages involved, to one of endemicity, predominantly affecting the under-5s.

Measles is the most contagious of all infectious diseases and no age is spared. In the Fijian outbreak in the 1870s, adults as well as children succumbed, so that whole families were affected at the same time, deprivation and starvation resulting in a high death rate. Now that adults have experienced measles as children, the age of infection is getting younger. This is explained by greater contact of communities due to improvement of communication, while the intense social contact at a very young age (babies carried on their mothers' backs) gives maximum opportunity for early transmissions.

Measles has a severe effect on the nutritional status of the child, so the healthy child will lose weight and the malnourished child will become critically ill. The peak of infection is between 1 and 2 years of age at the very time when breast milk alone is an inadequate source of food supply and weaning foods have probably not been introduced. The association of nutritional change and measles can be, and often is, a lethal combination.

There are a number of reasons for the nutritional depletion produced by measles. Any *disease process* puts extra demands on the body, increasing catabolism. Fever and the desquamation of all epithelial surfaces demands protein replacement, which is handicapped by a *sore mouth*, often secondarily infected by *Candida*, preventing the child from sucking properly, so that even breast milk is not taken. Then, from the other end, *diarrhoea*, which is such a common feature of measles in developing countries, further discharges the body reserves. But perhaps the greatest weight loss is due to *immunosuppression*, much of this taking place after the child has recovered from the acute attack.

The disease process attacks all epithelial surfaces, producing most of its complications in the respiratory tract. Pneumonia is the commonest complication, while laryngotracheobronchitis is serious, with a high mortality. ARI (see Section 13.1) are one of the leading causes of childhood ill health, and the sequelae of measles are responsible for a large component of this problem. If the acute pneumonia does not kill, the damage done makes the child more susceptible to further attacks of respiratory infection when the measles has long gone.

The effects on the eye can cause blindness. Corneal lesions result from epithelial damage, which can lead to ulceration, secondary infection and scarring. In severe cases, perforation or total disorganization of the eye can occur. These severe effects only result if there is concomitant vitamin A deficiency, so giving vitamin A to all measles cases is effective. Measles, through its nutritional and direct effects, has been regarded as the most important cause of blindness in a number of tropical countries.

13.2.1 Measles Vaccination

As measles is such an infectious disease, it can be reckoned that every child will develop it. Some 10% will either have a mild infection or be partially protected by maternal antibodies and will appear not to have been infected. A further 10–20% will not have measles until the following year due to the epidemic effect, so the expected number of cases of measles can be calculated from the birth rate minus 25%. If the birth rate in a developing country is 50 per thousand, 75% of this means that 37.5 cases of measles per thousand can be expected per annum, which represents 37,500 cases in an administrative unit of a million people. Calculations like these can be used to estimate the number of children to be vaccinated and hence the vaccine requirements.

Of susceptibles, 80% will need to be vaccinated to produce control of the disease, but a lower target may be acceptable in more isolated communities. This target will need to be achieved every year in rural areas, but as often as every 6 months in urban areas. Measles vaccine is 90% effective if the cold chain is not broken.

Maternal antibodies protect the newborn infant for the first 6 months of life, but thereafter it becomes readily susceptible to infection, with a peak around 1 year. Seroconversion rate is some 76% at the age of 6 months, 88% at 9 months and 100% at 1 year. Giving measles vaccination at 1 year would produce the best conversion, but, by that time in developing countries, some 50% will already have had the disease. Giving it at 6 months will be before all but a few have had the disease but the seroconversion rate is so poor that not many will be protected. The best compromise is a single vaccination at 9 months. In conditions of high infectivity, such as during an epidemic or admission to hospital, reducing

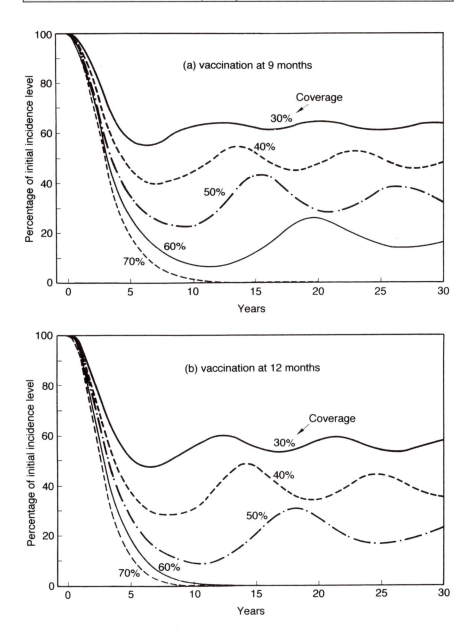

Fig. 13.1. Relative impact of immunization programmes on measles incidence in the age-group 0–19 years, according to age at vaccination and population coverage. (Reproduced, by permission, from Cvetanovic, B., Grab, B. and Dixon, H. (1982) *Bulletin of the World Health Organization* 60(3), 405–422.)

the age of vaccination to 6 months is justified. In this case another vaccination should be given at 9–12 months.

In developed countries vaccination is given at 12 months or older, as the time taken to reduce the incidence in the population will be less, as shown in Fig. 13.1. The greater the coverage the more rapidly this is achieved. For example, 60% coverage will theoretically take 12 years to reduce the incidence to zero if vaccination is given at 12 months, but never be achieved at 9 months. However, a 70% coverage will achieve zero incidence with vaccination given at 9 months, which is being achieved by an increasing number of developing countries.

Effective measles vaccination coverage will not only reduce the number of children developing the disease in an epidemic, but will have the secondary benefit of raising the age of developing the disease. This can be seen in Figure 13.2. Epidemics had occurred regularly every second year until 1978, when there was only a minor increase, the main epidemic being delayed until 1979. This meant that children born in 1977, who could have expected to become infected in their second year of life (1978), had their measles put off until 1979, when they were beyond the age of maximum mortality.

The chances of a susceptible child developing measles when admitted to hospital is very high, as he or she is already sick with another complaint. It is fortunate that measles vaccine can produce protective

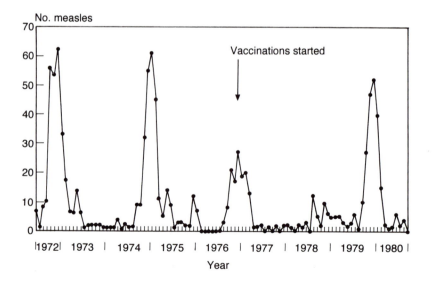

Fig. 13.2. Prolongation of the time interval between measles epidemics due to vaccination, Namanyere, Tanzania.

immunity quicker than the wild virus (about 8 days for the vaccine and 10 for the disease), so, as long as children are vaccinated within 48 hours of admission, they will be protected. Because of the severity of disease in the debilitated child, there are very few contraindications, and the malnourished and those with minor infection should all be vaccinated.

13.3 WHOOPING COUGH (PERTUSSIS)

Whooping cough is a serious disease if it occurs at a young age. *The severity of whooping cough is inversely proportional to age.* A mild infection in the older child, it becomes an important cause of death in the very young.

Whooping cough is due to infection with *Bordetella pertussis*. The *incubation period* is 7–10 days and the communicable stage from 7 days after first exposure until 3 weeks after the typical paroxysm starts. Isolation of cases, especially of young children and infants, should be instituted. Infective children should be kept from school, markets and any place where young children are likely to congregate. Known contacts of a case of whooping cough (e.g. in the extended family of a case) should be given a booster vaccination if they have been vaccinated before; otherwise they should receive prophylactic erythromycin and vaccine.

The classic 'whooping' disease is not seen in children under 3 months of age, when instead they have attacks of cyanosis and stop breathing. Erythromycin is only effective when given in the first week of the disease. Fluid loss is an important cause of mortality, so mothers should be encouraged to give extra fluids and breast-feed immediately after a coughing bout.

The opportunities for exposure of the young infant are high where the child is always carried around by its mother. In this way it comes into close contact with other children, who might be infectious. The median age for the disease is 2 years, but because of its severity immunization should be started at 1 month. Three doses are given, normally combined with tetanus and diphtheria as triple vaccine.

13.4 DIPHTHERIA

Diphtheria is a bacterial disease (*Corynebacterium diphtheriae*) which has both local and systemic effects. The organism can infect the tonsils, pharynx, larynx, nasal mucosa or skin, forming a membranous exudate. This exudate and the inflammatory reaction it produces in the respiratory tract can lead to obstruction. From the primary site, exotoxin is produced, which can cause myocarditis or neuropathy, especially cranial-nerve palsies.

Commonly a disease of children, it can occur in non-immunized adults, with serious results. Outbreaks of the disease are seen, but it is probably a much more frequent disease than realized, as subclinical transmission through skin and possibly nasal lesions maintains immunity.

The *incubation period* is 2–5 days and the period of communicability about 2 weeks. In an unimmunized population, there is a high incidence of carriers and a low incidence of cases, in a ratio of approximately 19:1. Between 6 and 40% of children are infected each year, so that by 5 years some 75% have been infected and by 15 years nearly all. This means that by 15 years of age the majority of children have developed immunity, either by an unapparent infection or by one in which clinical symptoms were revealed.

Diphtheria can be transmitted by the following.

- Direct contact.
- Indirect through fomites.
- Respiratory.
- Ingestion of contaminated milk.

Control is by immunization of all children with diphtheria toxoid. This is normally combined with pertussis and tetanus as triple vaccine in the first or second month of life.

In the event of an outbreak, previously immunized contacts can be given tetanus and diphtheria toxoids and those not immunized the toxoid and an antibiotic. Diphtheria antitoxin is given to cases and to immunized contacts if toxoid is not available. A test dose for hypersensitivity is given first.

13.5 BACTERIAL MENINGITIS

Meningitis is a widespread disease, which can occur as isolated cases or as epidemics. Infection of the meninges causes fever, headaches, neck stiffness and progressive loss of consciousness.

Many organisms can cause meningitis, but the most important are *Neisseria meningitidis*, *Haemophilus influenzae* and *Streptococcus pneumoniae* (pneumococci). Meningococcal meningitis (*N. meningitidis*) occurs in epidemics, especially in the Sahel part of Africa. These are markedly seasonal, with outbreaks in the early part of the year when the temperature is hottest and relative humidity at its lowest. With the arrival of the rains the epidemic abates (Fig. 13.3). The amount of rainfall delineates the southern boundary of the meningitis belt at 1100 mm rainfall, whereas the northern boundary is the desert. Within this band, stretching from Senegal to Sudan, major epidemics occur in 10–15-year cycles, with lesser ones in between.

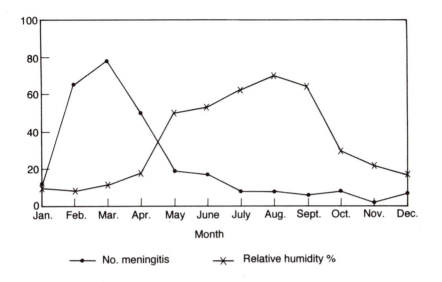

Fig. 13.3. The seasonal variation of meningococcal meningitis in relation to relative humidity.

Epidemic meningitis was first studied in cooler climates and an association found with overcrowding, especially in military institutions. When introduced into an overcrowded environment, the organism produced both cases and carriers (nasal). As the number of carriers increased, the number of cases of meningitis increased likewise. Transmission was considered to be by droplets and discharges from nose and throats, so the distance between people (bed space) was increased to reduce transmission.

In the African (Sahel) epidemic form, the heat makes people spend much of their time out of doors and overcrowding is not a phenomenon at this time of year (this occurs in the rains when the epidemic has ceased). It would seem unusual that meningococcal meningitis should use such opposing methods of spread, favouring a crowding together in cold climates and a dispersal pattern in hot climates.

The organism inhabits the nasal mucosa, within which it is anatomically very close to the meninges, although separated by formidable barriers of bone and membrane. The generally accepted theory is that the organism passes from this site into the bloodstream and then, for reasons unknown, crosses the blood–brain barrier and enters the cerebrospinal fluid (CSF). Experimental evidence does not substantiate this route unless there has been some trauma to the meninges. Difficult though the direct route may seem, it has been shown that minute passages through the bone of the skull do occur and transmission of organisms along this route is a possibility. Furthermore, if organisms are introduced directly into the subarachnoid space, infection will only occur if a critical level is exceeded (10^3 organisms in dogs), suggesting that this route could be frequently invaded but only when an excessive infection occured would meningitis develop. Therefore an alternative explanation is that the route of transmission is directly from the nose through the skull and that any traumatic insult to the nasal mucosa, such as the intense drying out and irritation of the Sahel hot season or upper-respiratory-tract infection in colder climates, potentiates a greater number of organisms to pass along these minute channels and overcome the defences of the meninges.

Epidemic meningitis is commonest in the age-group 5–15, with males more frequently affected than females. The organism is carried in the nose and throat of infected individuals for anything between 2 weeks and 10 months, but only a proportion, about one in 500, will develop meningitis. Overcrowding, especially in large, poor families, potentiates meningitis, suggesting a close dependent relationship.

13.5.1 Control

Overcrowding is a well-recognized feature in the transmission of meningitis; it encourages the transfer of the infecting organism and the carrier state as well as increasing the dose of bacteria that may be transmitted. All efforts should therefore be made to reduce overcrowding. It may be necessary to close schools and reduce collections of people, such as markets and religious gatherings. In the long term, improvement of housing and family planning will have an effect.

Chemoprophylaxis with sulphonamides used to be widely practised, but the appearance of resistant strains makes this largely a worthless exercise. In isolated outbreaks and where the organism is sensitive, prophylaxis to closed communities, using sulphonamides, antibiotics or rifampicin, can be given. Chemoprophylaxis is not recommended in large epidemics.

N. meningitidis is divided into at least 13 serogroups, but, of these, A, B and C are the most important in producing disease, while A and C predominate in epidemics. *Vaccines* have been developed against group A and group C, but it is preferable to use the combined (A and C) vaccine. Unfortunately, the very young have a poor response and those with acute malaria develop reduced immunity, as well as there being genetic variation. Due to these different factors, duration of immunity varies from 3 years or under in young children, and must be measured for each community when formulating a vaccination programme. Vaccine can be used to immunize those most at risk, concentrating on the 2–20-year age-group, or, in the face of an epidemic, communities in the affected area by mass vaccination. It has been suggested that an incidence of 15 cases per

100,000 in a well-defined population for 2 consecutive weeks heralds the beginning of an epidemic and the need to start mass vaccination. In endemic areas, vaccination can be given to household contacts of cases and those at special risk.

Every attempt should be made to identify the organism by lumbar puncture. A Gram stain is only reliable in some 50% of cases, so culture should be attempted wherever possible and sensitivity obtained. Countercurrent immunoelectrophoresis or the latex test is applicable where transport of samples is a problem.

Treatment may need to be organized on a massive scale when an epidemic occurs, by using dispensers, schoolteachers or other educated people to care for isolated communities. Temporary treatment centres (schools, churches, warehouses, etc.) may need to be set up, rather than bringing people into hospital. Benzyl penicillin 12–24 million units every 24 hours or chloramphenicol 100 mg kg^{-1} every 24 hours for 5 days should be used. Chloramphenicol is especially indicated when the suspected organism is *H. influenzae*. If the organism is unknown, use chloramphenicol. In epidemics, long-acting chloramphenicol in oil preparations, given as a single injection, can be used. Dehydration is common and intravenous fluids may be required initially, followed by frequent drinks administered by an attending adult.

13.6 ACUTE RHEUMATIC FEVER

Acute rheumatic fever (ARF) is a delayed non-suppurative sequel of upper-respiratory-tract infection with group A beta-haemolytic streptococci (GABHS). ARF derives its importance because it can lead to rheumatic heart disease (RHD), which causes considerable morbidity and mortality in such patients. ARF/RHD is the commonest form of heart disease in children and young adults in most tropical and developing countries.

The epidemiology of ARF mirrors that of streptococcal sore throat. The peak age incidence is 5–15 years, but both primary and recurrent cases can occur in adults. There is neither a sex predilection nor a racial predisposition. ARF results from an interaction of the bacterial agent, human host and environment. GABHS are transmitted from person to person through relatively large droplets, up to a distance of 3 m. ARF develops at a fairly constant rate of 3% following untreated epidemics of streptococcal pharyngitis. The attack rate is much lower (< 1%) following endemic or sporadic streptococcal infections. Healthy primary school-children are commonly found to be carriers of GABHS.

The M-protein in the wall of the streptococcus is responsible for its virulence and certain predominant serotypes, 1, 3, 5, 6, 14, 18, 19, 24, 27 and 29, have a much greater rheumatogenic potential. The most widely used serological marker of recent streptococcal infection is the antistreptolysin-O titre (ASOT). Cutaneous streptococcal infection (impetigo) is a frequent precursor of acute nephritis, but has not been shown to cause ARF.

Why only a small percentage of the youthful population develop ARF following infection with GABHS remains an enigma. ARF patients, as a group, show a higher antibody level to group A streptococcal antigens, suggesting that repeated exposure to GABHS may precipitate illness. Susceptibility is due to the immunological status of the host, including both humoral and cell-mediated immunity, with a 2% familial incidence of ARF. A larger proportion of children born to rheumatic parents contract the disease. The carditis of RHD might be the result of an autoimmune mechanism developing between group A streptococcal somatic components and myocardial and valvular components.

ARF is a disease of lower socio-economic groups, particularly those massed in the densely populated areas of urban metropolitan centres. It is widespread, with a high incidence in south Asia, Pacific islands, North and South Africa and urban Latin America. It has been estimated that RHD causes 25–40% of all cardiovascular disease in the Third World.

There is no permanent cure for RHD and the cumulative expense of repeated hospitalization for supportive medical care is a considerable drain on the meagre health resources of developing countries. The only reasonable solution is prevention of rheumatic fever. Prevention of the first attack (*Primary prevention*) is by proper identification and antibiotic treatment of streptococcal infections. The individual who has suffered an attack of ARF is inordinately susceptible to recurrences following sub-sequent streptococcal infection and needs protection (*Secondary prevention*). While primary prevention is preferable, the incidence of ARF as a sequel of streptococcal sore throat is never greater than 3% even in epidemics. A vast number of infections would need to be treated in order to achieve any meaningful reduction and, of the total number of sore throats, streptococci are responsible for only 10–20%.

Most cases of severe RHD would be prevented by adequate prevention of recurrences of ARF. No matter how mild the first attack of ARF, secondary prevention with intramuscular, long-acting benzathine penicillin G 1.2 million units should be given at monthly intervals. Penicillin V or sulphadiazine may be used for oral prophylaxis. Regular taking of prophylaxis is essential and compliance is a major problem. Patients with no evidence of cardiac involvement should receive prophylaxis for a minimum of 5 years after the last attack of ARF, while those with carditis should continue until they are 25 years old. Prophylaxis should be continued with penicillin in the pregnant woman.

The emphasis of a prevention programme should be on health education, early diagnosis and treatment of sore throats and the provision of treatment facilities at primary level. In developing strategies, baseline data on streptococcal epidemiology and ARF/RHD prevalence in high-risk groups should be collected. A fully established programme centre would operate a central register, coordinate case-finding surveys, run a system of secondary prophylaxis (especially follow-up) and promote health education. Community control of ARF and RHD is viable only if it is firmly based on existing health services, which are an integral part of the primary health-care activities in the country. It is especially relevant to school health services, for screening children and supporting those on secondary prophylaxis.

13.7 HISTOPLASMOSIS

Histoplasmosis is a systemic fungal infection of uncommon presentation. Sensitivity testing in some areas indicate that a large proportion of the population have had subclinical infection. It occurs in two forms – an American histoplasmosis caused by *Histoplasma capsulatum* and an African form due to infection with *H. duboisii*. The African form is restricted to West, East and Central Africa, whereas the American is found worldwide.

The *incubation period* is 5–8 days. Infection is acquired by inhaling airborne spores of *H. capsulatum*, found in bat-infested caves, chicken roosts and similar collections of decaying organic matter. There may be a mild respiratory illness, with malaise, weakness, fever, chest pain and cough, or a more serious progressive form, where almost any part of the body is affected. Diagnosis is made by finding the fungus in stained exudate, sputum or blood.

In *H. duboisii* infection the lesions are either large granulomatous subcutaneous masses or swelling and abscess development in bones.

Control is difficult and largely unnecessary, as the bulk of the population in an endemic area will develop immunity in early life. However, where a clustering of cases indicates a focus, efforts can be made to modify it, e.g. by spraying 3% formalin solution around chicken runs, or else warning people of the danger, for example, of entering certain caves.

13.8 TUBERCULOSIS

One of the major diseases in the world, tuberculosis is a considerable problem in developing countries. Not only are a proportion of the population infected with a debilitating and often fatal disease, but the period of infectiousness is prolonged (approximately 5 years in an untreated case), permitting transmission to many other persons. Indeed, in a number of countries an endemic balance has been achieved, whereby the number of cases that resolve spontaneously, are cured by medical treatment or die are replaced by an equal number of new cases entering the pool of tuberculosis. In India, for example, it is estimated that some five in every 1000 of the population are infected, which represents some 3 million cases of tuberculosis at any one time. In the world 10 million persons develop tuberculosis every year and 3 million die from it.

Tuberculosis infects people in a spectrum of severity, depending on the host response, the dose and the time. The *incubation period* between infection and development of the primary complex is 4–12 weeks. In the primary complex, the infection is localized to an area of the lung, with a corresponding enlargement of the hilar nodes. In the majority of people, this heals completely or with a residual scar and the person develops immunity to further challenge. If healing does not occur, the focus extends to cause glandular enlargement, pleural effusion or cavity formation. The third phase of the disease results from complications of the regional nodes. These may be obstructive, leading to collapse and consolidation, cause erosion and bronchial destruction or spread locally. The final stage is one of bloodstream spread, disseminating bacilli to all parts of the body, where they may produce tuberculous meningitis or a miliary infection. Longer-term complications are those of bones, joints, renal tract, skin and many other rare sites. These features are illustrated in Fig. 13.4.

The majority of people meet the tubercle bacillus in early life, acquire resistance and are quite unaware of ever having come into contact with it. A proportion, approximately 5%, will manifest the disease in varying levels of severity. It might be nothing more than an enlargement of the primary focus with a few systemic effects, only to resolve spontaneously. Others may have symptoms essentially in one phase, or may progress rapidly to bloodstream spread, presenting as a case of miliary or tuberculous meningitis. The type and severity of the disease are determined by the host response. This cannot be specified and why one person should develop tuberculosis and another not cannot generally be determined. (There is some evidence that susceptibility may be genetically determined, as people who have suffered from tuberculosis, even if adequately cured, are more likely to develop a new infection a second time.) The dose of bacilli might also be important because young children in close contact with an active case more commonly develop severe tuberculosis, (miliary or meningitis). Factors that are known to reduce resistance are the following.

- Young age, especially the first year of life.
- Pregnancy.
- Malnutrition.
- Intercurrent infections such as measles, whooping cough and streptococcal infection.

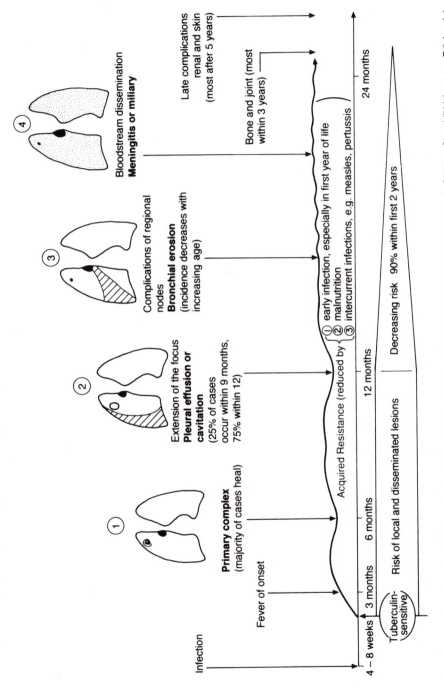

Fig. 13.4. The evolution of untreated primary tuberculosis. (Modified, by permission, from Miller, F.J.W. (1982) *Tuberculosis in Children*, Churchill Livingstone, Edinburgh.)

- Human immunodeficiency virus (HIV) infection.
- Occupations or environments that damage the lung (mining, dust, smoke).

The risk of developing local and disseminated lesions decreases over a period of 2 years. If the majority of cases are going to progress, they will do so within 12 months of infection or 6 months from the development of the primary complex. By the end of 2 years, 90% of complications will have occurred. Bone and other late complications are a very small proportion beyond this time.

As well as variation among individuals, there are also considerable differences in the susceptibility of populations. This can be measured by the annual tuberculosis infection rate, which compares the tuberculin reaction of non-vaccinated subjects of the same age every 5 years. With BCG vaccination at birth, this cannot be done, but data obtained before this became a universal policy are still valid. Countries of low prevalence are defined as those where less than 10% of children under 15 have a positive tuberculin test. These are largely the countries of Europe and North America. Nearly the whole of the tropical world has a high prevalence rate, with some countries experiencing over 50% of the under-15-year-olds tuberculin-positive. Also urban areas have higher rates than rural. There are high rates in Africa and parts of South America. In Asia, India, Myanmar, Thailand and Indonesia, all have high tuberculin-positive rates. In the Americas, the Indian peoples have a much higher rate than the non-indigenous. There is a high susceptibility in the Pacific islands, in which tuberculosis was an unknown disease until the arrival of explorers, who introduced the infection. Another method of estimating incidence is from tuberculosis notifications, as seen in Fig. 13.5.

There are clearly a number of compounding factors, and density is as important as susceptibility of the population. The dose of bacilli that the individual will meet is compounded by continued contact over a period of time. This dose/time factor is more likely to be found in conditions of poverty and overcrowding. If the dose is sufficiently large and maintained for long enough, even the defences of the immunologically competent individual may be broken down.

The risk of infection is greatest in the young and rises again in the old, so overcrowding increases the opportunity for infection to be acquired at a younger age. Since the young mix extensively, they will also have a greater opportunity for passing on the infection. At the other end of life, the elderly often form persistent foci in a community, a potent source of infection to the young.

Tuberculosis, then, is a disease of poor social conditions and over-crowding, as shown by the remarkable decline of the infection in industrialized countries prior to the advent of chemotherapy. In Europe at the turn of the century, tuberculosis was as bad as, if not worse than,

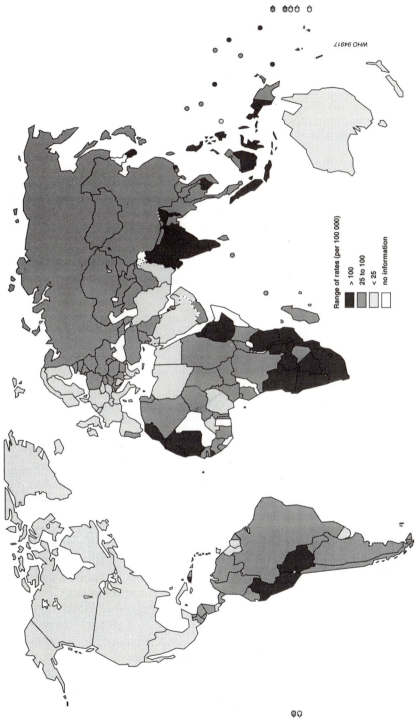
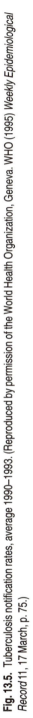

Fig. 13.5. Tuberculosis notification rates, average 1990–1993. (Reproduced by permission of the World Health Organization, Geneva. WHO (1995) *Weekly Epidemiological Record* 11, 17 March, p. 75.)

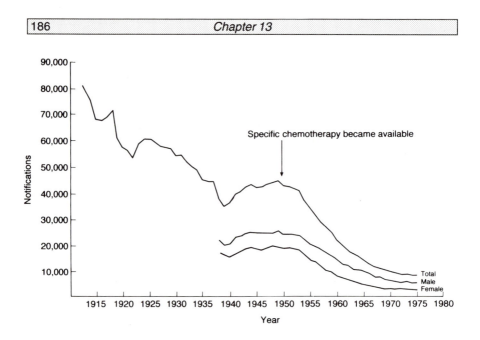

Fig. 13.6. The decline of respiratory tuberculosis in England and Wales, 1912–1975. (From DHSS (1977) *Annual Report of the Chief Medical Officer, Department of Health and Social Security for 1976,* Her Majesty's Stationery Office, London. Crown copyright, reproduced with the permission of the Controller of HMSO.)

in many developing countries now, but there was a progressive and continuous reduction of cases as living conditions improved (Fig. 13.6). As standards increased, there was a demand for improved housing with fewer people sharing the same room, so that overcrowding declined. Personal hygiene improved and such practices as spitting disappeared almost completely.

HIV infection has changed the epidemiology and presentation of tuberculosis, especially in Africa, leading to more lower-lobe and extrapulmonary disease. There are estimated to be more than 4 million persons worldwide with dual tuberculosis and HIV, with over 3 million of these cases in Africa. HIV infection may be adding a quarter of a million new cases of tuberculosis to those that would have been expected in Africa each year. Reduced host immune response has increased susceptibility and allowed reactivation or reinfection to take place, as well as increasing the likelihood of new infection from a contact or case. However, there is no evidence to suggest that HIV/tuberculosis patients are more infectious. Conversely tuberculosis patients are more likely to progress rapidly to full-blown acquired immune deficiency syndrome (AIDS) when infected with the HIV virus. Initially HIV-infected tuberculosis patients commonly present with pulmonary infection, similar to the HIV-negative case, but as the disease progresses extrapulmonary tuberculosis predominates and other manifestations of HIV disease, such as chronic diarrhoea, generalized lymphadenopathy, oral thrush and Kaposi's sarcoma are more common. All HIV-positive cases should therefore be investigated for tuberculosis and all tuberculosis cases tested for HIV. Despite the increase in extrapulmonary tuberculosis, it is still the sputum-positive case that is responsible for transmission of infection and this must remain the priority in searching for cases.

13.8.1 Chemotherapy

The functions of chemotherapy can be summarized as follows.

- Treatment of individual cases.
- Reduce the number and period of infectious cases.
- Provide a method of disease reduction in developing countries where the raising of social standards would take some time to achieve.

To prevent resistance developing multidrug therapy is used. The main drugs are:

- streptomycin;
- isoniazid;
- rifampicin;
- thiacetazone;
- pyrazinamide;
- ethambutol.

The usual procedure is to use a three-drug regime, streptomycin, isoniazid and thiacetazone, or rifampicin, isoniazid and pyrazinamide, for an initial period of 2–3 months. One of the three is then stopped and a two-dose regime is continued for a further 9–10 months. The majority of cases will be cured by this time, but in those where there is uncertainty therapy can continue for a further 6 months. Thiacetazone is cheap and favoured in many parts of the world, but in Mongoloid peoples it causes rashes and the occasional case of agranulocytosis, so a regime of fully supervised twice-weekly streptomycin plus isoniazid is preferred. Thiacetazone can also cause severe cutaneous hypersensitivity in patients who have both tuberculosis and HIV infection, and where the latter is suspected it should not be used.

This standard regime is effective if taken consistently and for the complete length of treatment, but unfortunately this does not always happen. As soon as the patient begins to feel better, he/she defaults and does not complete the course. This has two very serious consequences.

- The patient will relapse and infect other people in the community.
- Resistant organisms will be encouraged to develop.

In the search to overcome this problem a more intensive short-course therapy has been developed. Four drugs are given for an initial intensive phase of 8 weeks in hospital, continuing on a two-drug regime for 4–6 months after discharge. The regimen for an adult is:

Streptomycin	1 g daily	
Isoniazid	400 mg daily	for 8 weeks,
Rifampicin	600 mg daily	
Pyrazinamide	2 g daily	

then:

Isoniazid	300 mg daily	for a further 16–24 weeks.
Thiacetazone	150 mg daily	

If satisfactory follow-up is achieved, a 6-month period is a considerable saving. So, while the drug regime is more expensive, this is offset by a shorter follow-up period. The four-drug therapy should be used in cases of simultaneous tuberculosis/HIV infection, but it may be necessary to prolong treatment.

13.8.2 Follow-up and Registration

A system of following up all diagnosed cases of tuberculosis discharged from hospital or health centre is required on the following lines.

- Register the case with a central registry on diagnosis.
- When the patient is discharged inform the registry, the nearest clinic to the person's home and the supervising health worker.
- The clinic ensures the patient receives regular follow-up treatment or goes and finds the patient if he/she defaults.
- The supervising health worker visits on a regular basis to check the clinic records and make sure that the registered patients are receiving treatment.
- When the full course of treatment is completed and the health worker is satisfied that the patient is cured, the central registry is notified. Reminders and double checks can be built into the system, such as the central registry sending out quarterly checks on each patient.

The sophistication of the system depends upon the resources of the country, but lack of resources is never an excuse not to have a system at all. Not following a partially treated patient is a waste of expensive hospital treatment, encourages the development of resistant organisms and increases the risk to the community. Follow-up is always cheaper than rediagnosis and treatment. A national registration and follow-up system for tuberculosis is suitably combined with one for leprosy, and many countries have adopted this joint registry system.

13.8.3 Diagnosis and Community Search

Tuberculosis is spread by droplet infection, so only sputum-positive cases transmit the disease. The risk to the community is therefore from pulmonary tuberculosis and the emphasis of the programme should be on finding these cases. Sputum-positive tuberculosis is diagnosed by taking a sputum smear, not an X-ray. The comparative costs of diagnostic techniques are as follows.

Smear	0.02
Culture	0.20
Sensitivity	0.40
Full-plate X-ray	1.00

Fifty sputum smears can be made for the equivalent cost of one X-ray. Sputum examination is used for diagnosing cases in the community. Areas can be surveyed regularly and anybody with a productive cough asked to produce some sputum and a smear made. This is dried and stained with Ziehl–Neelsen for acid-fast bacilli. A simpler form of search is made in the village of a newly diagnosed case. The contacts are examined to see if there is anybody with a productive cough or clinical signs, and a smear is made. Contacts should be followed up at regular intervals. This can all be included in the national registration system.

A productive cough, especially if sputum-positive, is the most important sign of tuberculosis, but loss of weight and anaemia are often present and can be adequately judged on clinical examination.

13.8.4 BCG Vaccination

Vaccination by BCG induces cell-mediated immunity to the mycobacteria and does not generate humoral immunity, as do other vaccines. BCG vaccination therefore alerts the body's defences rather than inducing antibody formation. After a BCG vaccination, a primary infection will still take place, but the progressive or disseminated infection will be reduced.

Effectiveness of BCG varies considerably in different countries. In Europe there is a good response, while in India it is marginal. This is thought to be due to atypical mycobacteria circulating in the environment, so BCG should be given at birth or as soon after as possible. BCG should be administered to all infants, including those born to mothers with HIV infection. It should not, however, be given to those with symptomatic HIV.

BCG is a freeze-dried vaccine, given intradermally. Other methods, such as multiple puncture, jet injection or scarification, have been found to be less satisfactory. The vaccine is sensitive to heat and light and so must be carefully protected.

13.8.5 Evaluation of Tuberculosis Control Programmes

The following indicators can be used.

- Annual rate of new tuberculosis cases diagnosed.
- Rate of sputum–positive cases diagnosed.
- Proportion of children under 5 diagnosed.
- Proportion of cases of miliary and meningeal tuberculosis.
- Rate of sputum smears examined.
- Rate of BCG scars, on survey.
- Relapse rate.
- Rate lost to follow–up.

The proportion of sputum–positive cases out of the total new cases can give a good indication of level of infection, provided there has not been a reduction in the number of smears examined. A decrease in the proportion of children under 5 diagnosed and those with miliary and meningeal tuberculosis will add support; however, this will need to be confirmed by a survey of either sputum smears or tuberculin testing.

14

Leprosy: a Disease of Uncertain Means of Transmission

Leprosy is a major disease problem, with an estimated 11–15 million patients in the world. Some 2000 million people are living in areas of sufficient endemicity for transmission to occur. As with tuberculosis and other major diseases, the majority of the problem falls on the tropical world (Fig. 14.1).

Leprosy, more dramatically than other diseases, illustrates the conflict between infecting organism and host. It is evident that *Mycobacterium leprae* is widespread, and yet only a small proportion of people ever show clinical symptoms of the disease.

The generation time from inoculation to multiplication of a stable number of *M. leprae* is only 18–24 days, but the development of the disease will take anything from 7 months to in excess of 7 years (mean 3–6 years). The first lesion is described as *indeterminate* (Fig. 14.2) because at this early stage it is impossible to decide to which place in the spectrum of disease it will develop. There is either a single ill-defined, slightly hypopigmented macule, commonly seen on the face, trunk or exterior surfaces, or there may be a small anaesthetic patch. The lesion will develop into a *lepromatous* or *tuberculoid* type or oscillate in the transitional state of *borderline* leprosy.

14.1 LEPROMATOUS LEPROSY

Lepromatous leprosy (LL) reflects the complete breakdown of the host's immune responses and the maximum infection with *M. leprae*. In the early stages, signs of disease may be very few but a skin smear will reveal large numbers of mycobacteria (multibacillary). Two early signs that

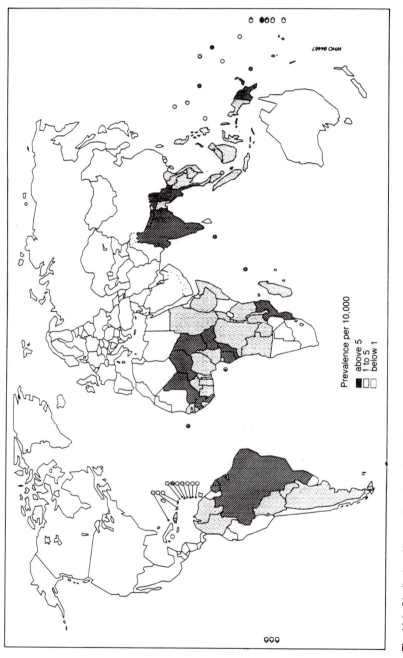

Prevalence per 10,000

■ above 5
▨ 1 to 5
□ below 1

Fig. 14.1. Distribution of leprosy throughout the world, 1994. (Reproduced by permission of the World Health Organization, Geneva.)

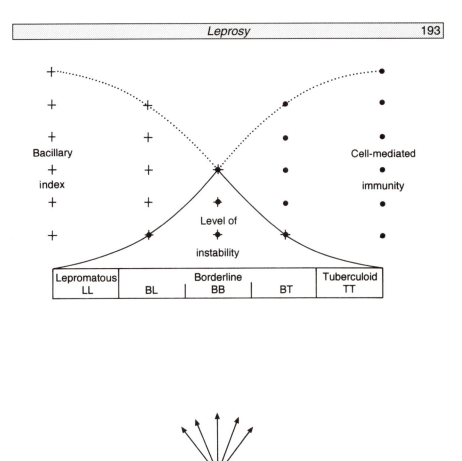

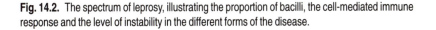

Indeterminate

Fig. 14.2. The spectrum of leprosy, illustrating the proportion of bacilli, the cell-mediated immune response and the level of instability in the different forms of the disease.

have been described but rarely observed are oedema of the legs and a collection of nasal symptoms – stuffiness, crust formation and blood-stained discharge. These are unlikely to be recognized as leprosy, and it is generally not until the more obvious skin lesions become apparent that the diagnosis is made.

Leprosy lesions favour the cooler parts of the body, so the buttocks, trunk, exposed limbs and face are the more likely sites. Lesions may be macules, papules or nodules, with or without a colour change, and they often show lack of sweating when the patient becomes hot. The diagnostic criterion is the presence of mycobacteria, and a skin smear must be taken from any suspicious skin lesions. The signs of nerve damage do not appear until much later in LL with a concurrent thickening of the skin of the forehead, loss of eyebrows and damage to the cartilage of the nose.

The eyes are also attacked with an infiltrative keratitis, iritis and eventually blindness.

14.2 TUBERCULOID LEPROSY

Tuberculoid leprosy (TT) is at the opposite end of the spectrum, showing the full response of cell-mediated immunity to the attacking organism (Fig. 14.2). M. leprae has a predilection for nervous tissue and it is within this nervous tissue that the cell-mediated response takes place, causing early damage to the nerves. The tuberculoid patient therefore tends to present early with signs of weakness or loss of sensation. Palpation of the nerves will often demonstrate a thickening, with loss of sensation or motor power in the distribution of the affected nerve. The ulnar nerve, as it bends over the medial epicondyle at the elbow, or the lateral popliteal nerve, where it curves round the neck of the fibula, are good places to palpate nerves for thickening. Dermal lesions are not raised, often appearing as apparently normal areas of skin, lacking sensation or sweating when the patient exercises. Occasionally, though, they are well defined and scaly, with raised edges, but quite different from the succulent macules and papules of LL. Loss of sensation should be elicited with a pin as well as a light touch. A skin smear in TT is nearly always free of bacilli (paucibacillary), so the diagnosis depends upon the detection of nerve damage. Confirmation can be made by skin or nerve biopsy.

14.3 BORDERLINE LEPROSY

Borderline leprosy, as its name suggests, is on the border between the two extremes of LL and TT. True borderline (BB) is uncommon, with the disease tending to progress to either the lepromatous (BL) or tuberculoid (BT) part of the spectrum. Signs therefore vary between the two extremes with features of each, but predominating in one or the other. Borderline leprosy is common, but its instability leads to reaction and nerve damage, which can often be severe.

14.4 DIAGNOSIS

A *skin smear* is the most important method of diagnosis and is made from every suspected case of leprosy. A negative smear does not mean that a case is not leprosy, as tuberculoid cases rarely have mycobacteria. The method of making a smear is illustrated in Fig. 14.3. The incision should be neither so deep as to enter the subcutaneous layer, which will bleed,

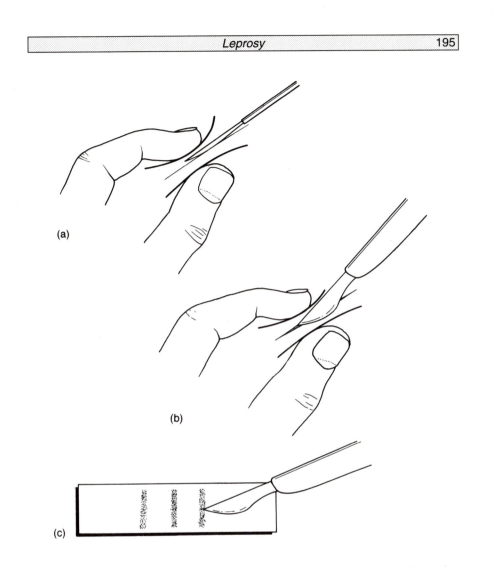

(a)

(b)

(c)

Fig. 14.3. Making a skin smear for leprosy. (a) Pinch up the skin, clean it and then make a shallow cut into the dermis without drawing blood. (b) Turn the knife sideways and scrape dermal tissue from the cut with the point. (c) Spread the dermal tissue on to a microscope slide. Several smears can be made on the same slide.

or so superficial that only the epidermis is cut. (Dermal tissue is white and spongy.) Smears should be protected from sunlight and stained as soon as possible with Ziehl–Neelsen stain. After staining, the slide is examined with a ×100 oil immersion lens. Mycobacteria are red-staining rods and their presence or absence is recorded after examining 100 fields.

Mycobacteria are counted and expressed as the *bacterial index.*

6+	Over 1000 bacilli in an average field
5+	100 to 1000 bacilli in an average field
4+	10 to 100 bacilli in an average field
3+	1 to 10 bacilli in an average field
2+	1 to 10 bacilli in 10 fields
1+	1 to 10 bacilli in 100 fields

After the diagnosis is made and treatment started, further skin smears are made to assess progress. Under treatment mycobacteria gradually break up and show irregular outlines or become beaded. These are dead mycobacteria and are differentiated from solid-staining live bacilli. The proportion of solid-staining to dead bacilli, known as the *morphological index*, gives an indication of the progress of treatment. In a lepromatous case it may fall from 50% to zero in 6 months on dapsone therapy, or only a matter of 5 or 6 weeks with rifampicin. If the morphological index rises, it indicates that the bacilli are resistant or the patient has not been taking treatment. The morphological index is not recommended in control programmes due to difficulties in standardization.

Nasal scrapings are a valuable aid in assessing the infectiousness of a patient. They are not made from the septum, but from the inferior turbinate where it juts into the nasal cavity. Nasal secretions from nose blows are an alternative means of obtaining bacilli. Smears are made and stained in the same way as for skin. Care must be taken to differentiate *M. leprae* from commensal acid-fast bacilli that occasionally inhabit the nose.

Skin biopsy is the only method of confirming a tuberculoid case and is required to classify borderline patients. A small portion of the lesion is excised, down to and including subcutaneous tissue, with a scalpel or biopsy punch under proper aseptic conditions. Care must be taken not to damage the biopsy specimen, which is preserved in 10% formal saline, in formaldehyde, mercuric chloride and acetic acid (FMA) or in the preservative specified by the histologist.

Nerve biopsy is required when there is no skin lesion. A thickened sensory nerve is suitable. A piece no longer than 1 cm is adequate, which is similarly handled with great care (not squeezed by dissecting forceps) and preserved in the same way.

The *lepromin test* is not a diagnostic test but can be useful in classification. It measures the degree of cell-mediated immunity. For the test, 0.1 ml of an autoclaved suspension of tissue infected with *M. leprae* (Mitsuda antigen) is injected intradermally and the response measured in 4 weeks. An erythematous papule larger than 3 mm indicates a positive test. The degree of positivity is further classified.

+	3–5 mm diameter papule
++	6–10 mm diameter papule
+++	Larger than 10 mm papule
U	An ulcerating lesion

The results of the test classify types of leprosy.

Tuberculoid (TT)	+++ or U
Borderline tuberculoid (BT)	++ or +
Borderline or lepromatous (BB, BL or LL)	Negative

A similar reaction, but occurring after only 48 hours, is elicited by the Dharmendra lepromin (commonly used in India). Research is continuing for a more purified protein derivative of *M. leprae*. The other value of the lepromin reaction is in community surveys to assess the susceptibility of the population.

14.5 TREATMENT

Since its introduction in 1941 dapsone has been the main drug for treatment of all types of leprosy. However, the development of dapsone resistance stimulated alternative methods of treatment along similar lines to tuberculosis, with the introduction of multiple drug treatment (MDT). The drugs available are:

- dapsone;
- rifampicin;
- clofazamine;
- ethionamide;
- prothionamide;
- ofloxacin;
- minocycline;
- clarithromycin.

The dose of *Rifampicin* (150 mg capsules) is:

- less than 35 kg body weight – three capsules (450 mg);
- 35 kg or more – four capsules (600 mg).

The type and duration of therapy is determined by the bacterial index of the case.

1. High-risk (multibacillary) LL and BL cases. A three-drug regime consisting of:

- rifampicin 600 mg once a month, supervised;

- dapsone 100 mg daily, self-administered;
- clofazamine 300 mg once a month, supervised, and then 50 mg daily, self-administered.

Treatment should be continued for at least 2 years or until smear negativity.

2. Non-bacillary BT or TT cases:

- rifampicin 600 mg once a month, supervised, plus dapsone 100 mg daily, self-administered, for 6 months.

3. Old cases of LL or BL which have been treated for 5 years or more and still have a bacterial index of 2 or greater, or those cases suspected of dapsone resistance should be treated as in **1.**

4. Multibacillary cases resistant to rifampicin or exhibiting toxic effects:

- clofazamine 50 mg, plus ofloxacin 400 mg, plus minocycline 100 mg daily for 6 months;
- then clofazamine plus either ofloxacin or minocycline in the same dosage for an additional 18 months (clarithromycin can be used instead of ofloxacin or minocycline in the first 6 months).

All patients with positive skin smears at start of treatment should have repeat skin smears at 6, 12, 18 and 24 months. Dapsone resistance has been found to be potentiated by starting therapy with small doses, so full-dose regimes are used. Clofazamine has the advantage of being anti-inflammatory as well as bacteriostatic, so it can be used in reactions at a dose of 100 mg three times a week.

14.6 HOST RESPONSE AND REACTIONS

The response to *M. leprae* by the host decides the type of leprosy that will develop. Where the response is adequate and cell-mediated immunity high, the disease tends towards the tuberculoid end of the spectrum. In contrast, in LL there is a surprising absence of host response. BL and BB cases can move towards the lepromatous end if untreated and to the tuberculoid if treated. Simultaneous human immunodeficiency virus (HIV) infection will shift the host response from the tuberculoid towards the lepromatous.

It is the unstable nature of the *M. leprae* host response that leads to reactions. These have been described as either upgrading (towards the tuberculoid end) or downgrading (towards the lepromatous). These are type 1 reactions. The nearer the case is to the centre of the spectrum the more severe the reaction. They may affect all tissues, skin and nerves or produce a systemic reaction.

A different type of reaction (type 2) is found in lepromatous and borderline lepromatous cases and is associated with massive destruction of bacilli. Immune complexes are formed in the tissues and these lead to an increased reaction in existing lesions. The characteristic finding is erythema nodosum leprosum, which appears on the skin as painful red nodules, commonly on the face and exterior surfaces.

Both types of reaction require admission and bedrest, with protection of vulnerable structures. Clofazamine, steroids and thalidomide are useful in the treatment of reactions.

14.7 EPIDEMIOLOGY

Leprosy can occur in an epidemic as well as an endemic pattern, but due to the incredibly protracted life history of the disease, the epidemic form is rarely seen. Between 1921 and 1925 there was an epidemic on the island of Nauru, 30% of the population were infected and the disease was notably non-focal. Most people developed tuberculoid (BT–TT) leprosy which healed spontaneously. All ages were susceptible and contact with lepromatous patients did not potentiate spread. The findings from this rare natural event are supported by lepromin studies, where the majority of the population are found to be naturally positive although they have seemingly not come into contact with the disease. Even in areas of high endemicity a very small proportion of lepromin-positive individuals will develop leprosy and then of the tuberculoid type, whereas a much higher proportion of lepromin-negative individuals will develop the disease and it will be the lepromatous end of the spectrum. It has been estimated that as much as 5% of the population are susceptible to LL and contact with a lepromatous case increases the risk of infection. Children and young adults are more commonly affected, but the children of leprosy patients do not develop LL any more frequently than the general population. It would seem that leprosy is very similar to tuberculosis in that the organism is more common than realized and asymptomatic or subclinical infections occur, but it is only those people who are susceptible that develop the disease.

LL is more common in Asia and TT in Africa. This differing susceptibility might help to explain the response to bacillus Calmette-Guérin (BCG) in these two peoples. BCG given at birth can produce a hypersensitivity and change the lepromin reaction from negative to positive, but some people are inherently lepromin-negative and remain always susceptible to the lepromatous form of the disease. BCG protected over 80% of schoolchildren in Uganda, but only 40% of children under 5 in Myanmar.

There is only one form of *M. leprae* and organisms cultured from all the different types of leprosy react in exactly the same way, showing that the kind of leprosy is determined by the host response. The route of transmission is still uncertain, but much evidence suggests that nasal discharges are the most likely. Certainly lepromatous patients are more infectious than any others, but, despite the large number of bacilli in the skin, none are shed this way. There are, however, considerable numbers in the nasal mucosa and these may be disseminated in an aerosol by the respiratory route. M. leprae has been found to survive from 2 to 7 days outside the body in nasal secretions. Tuberculosis and leprosy may have more in common than being conveniently combined together in joint control programmes.

If M. leprae is discharged through nasal secretions, what is the portal of entry? In epidemic leprosy and the case that occurs by transient contact, the organisms are abundant and easily absorbed. Since they are mainly disseminated by the respiratory system, could this not also be the most likely route to enter the body? The observation that lesions are found more commonly on exposed parts of the body suggests that they might enter the skin directly or, once inside, gravitate to these more traumatized areas of the body. A more general observation is that leprosy has declined spontaneously in Europe and North America with increasing standards of hygiene (similar to tuberculosis), but persists in areas of the USA where standards have not improved. Nasal secretions, poor personal hygiene and close contact appear to be the most important links in a chain of transmission that has still not been adequately explained. Perhaps leprosy has been correctly placed here, next to the group of respiratory diseases.

14.8 CONTROL

The control of leprosy can be considered in three phases: the immediate, the intermediate and the long-term. The immediate method is a reduction of the leprosy reservoir by case finding and contact follow-up. Case finding is the identification and treatment of all cases of leprosy, especially those with the lepromatous form of the disease. A small proportion of cases will present themselves, but an active search must be made by all health workers for others. This can be done systematically from village to village or in selective groups. A particularly important group are schoolchildren, as they are likely to contain a quarter of all cases and a higher proportion of new ones. Once cases are found, they must be treated adequately, preferably by MDT to reduce the time of infectivity and follow-up.

Contact tracing is undertaken, as leprosy is more common in those people that have prolonged contact with a leprosy case. The names of contacts are taken, and they are examined at frequent intervals.

BCG immunization is used for the intermediate control of leprosy. It appears to induce hypersensitivity and increased resistance to developing leprosy in some ethnic groups. BCG immunization is given at birth or soon after, as explained under tuberculosis (Section 13.8). Vaccines based on *M. leprae* are under trial in several countries, with promising results. The long-term reduction of disease will require an improvement in general hygiene, better housing and less overcrowding.

Part of any leprosy programme is the development of a *rehabilitation service*. This not only encourages leprosy patients to present themselves for treatment, but helps to return them as participating members of the community. Much can be done from limited resources, such as making sandals out of old tyres and pieces of wood. The elements of rehabilitation are to protect anaesthetic limbs, actively treat sores and ulcers and provide support (including surgery) to restore function. The eyes are also damaged in leprosy and supportive treatment can do much to prevent blindness from developing.

Organization of leprosy control is often managed as a combined programme with tuberculosis, and Section 13.8.2 on follow-up and registration is equally applicable to both.

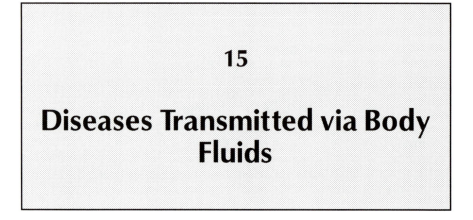

15

Diseases Transmitted via Body Fluids

This category includes infections transmitted from one human to another by the physiological fluids of the body: blood, serum, saliva, seminal fluid, etc. Transmission is normally direct, but indirect transmission, via fomites or flies, can occur in some cases. It includes the treponematoses, both the sexually and the non-sexually transmitted. Sexual transmission accounts for the largest number of persons affected by these diseases.

These are the diseases of close personal contact, thriving either in conditions of poor hygiene or in the most intimate contact of all, sexual intercourse. They are therefore social diseases, determined by the habits and attitude of people, and it is only by effecting change in these values that any permanent improvement will occur.

15.1 YAWS

Yaws is a non-venereal treponemal disease affecting both the skin and bone. It is restricted to the moist tropical areas of the world in a band that passes through the Caribbean, South America, Africa, South-East Asia and the Pacific islands (Fig. 15.1).

The disease commences as a primary papule after an *incubation period* of 2–8 weeks. The initial lesion starts to heal, but after a period varying from a few weeks to several months it is followed by generalized lesions, multiple rounded papules scattered all over the body. These lesions exude serum which is highly infectious. There is also a mild periostitis in focal bony sites but these and the skin lesions normally heal with little residual damage. It is the tertiary stage, which appears after an asymptomatic period and some 5 years after initial infection, that results

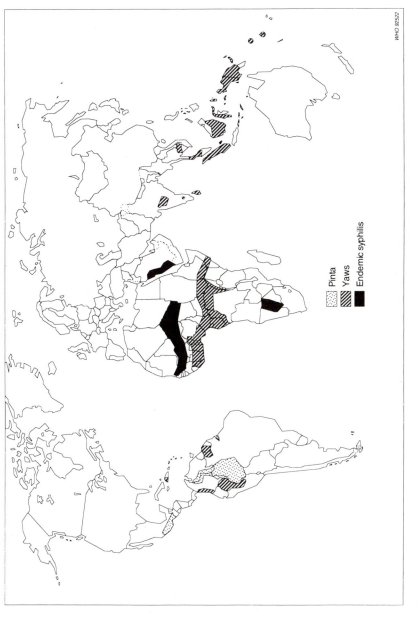

Pinta

Yaws

Endemic syphilis

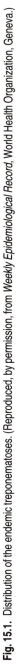

Fig. 15.1. Distribution of the endemic treponematoses. (Reproduced, by permission, from *Weekly Epidemiological Record*, World Health Organization, Geneva.)

WHO 92522

in gross damage to skin and bone, leading to hideous deformities. The opposite ends of the body are affected with destructive lesions of the nasal bones (gangoza) and scarring and deformity (sabre tibia) of the lower limbs.

The infection is *diagnosed* by finding *Treponema pertenue* in the exudates of lesions. In the motile state it can be seen by dark-ground microscopy or stained by Giemsa or silver salts. The serological tests for syphilis (see below) are positive.

Treatment is with procaine penicillin in 2% aluminium monostearate in oil (PAM) in a dose of 2,400,000 units for an adult. Response is very satisfactory and lesions heal within 2–3 weeks.

Yaws is a disease of poor hygiene, with close bodily contact being the manner in which infection commonly takes place. Flies may be involved in transmission from clothing and dressings that have become contaminated by fluid from sores. The spirochaete cannot penetrate broken skin but requires a minor skin abrasion or cut by which to enter. Yaws is predominantly an infection of children, with the mother becoming infected if she did not acquire her infection in childhood. The large overcrowded family with a poor standard of hygiene is the characteristic environment in which yaws so readily spreads. The need to stay indoors and keep close together for warmth in the rainy season might be the reason why the disease is more common at this time of year.

Yaws, with its rapid response to a single injection of procaine penicillin has been the subject of successful mass treatment campaigns in the endemic parts of the world. Treatment in a mass campaign is given to the following.

- All those with clinical signs of yaws.
- Household, school and other close contacts.
- Any person suspected of incubating the disease.

The campaign is preceded by health education encouraging all people to come forward with any suspicious lesions. Each village is visited in turn, everyone examined and treatment given to cases, contacts or suspects. A follow-up surveillance service treats missed cases or new infections. This can readily be done by an effective rural health service.

The success of the World Health Organization (WHO) mass campaigns against yaws resulted in the virtual disappearance of the disease from many areas, but unfortunately there is now a resurgence. Newly trained health personnel are unaware of the disease and penicillin has been replaced by other antibiotics in the treatment of common infections.

15.2 PINTA

A non-venereal treponematosis, pinta is restricted to Central America (Fig. 15.1). The disease has many similarities to yaws, commencing as a primary lesion after an *incubation period* of 1–3 weeks. Secondary lesions are flat and erythematous but cover large areas of the body. Tertiary lesions result in pigmentary changes, with – often large – patches of leucoderma. Only the skin is involved in pinta.

Diagnosis is made on clinical grounds, with supporting evidence from positive serological tests for syphilis. *Treatment* is with penicillin, as for yaws.

The organism, *Treponema carateum*, can be found in the serous exudates from lesions. Direct contact or carriage by flies has been suggested as the means of transmission. The disease occurs in moist tropical areas in communities with poor hygiene. Mass treatment and control are the same as for yaws (see above).

15.3 ENDEMIC NON-VENEREAL SYPHILIS

The non-venereal form of syphilis is found in localized foci in Africa and the Arabian peninsula (Fig. 15.1). It resembles venereal syphilis in many of its features, except that it is not spread venereally. The primary lesion is commonly found at the angle of the mouth and appears as a raised mucous plaque. A more florid skin infection follows, with tertiary signs in the bones and cardiovascular system.

Diagnosis is made on clinical grounds in endemic areas with the assistance of serological tests. *Treatment* is with penicillin in the same manner as yaws.

Because of the site of the primary lesion on the mouth, transmission by shared drinking vessels is considered a possibility. It is a disease of low personal hygiene where crowding together and contact with lesions readily occurs. The organism appears to be identical to the *Treponema pallidum* of venereal syphilis, with which cross-immunity is shared. With people living in conditions of low hygiene and poor education, to eradicate the disease by mass treatment generally means a replacement by the more serious and devastating venereal syphilis. Improving the general standard of hygiene might be a preferable control strategy in such situations.

15.4 VENEREAL SYPHILIS

The venereal diseases are totally cosmopolitan, taking no account of climate, ethnic group or social class: wherever sexual contact occurs, the venereal diseases can occur also.

Because of the identical nature of the *Treponema pallidum* of endemic syphilis and venereal syphilis, it has been considered by some authorities that venereal syphilis developed from this more benign form. Once a venereal method of transmission had evolved, the disease was able to extend its boundaries from the Tropics to the Arctic. Fortunately, syphilis has not seen the same rapid increase as other venereal diseases in recent years, but it is estimated that there are some 50 million cases in the world today, with a very large proportion of these in the Tropics.

The primary lesion of syphilis is the chancre developing after an *incubation period* of 9–90 days (usually 3–4 weeks). This lesion is normally found on the genitalia of males and females, but can occur in the mouth, on the breast or in the anorectal region. The primary lesion heals spontaneously after a few weeks, but 6 weeks to 6 months later the signs of secondary syphilis appear. These may take several forms, but the commonest are a cutaneous maculopapular rash and mucocutaneous condylomata around the genitalia and anus. As the infection is systemic, a generalized lymphadenopathy and splenomegaly can occur, often accompanied by fever. Following the period of secondary syphilis, there is a latent phase, after which the destructive cardiovascular and central nervous symptoms occur, often many years later. Should a woman be pregnant while she has syphilis, her fetus may be seriously affected. If she is pregnant during early syphilis, the child is likely to be stillborn, while the later stages of the disease are more likely to produce a live-born child suffering from congenital defects.

Diagnosis is confirmed by finding *T. pallidum* in the serous exudate from a chancre or by gland puncture. This can be examined by dark-ground microscopy or immunofluorescent staining. Serological tests can assist in the diagnosis or be used in epidemiological studies. The rapid plasma reagin (RPR) is a sensitive test, while specific tests such as treponemal immobilization (TPI) or the fluorescent treponemal antibody (FTA) test are more difficult and expensive to perform. Cross-reaction between the *Treponema* of yaws, pinta and endemic syphilis negate the differential diagnosis of these diseases. All patients with syphilis should be encouraged to have a human immunodeficiency virus (HIV) test, because of the high frequency of dual infection.

Treatment is with penicillin: for primary and secondary syphilis, either benzathine benzylpenicillin 2.4 million units as a single dose (but often given intramuscularly at two different sites) or procaine benzylpe-nicillin 1.2 million units daily intramuscularly for 10 days. Tetracycline can be used in the non-pregnant and erythromycin in the pregnant patient allergic to penicillin.

Syphilis is transmitted by direct contact from an infectious lesion or body fluids and secretions (saliva, semen, blood, vaginal discharges). The spirochaete can pass through the unbroken skin, although it more commonly penetrates the mucous membrane. Kissing as well as sexual intercourse can transmit the spirochaete.

Syphilis is predominantly a disease of urban areas and in conditions of sexual imbalance, such as mines, military establishments and among seamen. With the rapid urbanization that has occurred in the developing world and large movements of migrant labour, syphilis has been on the increase in the Tropics. When the migrant workers return to their homes and families, they bring venereal disease back with them. The main reservoir of infection is generally in commercial sex workers or deserted women forced into prostitution to support their children. Due to the prolonged incubation period, the hidden site of the primary lesion within the vagina and the latent period of the disease, syphilis is either not suspected or purposely hidden. A large number of contacting males can be infected by a single female.

Contact tracing, so widely practised but only moderately successful in developed countries, is largely an impossible task in developing countries. In restricted communities, such as mines or plantations, it can be used with considerable value, but in the vast, sprawling urban slums, where people come and go and addresses are not known, it is a hopeless task. The prohibition of commercial sex workers only drives the practice underground, and it is generally not acceptable in developing countries as they are a recognized segment of society in many cultures. A preferable answer is to try and examine known commercial sex workers at regular intervals and encourage them to bring in others for check-ups. A commercial sex worker aware of the damage that can be caused by the disease, once converted, can be a greater proponent of health education than any trained worker.

Antenatal and family planning clinics provide an important opportunity to examine a large number of women and also prevent cases of congenital syphilis. Routine RPRs should be performed and all positive cases fully investigated and treated.

15.5 GONORRHOEA

The number of cases of gonorrhoea in the world today is estimated to be some 200 million, making it one of commonest communicable diseases. There has been a rapid increase of the infection in all parts of the world.

Gonorrhoea is a bacterial disease caused by *Neisseria gonorrhoeae* (the gonococcus). In the male it commences as a mucoid urethral discharge after an *incubation period* of 2–7 days (average 3), which soon changes to a profuse, purulent secretion (as opposed to non-gonococcal urethritis where it is scanty, white, mucoid or serous). The discharge is best seen first thing in the morning (dewdrop) and a smear should be made from this before the patient urinates. The main symptom is pain on micturition, but the degree of discomfort is very variable.

In the female, the infection generally passes unnoticed, but may present with urethritis or acute salpingitis. It is this latter presentation of the disease that can lead, in an acute or chronic form, to sterility in the female. This is a serious problem in the unmarried woman and a cause of divorce in the married. In the male, untreated or improperly treated infection can result in urethral stricture, while generalized symptoms of arthritis, dermatitis or meningitis can rarely occur in either sex. In the pregnant woman there is a danger of the newborn infant developing gonococcal conjunctivitis at the time of delivery. The discovery of this infection in the newborn infant may be the manner in which the infection is found in the woman.

Diagnosis is ideally made by finding the intracellular diplococci in urethral or high vaginal smears. Smears are easily made at any level of health institution and should always be taken if microscopy services are available. If intracellular diplococci (ICD) are found the patient is treated for gonorrhoea and chlamydial infection, if no ICD but more than five polymorphonuclear leucocytes (PMN) per oil-immersion field the patient is treated just for *Chlamydia* and if less than five PMN per field no treatment is given. If microscopy services are not available, all confirmed urethral or cervical discharges should be treated for gonorrhoea and chlamydial infection. Where facilities permit, the discharge should be cultured, but as the organism is very sensitive it must be inoculated on to a culture plate or placed in transport medium (less satisfactory) as soon as possible.

Treatment, which used to be a simple matter with penicillin, is now fraught with problems of resistance not only to this antibiotic, but to many others that have subsequently been tried. Any recommended treatment regime may be ineffective in certain parts of the world and local expertise must be consulted to develop routines that are compatible with the resistance patterns and available resources. Recommended regimens are:

- cetriaxone 250 mg by single intramuscular injection, or
- ciprofloxacin 500 mg as a single oral dose (but not in pregnant women or children), or
- spectinomycin 2 g by single intramuscular injection.

Where gonococci remain fully sensitive, the following regimens are cheaper and more available:

- procaine benzylpenicillin 4.8 million units intramuscularly, plus probenecid 1 g orally as a single dose, or
- amoxicillin 3 g orally, plus probenecid 1 g orally as a single dose, or
- tetracycline 500 mg four times daily for 7 days, or
- doxycycline 100 mg orally, twice daily for 7 days.

N. gonorrhoeae is unable to penetrate stratified epithelium but has a predilection for mucous membranes. Here it produces an accumulation of PMN and outpouring of serum to give the characteristic discharge. Transmission is by sexual contact.

The epidemiologically important features are as follows.

- The short incubation period.
- The often asymptomatic disease in women.
- Promiscuous sexual intercourse.
- Urbanization and changing social values.
- Use of contraceptives.
- Inadequate treatment.

The combination of a short incubation period and promiscuous sexual activity means that a large number of people can become infected in rapid succession. Since women are often largely unaware of their infection, they provide a continuous reservoir of the disease. Urbanization changes the social balance that occurs in the village, traditional values and taboos are lost and promiscuity develops. Contraceptives allow increased opportunity for sexual intercourse, although the condom provides limited protection. The contraceptive pill, by reducing the acidity of genital secretions, removes some of the natural defences, while the intrauterine contraceptive device encourages mechanical spread to the uterus and tubes. Improper treatment by both doctors and quacks, usually with grossly inadequate doses of antibiotics, has led to chronic infections and the development of resistant organisms.

The continuing increase of gonorrhoea demonstrates the inability of control measures, even in developed countries. Under-reporting, illegal treatment and the protection of contacts make any standard methods of case treatment and contact tracing quite inadequate. Gonorrhoea is not so much found as a reservoir in commercial sex workers as more widely distributed among the promiscuous under-25s. Where possible, cases presenting at sexually transmitted disease (STD) clinics should be encouraged to bring their partners or provide information so that they can be traced, to give them counselling and treatment. Alternatively, contact cards can be sent anonymously to all contacts of a case, recommending them to present at a clinic. Condoms can be given out at the same time as a person presents at a clinic. Health education concentrating on the dangers of STD is the main preventive action (see below).

15.6 NON-GONOCOCCAL URETHRITIS (NGU)

A low-grade urethritis with mucoid rather than purulent discharge in the male, in which intracellular diplococci are not found in the smear, suggests non-gonococcal urethritis (NGU). In areas where gonococcal urethritis is common, the prevalence of NGU is also high, so treatment should be given for both conditions.

A number of organisms have been found to be responsible, including *Chlamydia trachomatis*, *Trichomonas vaginalis*, *Mycoplasma hominis*, *Candida albicans* and non-*Neisseria* bacteria, but, even so, no organism is discovered in over half of the cases.

Infection is generally transient or asymptomatic in the female, in whom a reservoir of infection can occur if simultaneous treatment to the sexual partner is not given. Incubation period is 1–2 weeks.

Where possible, diagnosis should be made by smear and culture, with specific treatment for the organism if one is found. In the majority of cases, no organism will be elicited and *Chlamydia* is the most likely cause. Treatment is with tetracycline 500 mg four times daily for 7 days or doxycycline 100 mg daily for 7 days (erythromycin can be used where tetracyclines are contraindicated). Sexual intercourse must be avoided until both partners are free of signs. The epidemiology and control of gonorrhoea are applicable to NGU.

15.7 LYMPHOGRANULOMA VENEREUM (CHLAMYDIAL LYMPHOGRANULOMA)

Lymphogranuloma venereum is a chronic infection caused by *Chlamydia trachomatis*. The primary lesion is a small painless papule, vesicle or ulcer, which is often not noticed, lymphadenitis being the presenting sign. The lymph nodes become grossly enlarged and generally suppurate. Fistulas and fibrosis occur, especially in the rectal area, if treatment is delayed. Differential diagnosis is from bubonic plague, tuberculosis and other causes of lymphadenitis. The Frei test can be of assistance. Treatment is with tetracycline 500 mg four times daily for 14 days, or doxycycline 100 mg daily for 14 days.

Although sexual intercourse is considered the main means of transmission, extragenital lesions suggest that other means can also occur. Control methods are discussed in Section 15.11.

15.8 GRANULOMA INGUINALE

A chronic, progressive, ulcerating disease of the anogenital area, granuloma inguinale is caused by an encapsulated bacillus, *Calymmatobacterium granulomatis*. An initial lesion on the genitalia becomes eroded and ulcerates with new nodules forming at the margins as the lesion extends. Ulceration can continue to produce extensive destruction. Carcinoma of the vulva has been reported to be associated with granuloma inguinale.

Diagnosis is made from smears or scrapings of the lesions, in which are found the characteristic intracellular organisms. *Treatment* is with trimethoprim (80 mg)/sulphamthozole (400 mg) two tablets twice daily for 14 days, or doxycycline 100 mg daily for 14 days, or tetracycline 500 mg four times daily for 14 days plus streptomycin 1 g intramuscularly daily for 14 days.

The disease is transmitted by sexual intercourse although other methods have also been suspected. It is frequently associated with anal intercourse.

Control is the same as with other STD.

15.9 CHANCROID

Chancroid is an acute venereal infection characterized by a soft chancre on the external genitalia and regional lymphadenopathy. The organism is *Haemophilus ducreyi*, which can be identified with Giemsa or Wright's stain. The lesion has an indurated base of the chancre, which differentiates it from syphilis. Chancroid can be treated with one of the following regimes:

- ceftriaxone 250 mg intramuscularly as a single dose, or
- erythromycin 500 mg orally three times daily for 7 days, or
- trimethoprim (80 mg)/sulphamethoxazole (400 mg) two tablets twice daily for 7 days.

The epidemiology and control are similar to those for syphilis.

15.10 HUMAN IMMUNODEFICIENCY VIRUS (HIV) INFECTION

HIV infection leads to a disruption of the helper T4 cell-mediated immune mechanisms, resulting in an increased susceptibility to opportunistic infections. This breakdown of the body's defence system and the range of symptoms produced is called acquired immune deficiency syndrome (AIDS). Presentation is generally by the symptoms of the opportunistic infection so can be many and varied.

15.10.1 Evolution of a New Disease

In June 1981 the Centres for Disease Control (CDC) in the USA reported five cases of *Pneumocystis carinii* pneumonia. In the following month 15 more cases of this normally rare disease were reported, as well as 26 cases of Kaposi's sarcoma, an unusual tumour. The common feature was that all these cases were in homosexual men. On more detailed enquiry, the

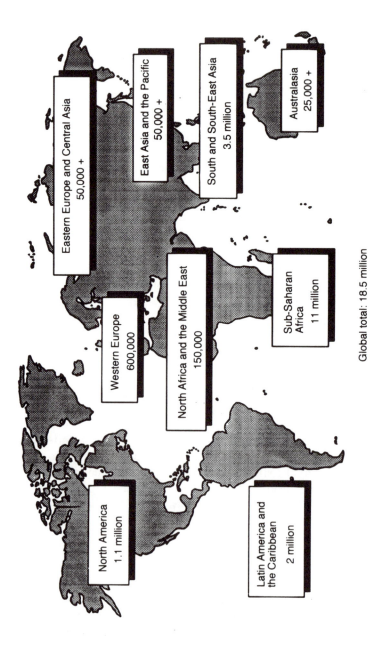

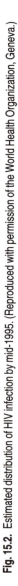

Fig. 15.2. Estimated distribution of HIV infection by mid-1995. (Reproduced with permission of the World Health Organization, Geneva.)

first cases could be traced back to 1978.

By the end of 1981 AIDS was being reported from countries in Europe. In Belgium and France an AIDS-like illness was also noted among people originating from Africa. These observations led to investigations in Rwanda and Zaire, where many AIDS patients were found. At the same time, an aggressive form of Kaposi's sarcoma was reported from Zambia and a new disease, called slim disease, described in Uganda. These were found to be manifestations of AIDS.

HIV infection has now spread to most parts of the world, but is particularly prevalent in Africa, the Americas and Europe. There are foci in South and South-East Asia from which the infection is spreading. Australia and New Zealand show a North American pattern of infection, while the disease is now being reported from Pacific islands (Fig. 15.2).

WHO estimates a prevalence rate of one in 40 for Africa, Central and East Africa having rates of over 20% in the adult population of some large cities. Parts of Latin America and some Caribbean islands have very high incidence rates. Prostitution and injecting drug use are responsible for very high rates in parts of Thailand and India, from which spread is being encouraged through illegal networks.

15.10.2 Organism

HIV is a lentivirus, a subgroup of the retroviruses, of which at least two types have been described. HIV-I is common in the Americas, Europe and Central and East Africa, whereas HIV-II is found in West Africa or in people that acquired their infection there. HIV-II is now spreading from its origin to other countries, such as Mozambique. It is thought that there is a whole family of the HIV viruses.

Serological tests are available to detect infection and the type of virus, but they do not become positive until 3 months after the person became infected. It is therefore possible for a person to transmit infection before he/she is shown to be positive.

15.10.3 Clinical Features

The HIV-positive individual may show no clinical signs of the disease when first diagnosed, and then progress to a generalized lymphadenopathy, weight loss, recurrent upper-respiratory-tract infection and minor mucocutaneous manifestations, such as seborrhoeic dermatitis, prurigo or oropharyngeal ulceration. Chronic diarrhoea for more than a month and prolonged fever (intermittent or constant) for over a month indicate that the person is entering the third clinical stage, when he/she is likely to require hospital treatment or be confined to bed for much of the time.

The final stage will depend on the opportunistic infections that the immunocompromised patient falls prey to, so the clinical signs are variable. The opportunistic infections in increasing order of seriousness are as follows.

- Oral candidiasis.
- Oral hairy leucoplakia.
- Pulmonary tuberculosis.
- Severe bacterial infections such as pneumonia or pyomyositis.
- Vulvovaginal candidiasis (chronic or not responding to treatment).
- *Pneumocystis carinii* pneumonia.
- Toxoplasmosis of the brain.
- Cryptosporidiosis with diarrhoea.
- Isosporiasis with diarrhoea.
- Cryptococcosis, extrapulmonary.
- Cytomegalovirus of an organ other than liver, spleen or lymph nodes.
- Herpes simplex, visceral or non-resolving mucocutaneous.
- Progressive multifocal leucoencephalopathy.
- Disseminated mycosis such as histoplasmosis or coccidioidomycosis.
- Candidiasis of the oesophagus, trachea, bronchi or lung.
- Atypical disseminated mycobacteriosis.
- Non-typhoid *Salmonella* septicaemia.
- Extrapulmonary tuberculosis.
- Lymphoma.
- Kaposi's sarcoma.
- HIV encephalopathy.

15.10.4 Epidemiology

The *incubation period* to full-blown AIDS has not been fully established, but from studies on people who were given infected blood it ranges from 12 months up to 8 years, but could be as long as 18 years. In perinatal infection the incubation period is often shorter than 12 months.

The routes of transmission are as follows.

- Sexual contact with an infected person.
- Inoculation with infected blood or blood products (including non-sterile needles and syringes).
- From an infected mother to her child before, during or shortly after birth.
- From tissue transplants (rare).

Sexual contact is the commonest method of transmission, with both heterosexual and homosexual practice. The important epidemiological factor is number of sexual contacts, so that prostitutes or promiscuous homosexuals with hundreds, if not thousands, of new contacts annually are at greatest risk. However, one contact with an infected person is able to produce infection. Anal intercourse carries a higher risk of infection than vaginal. There is no evidence of increased risk during menstruation. There is an association with other STD, particularly genital ulcers. Other STDs may potentiate infection.

Blood transfusion of infected blood will virtually always transmit AIDS. Pooled blood, such as for producing factor VIII for the treatment of haemophilia, is particularly dangerous, because it contains donations from many people, any of which could be infected. Syringes and needles, if they are not properly cleaned and sterilized, can contain small quantities of blood sufficient to transmit infection. This method may be responsible for many infections in developing countries and is an important way of transmitting infection among drug abusers. Transmission by needle-stick injury can occur among health workers, but is uncommon.

The infected mother can pass on infection to her child. Infection can be transmitted congenitally, but it is more likely to occur from a mixing of the mother's and infant's blood at the time of delivery. HIV is found in breast milk and infants can be infected via this route.

Any process which puts stress on the immune mechanism will accelerate progression to AIDS. The seropositive woman who becomes pregnant or suffers repeat infections, such as diarrhoea, may have accelerated symptoms of disease.

Tuberculosis and leprosy are affected by the disruption of the immune process. Any person with tuberculosis who develops AIDS is likely to have a more florid disease, while tuberculoid leprosy cases can convert to lepromatous. There is an increase in both tuberculosis and leprosy, as these infections can easily attack the immunocompromised seropositive person.

15.10.5 Control

Methods of control and prevention are aimed at the three routes of transmission, sexual, blood and perinatal. Vaccines are under trial, but it is likely to be many years before an effective vaccine has been developed, so until that time other control measures are required.

To prevent *sexual* spread:

- limit the number of sexual partners, encouraging monogamous relationships;
- avoid sexual contact with persons at high risk, such as commercial sex workers, bisexuals and homosexuals;
- discourage the practice of anal intercourse;

- encourage condom use (certain spermicides can inhibit HIV);
- provide adequate facilities for the detection and treatment of STD.

To prevent *blood* spread:

- screen all blood for transfusions;
- test donors before they give blood;
- only use blood transfusions when essential;
- discontinue paid blood donors;
- use disposable syringes, needles, giving sets, lancets, etc. or ensure they are properly sterilized.
- injecting drug users should be discouraged from sharing equipment, e.g. by instituting needle-exchange schemes;
- medical workers should wear gloves when dealing with possible infected blood, e.g. at delivery and in the laboratory.

To prevent *perinatal* spread:

- advise infected women about the possible risk to their infant and themselves if they become pregnant;
- good obstetric practice, especially reducing trauma and only cutting the cord when it has stopped pulsating.

Caesarean section should not be encouraged in developing countries as the risk to the mother in subsequent pregnancies is considerably increased. Breast-feeding should not be discouraged as the chance of the infant dying from diarrhoea or malnutrition is far greater than that of dying from AIDS. WHO recommend that no change should be made in the vaccination programme to mothers and children, even though they may be infected with AIDS, except in the child with clinical AIDS, who should not be given bacillus Calmette–Guérin (BCG).

AIDS is *not* spread by:

- mosquitoes;
- casual contact, such as shaking hands, or lavatory seats;
- food, water or the respiratory route.

Control programmes

The main method of control is health education. This can be to the general public to supply them with the correct information, or to specific groups. The most cost-effective health education will be to high-risk groups, such as commercial sex workers, homosexuals, single workers, etc.; however, they are difficult to motivate and it is probably better to concentrate effort on schoolchildren. A combination of sex education as part of the school curriculum, followed by specific instruction on STD is preferable. There needs to be improved diagnosis and treatment facilities for STDs, providing early and adequate treatment. Condoms can be dispensed at STD clinics.

15.11 EPIDEMIOLOGY AND CONTROL OF SEXUALLY TRANSMITTED DISEASES

There has been an astronomical increase in STD over the past four decades. The relative importance of these diseases has also changed and new STDs are appearing. Some of the reasons for these changes are as follows.

- Increasing world population, especially of younger age–groups.
- Urbanization and migrant labour.
- Increasing travel and mixing of populations.
- Alteration of social values and increasing promiscuity.
- Development of contraceptive practice.
- Inadequate treatment and development of resistant organisms.
- Ignorance of STD.

International travel has allowed a mixing of cultural groups that would otherwise have remained isolated, potentiating the spread of different types and strains of STD. The development of resistant strains has posed a problem of imported cases to the developed world, but has left the developing world with an intolerable situation, which they are economically unable to deal with.

STD are more prevalent in young people, and yet with an increasing world population it is predominantly these younger age–groups that are expanding at a more rapid rate than others. This increase in the youth of the world has thrown a greater strain on the education services, so that health education, especially regarding STD, is neglected.

Perhaps STD can be described as the greatest pandemic affecting the world at this time. What has occurred is a revolutionary change in social structure, where traditional values and the monogamous married couple are no longer regarded as the norm. However, the risk of developing STD is more recognized, rather than the shock that previously led to concealment or recourse to treatment from a medical quack. Neither should contraceptive practice be discouraged, for it is the problem of the rapidly expanding young population that is a major contributory factor. The key is health education with a combined approach of contraceptive advice and STD information. If this is to succeed, there must be a considerable increase in treatment facilities, especially in urban areas. Standard regimes should be decided by specialists and administered by primary health-care workers. Improved treatment facilities, training of health workers and more effective drugs will not only reduce the prevalence and seriousness of STDs, but also of HIV infection.

15.12 HEPATITIS B (HBV)

Hepatitis B (HBV) is a more severe disease than hepatitis A and quite distinct in its epidemiology and means of spread. With a much longer *incubation period* of 2 weeks to 6 months (usually 9–12 weeks), symptoms of jaundice are more persistent and liver damage common. HBV infection can become a chronic active disease or develop into frank cirrhosis. Hepatoma is associated with HBV injection.

Diagnosis can be made by finding the surface antigens (HBsAg). There are four subtypes, adw, ayw, adr and ayr, which vary in their geographical distribution, providing useful epidemiological markers. A further antigen e (HBeAg) is a marker of increased infectivity, as well as indicating active viral replication in hepatocytes (which may result in liver damage).

Transmission can occur from blood, serum, saliva and seminal fluid. It is a hazard of blood transfusions, renal dialysis, injections and tattooing. It can be transmitted by sexual intercourse and during delivery. The virus has been found in some bloodsucking insects (e.g. bedbugs), but transmission by this means has not been shown. As mentioned above, certain people are more infectious than others and this period of time can be considerable. The carrier state has been estimated to be present in over 176 million people with varying rates in different parts of the world: Western Europe 1%, USA 6–8%, and Africa, Asia and Western Pacific 10–25%. Infection is thought to occur commonly at birth in the more endemic areas.

The risk of an infant becoming infected from a carrier mother can be 50–60% in some ethnic groups. There is a greater likelihood of the mother passing on the infection if she has acute HBV in the second or third trimester or up to 2 months after delivery. A high titre of HBeAg or a history of transmission to previous children increases the risk of a mother infecting her infant. The carrier state is more common in males and in those that acquired their infection in childhood.

There is no specific treatment and corticosteroids are contraindicated. Interferon has a place in the treatment of chronic hepatitis.

HBV vaccine can be given to those at risk and as part of the EPI (Expanded Programme of Immunization) in countries with a high carrier rate. There is convincing evidence that reduction of carriers can prevent hepatoma.

Preventive methods are strict aseptic precautions in giving blood transfusions and injections and in the handling of blood. All blood donors should be screened, contributions to pooled blood being particularly dangerous. The control of STD has been covered above. Homosexual practice is particularly liable to lead to HBV infection. Persons at risk should be vaccinated.

Another hepatitis virus, *delta hepatitis* (HDV), is associated with a coexistent HBV infection. It may co-infect or be superimposed on the HBV carrier state. Fulminant hepatitis can result from superinfection. Transmission, control and prevention are the same as for HBV.

15.13 HEPATITIS C (HCV)

Similar in many respects to HBV, HCV produces a milder disease, but as many as 30–50% will progress to chronic liver damage in later life. It has been found to occur in many parts of the world.

The main method of transmission is by blood rather than the sexual route or during delivery. It is, however, less transmissible than HBV. The epidemiology and control of HCV are similar to those for HBV.

15.14 LASSA FEVER

A highly infectious disease with an appalling mortality in epidemic form, Lassa fever first appeared in Lassa in Nigeria in 1969. Since then, there have been outbreaks in Liberia and Sierra Leone affecting all age-groups. The disease appears to be endemic in West Africa.

The reservoir is *Mastomys natalensis*, the multimammate or grey rat, but human-to-human transmission results in the more serious disease. Initial infection from rodents is by contamination of food or dust with animal urine. This is probably the method of spread in the endemic area. Once a person is infected, the organism is found in his/her blood, urine, pharyngeal secretions and the aerosol produced by a coughing bout. Any of these routes can very easily infect other people.

The *incubation period* is 5–15 days, followed by an insidious onset of malaise, fever, headache, sore throat, cough, diarrhoea and body pains. By the second week, there is lymphadenopathy, pharyngitis and a maculo-papular rash on the face or body. In severe cases, pleural effusion, encephalopathy, cardiac and renal failure can develop, with a mortality of 30–50%.

Diagnosis is made by isolating the virus from blood, urine or throat washings, using extreme care. Complement fixation or immunofluor-escent tests are also available. *Treatment* is with ribavirin (Virazole).

Control is by the following.

- Rigorous isolation of the patient by the most secure means possible.
- Careful sterilization of syringes, needles and all reused equipment (5% chlorous antiseptic can be used).
- Extreme precautions with any oral secretions, blood, faeces and urine. Blood must be handled with the utmost caution, using, as a minimum, holeless rubber gloves. Faeces and urine should be placed

in plastic bags, which are boiled or burnt.
- Terminal disinfection, with formaldehyde fumigation of all articles used by the patient.
- All case contacts should be quarantined for 3 weeks and isolated if they show any signs of fever.

15.15 EBOLA HAEMORRHAGIC FEVER

This is an acute haemorrhagic illness of viral origin and high fatality. Illness presents with sudden onset of fever, headache, muscle pains, sore throat and profound weakness. This progresses to vomiting, diarrhoea and signs of internal and external bleeding, with generally liver and kidney damage.

The *incubation period* is 2–12 days. Confirmatory diagnosis can only be done in special laboratories and all specimens should be handled with extreme caution. There is no specific therapy.

Outbreaks have occurred in Zaire and Sudan. Monkeys have been found infected and a rodent reservoir is suspected; however, no reservoir has yet been confirmed, although some persons in the endemic area show antibodies to the virus.

The disease is transmitted by person-to-person contact via blood, secretions, semen or droplet infection. Infected blood, especially via syringes, causes the most serious infections, while transmission has occurred via semen up to 7 weeks after clinical recovery. Control measures are similar to Lassa fever, with strict quarantining of patients and their secretions. Sexual intercourse must be stopped until the semen is free of infection.

Outbreaks should be reported so that neighbouring countries and those with air connections can mount surveillance on travellers.

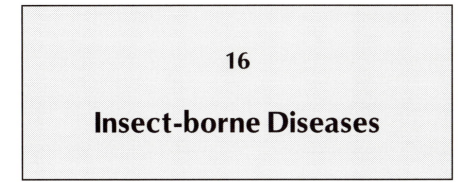

16

Insect-borne Diseases

By adopting a more specific means of transmission, some parasitic organisms have become dependent on vectors for carriage from the reservoir to a new host. This restriction to a particular vector would at first appear to reduce the chance of infection, but the parasite is carried right to the new host and in many cases directly introduced. Instead of the haphazard method of scattering large numbers of organisms into the environment, using a vector can have a greater chance of success. Often a development stage takes place in the vector and the infective stage continues for the rest of its life. Transmission depends on the vector being able to find a new host, a vulnerable step in the life cycle and one where control methods are most likely to succeed.

16.1 MOSQUITO-BORNE DISEASES

The mosquito is the most important vector of disease, because it is abundant, lives in close proximity to humans and needs to feed on blood (the female must have a blood meal for the development of its eggs). Incredibly, it is a very delicate insect, being easily blown by the wind, is a weak and slow flyer and is susceptible to climatic change. Its success lies in its opportunism and rapid developmental cycle, allowing large numbers to be produced in a short time. Once a suitable breeding place appears, be it a few puddles after a rainstorm or a human-made water storage tank, mosquitoes will quickly lay eggs, which will develop within a short period into a large number of adults. Each of these adults may become a vector and, although many will die, there will be sufficient to seek out suitable blood meals. An infected mosquito must survive long enough for any developmental stage to be completed before it can infect a new host.

Some parasites are specific to certain types of mosquitoes, e.g. malaria

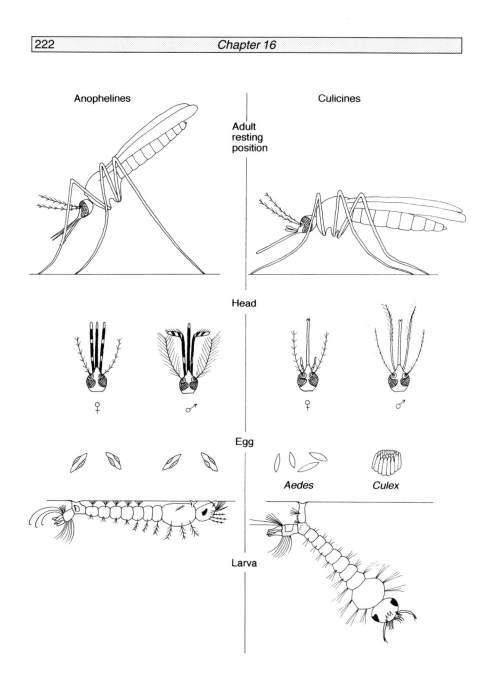

Fig. 16.1. The main differences between anopheline and culicine mosquitoes.

and the anophelines, while others, like the arboviruses, are less selective and utilize many different species. Different kinds of mosquitoes may be required in a complex transmission cycle, such as yellow fever.

Development of the parasite within the mosquito may be morphological without multiplication (as with filaria), asexual (arbovirus) or sexual reproduction (malaria).

Mosquitoes may be specific in their habits, preferring to take blood meals on humans (*anthropophilic*) or on animals (*zoophilic*), or be non-specific depending on which is most readily available. They also have particular habits, like preferring to bite indoors or outdoors.

See Fig. 16.1 for the main morphological differences between anopheline and culicine mosquitoes.

16.2 ARBOVIRUSES

Arthropod-borne virus (arbovirus) infections occur in epidemic form in a number of different parts of the world. Many viruses have been identified (see Section 19.1), but they are best grouped into three symptom complexes.

16.2.1 Arboviruses Producing Mainly Fever or Arthritis: Chikungunya, O'nyong-Nyong, West Nile, Orungo, Oropouche and Ross River

This group of infections is summarized in Table 16.1. They present as a dengue-like disease (see below) with headache, fever, malaise, arthralgia or myalgia, lasting for a week or less. Rashes are common in Chikungunya, O'nyong-Nyong and West Nile. Chikungunya may present as a haemorrhagic fever in India and South-East Asia (see below) and West Nile and Oropouche as encephalitides. Ross River predominantly presents as a polyarthritis and rash. There are many other arbovirus infections presenting as fever, listed in Section 19.1.

The *incubation period* is from 3 to 12 days. Susceptibility is general but infection leads to immunity, probably lifelong. In endemic areas they are diseases of children; otherwise they are epidemic, affecting all age-groups and both sexes.

16.2.2 Arboviruses Presenting as Fever and Encephalitis: Western Equine, Eastern Equine, St Louis, Venezuelan, Japanese, Murray Valley and Rocio

This group of diseases presents with a high fever of acute onset, headache, meningeal irritation, stupor, disorientation, coma, spasticity and tremors. Fatality rates are variable, with up to 60% in Japanese, eastern equine and Murray Valley. Their distribution, vectors and reservoirs are summarized in Table 16.1.

The *incubation period* is from 5 to 15 days. Susceptibility is highest in

Table 16.1. The important arbovirus infections of humans.

Virus	Distribution	Vectors	Reservoir
1. Causing mainly fever or arthritis			
Chikungunya	Africa, India, Sri Lanka, S.E. Asia	*Ae. aegypti, Ae. africanus, Ae. luteocephalus, Culex* spp. *A. gambiae, A. funestus*	Baboons, bats, rodents, monkeys
O'nyong-Nyong	E. Africa, Senegal		Humans?
West Nile	Africa, Asia, Europe	*Culex* spp.	Birds
Oropouche	Trinidad, S. America	Mosquitoes, possibly *Culicoides*	Monkeys, sloths, birds
Orungo	W. Africa, Uganda	*Ae. dentatus, Anopheles* spp.	Humans?
Ross River	Australia, New Zealand, Pacific Is.	*Ae. vigilax, C. annularis*	Rodents
2. Causing fever and encephalitis			
Western equine	Americas (Canada to Argentina)	*C. tarsalis, C. melanura*	Birds
Eastern equine	Americas, Caribbean	*C. melanura, Aedes* and *Culex* spp.	Birds, rodents
St Louis	Americas, Caribbean	*C. tarsalis* and other *Culex* spp.	Birds
Venezuelan equine	Central and S. America, Caribbean, parts of USA	*C. tarsalis* and other *Culex* spp.	Birds
Japanese	East Asia, S.E. Asia, India, Sri Lanka, former USSR	*C. tritaenio rhynchus, C. gelidus, C. vishnui*	Birds, pigs
Murray Valley	New Guinea, Australia	*C. annulirostris*	Birds
Rocio	Brazil	Probably mosquitoes	Birds?
			Rodents

3. Causing haemorrhagic fevers

Disease	Region	Vector	Host
Yellow fever	S. America and Africa	*Ae. aegypti, Ae. africanus, Ae. simpsoni, Ae. furcifer/taylori, Ae. luteocephalus, Haemagogus* spp.	Monkeys and humans (mosquitoes)
Dengue 1, 2, 3 and 4	Asia, Pacific, Caribbean, Africa, Central and S. America	*Ae. aegypti* (urban) *Ae. albopictus, Ae. scutellaris* group	Humans (Monkeys in jungle cycle)
Rift Valley	Africa	*Ae. caballus, C. quinquefasciatus, C. theileri* and other *Culex* and *Aedes* spp.	Domestic animals
Kyasanur Forest disease	S. India	*Haemaphysalis* spp. (Hard ticks)	Rodents, monkeys
Crimean/Congo HF	Europe, Africa, Central Asia, S.W. Asia	*Hyalomma* spp. (Hard ticks)	Domestic animals

HF, haemorrhagic fever.

the very young and old, with unapparent infection occurring in other age-groups.

Japanese encephalitis is particularly associated with rice fields and the keeping of domestic pigs. Birds spread the virus from rural to urban areas. There is a marked seasonality with a peak period in Thailand in July and August, in China in August, and in India/Nepal in September and November. It is endemic in the remainder of the area. Vaccination of children and susceptible adults has been found to be a successful control method in Taiwan and Korea.

16.2.3 Arboviruses Presenting as Haemorrhagic Fevers: Yellow Fever, Dengue, Rift Valley, Kyasanur Forest Disease, Crimean/Congo and Chikungunya

Apart from yellow fever, which will be covered in more detail below, a group of generally mild viral fevers, including dengue, Rift Valley, Kyasanur Forest disease and Chikungunya, at certain places and occasions, take on a severe form, resulting in vascular permeability, hypovolaemia and abnormal blood clotting. Infection commences as an acute fever, malaise, headache, nausea or vomiting, with petechial rashes, severe bruising, epistaxis and bleeding from various sites. After a few days sudden circulatory failure and shock may occur, producing a mortality of up to 50%. (For Kyasanur Forest disease and Crimea/Congo, see Section 17.6.)

16.2.4 Control of Arbovirus Infections

The main method of control is the destruction of vector mosquitoes and their breeding places. The most important is *Ae. aegypti*, which lives in collections of water close to the home. A search is made for larvae and all breeding places are destroyed. A simple method is to use schoolchildren, making a game or giving a reward for the number of breeding places found. Water tanks, discarded tin cans or old tyres are favourite breeding places. Large breeding areas (such as water tanks) can be covered, screened or treated with insecticides, or natural predators can be introduced (e.g. fish or dragonfly larvae).

Where there is an epidemic in a compact area, such as a town, the quickest and simplest (although expensive) method of bringing the epidemic to an end is to use fogging or ultra-low-volume (ULV) aerial spraying. Compared with lost working hours, this can be a cost-effective procedure.

Where an animal reservoir is involved, some restriction of animals or reduction of rodents can be of value. In Rift Valley fever special precautions should be taken in handling domestic animals and their products. All animals should be vaccinated. Personal prevention with nets and repellents can protect the individual. The infected case should be nursed under a mosquito net so as not to infect mosquitoes.

16.3 DENGUE

Dengue presents as a sudden onset of fever, retro-orbital headache and joint and muscle pains. A maculopapular or scarlatiniform rash usually appears after 3–4 days. Depression and prolonged fatigue often occur after the acute manifestations.

The *incubation period* is 3–15 days (commonly 5–6). Four separate viruses have so far been identified (1, 2, 3 and 4) with *Aedes* species, especially *Ae. aegypti*, *Ae. albopictus* or a member of the *Ae. scutellaris* group, responsible for transmission (Fig. 16.2). Dengue is now endemic in many parts of the world, so children are the main sufferers. Large epidemics have occurred, especially in island countries of the Caribbean and Pacific, with devastating effect. The epidemic can be so massive as to immobilize large segments of the population, disrupt the workforce and cause a breakdown in organization. The development of haemorrhagic disease has been variable, producing a number of deaths.

With infection, immunity develops to the dengue virus. However, there is no cross-immunity to the other three viruses so a new epidemic can occur. It was noticed that epidemics with haemorrhagic cases followed an epidemic of dengue in which there were no haemorrhagic cases, suggesting that the first virus sensitized some individuals. On repeat infection they had a profound reaction, which resulted in vascular damage and upset of the clotting mechanism. There is also a difference in virulence, with dengue 2 strains associated with the severe epidemics in South-East Asia and the Caribbean. Differential effects on racial groups suggest that host factors may also have a role. Outbreaks of haemorrhagic dengue have occurred principally in Sri Lanka, China, South-East Asia, Caribbean countries and Pacific islands.

Virus can be isolated from the blood in acute cases, or a rising antibody level may assist in diagnosis. There is no specific treatment, but hypovolaemic shock must be treated with rapid fluid replacement and oxygen therapy.

16.4 YELLOW FEVER

One of the haemorrhagic group of arbovirus infections, yellow fever presents with a sudden onset of fever, headache, backache, prostration and vomiting. Jaundice commences mildly at first and intensifies as the

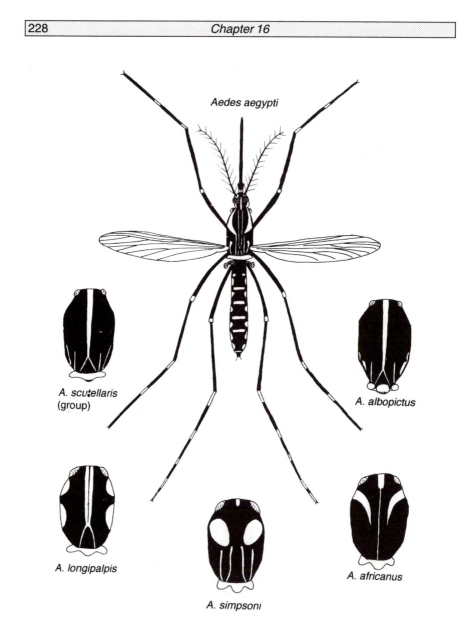

Fig. 16.2 Aedes, the black and white mosquitoes.

disease progresses. Albuminuria and leucopenia are found on examination, while haemorrhagic symptoms of epistaxis, haematemesis, melena and bleeding from the gums can all occur. In endemic areas the fatality rate is low except in the non-indigenous. The death rate may reach 50% in epidemics.

Diagnosis is made on clinical grounds and in fatal cases by liver

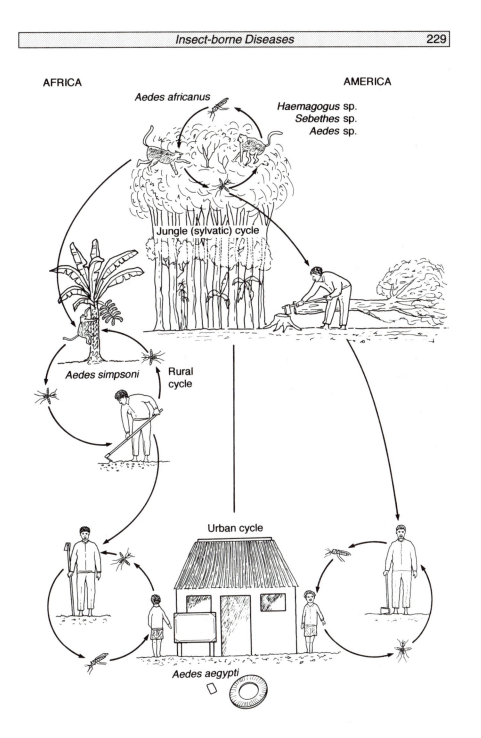

AFRICA

AMERICA

Aedes africanus

Haemagogus sp.
Sebethes sp.
Aedes sp.

Jungle (sylvatic) cycle

Aedes simpsoni Rural cycle

Urban cycle

Aedes aegypti

Fig. 16.3. Yellow fever transmission cycles.

biopsy. Blood must be sent to a viral laboratory so that the virus can be isolated. Paired serum can be taken for the neutralization test. There is no specific treatment, but supportive therapy is given to combat shock and renal failure.

The *incubation period* is 3–6 days. The period of communicability is from before the fever commences to 5 days after, so the patient should be nursed under a mosquito net to prevent new mosquitoes from becoming infected.

Yellow fever is a disease of the forest, maintained in the monkey population by *Haemagogus* mosquitoes in America and *Ae. africanus* in Africa. The monkeys are generally not affected by the disease but occasionally they start dying, indicating that spread to the human population may soon begin. In South America it may be a reduction in the monkey population that makes the canopy mosquito look for another blood meal and perhaps feed on humans. More commonly, it is those who go into the forest to cut wood, who are bitten incidentally. When they return to their village or town, they are fed on by *Ae. aegypti* and an urban yellow fever transmission cycle is set up (Fig. 16.3). In Africa three different kinds of mosquitoes are involved. *Ae. africanus* remains in the jungle canopy and rarely feeds on humans, but should the monkey descend to the forest floor or even enter areas of human habitation it is fed on by *Ae. simpsoni*. This mosquito then bites humans on the edge of the forest, from where they return to their village and the peridomestic mosquito *Ae. aegypti* can become infected (see Fig. 16.2). The extrinsic cycle of infection takes 5–30 days in the mosquito, depending on temperature and type of mosquito. Transovarian infection can also occur.

The most important part of the complex mosquito transmission cycle is *Ae. aegypti*. With its proximity to humans, it is capable of infecting a large number of people, as well as being the most easy to control. It breeds in small collections of water near to people's houses, so a careful search for larvae and the destruction of breeding places can do much to reduce the danger. A useful indicator of the prevalence of this mosquito is the *Ae. aegypti* index, which is the number of houses with breeding sites within a specified area of 100 houses. Alternatively, the Breteau index, which is the number of positive containers out of 100 samples, can be used. If these are kept below 5% or preferably 1%, the danger of an epidemic is minimized. Simple clearance is the most effective method of reducing the mosquito population, but insecticides, such as temephos (Abate) can be used where collections of water cannot be destroyed. In the event of an epidemic, emergency reduction by fogging or ULV sprays from aircraft will rapidly destroy the adult population (but not the larvae).

One attack of yellow fever confers immunity for life if the person survives the disease. Unapparent infections also occur. However, a very effective vaccine has been developed which provides immunity for at least 10 years and probably longer. The endeavour should be to vaccinate all those at risk in the known endemic areas (see Fig. 6.1). This has been attempted by offering vaccination at markets and meetings or systematically to schoolchildren. In the event of an epidemic, ring vaccination can be performed; the epidemic is surrounded by a circle of vaccinated persons, progressively closing in on the centre of the outbreak. Areas of Africa and South America have been designated as yellow fever areas (see Fig. 6.1) and vaccination is required by all visitors. Yellow fever is an internationally notifiable disease.

In these days of rapid air transport, it has always been surprising that yellow fever has not been transported to Asia, where there are the vectors and conditions for transmission. A suggested reason is that there is some cross-immunity with other similar viruses and the level of such induced immunity may be sufficient to prevent epidemic spread. A precaution is to spray all aircraft coming from a yellow fever area.

16.5 MALARIA

Malaria is probably the most important parasitic infection of humans. Each year some 300 million cases occur, of which 3 million die.

The epidemiology of malaria (Fig. 16.4) can be divided into persons, parasite, vector and environment.

16.5.1 Persons

In a non-immune population, children and adults of both sexes are affected equally. In areas of continuous infection, malaria mortality in childhood can be considerable while the immune response is being developed. The survivors acquire immunity, which is only preserved by a maintenance of parasites in the body due to reinfection. Should the individual leave an area of continuous malaria, immunity may be reduced. The other time when immunity is reduced is during pregnancy, and severe malaria can occur in the pregnant woman, even one that has lived in an endemic area. This is more severe in the first pregnancy than subsequently.

The body responds to malaria by an enlargement of the spleen. The degree of enlargement and the proportion of the population with palpable spleens have been used as a measure of endemicity.

- *Hypoendemic.* Spleen rate in children (2–9 years) not exceeding 10%.
- *Mesoendemic.* Spleen rate in children between 11% and 50%.
- *Hyperendemic.* Spleen rate in children constantly over 50%. Spleen rate in adults also high (over 25%).

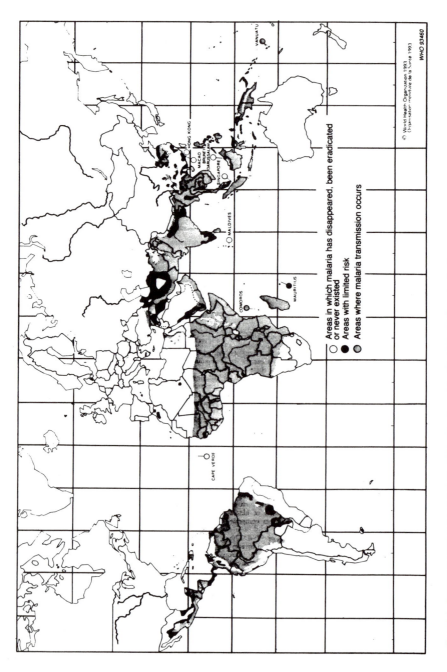

Fig. 16.4. Epidemiological status of malaria, 1991. (Courtesy of the World Health Organization.)

Areas in which malaria has disappeared, been eradicated or never existed

Areas with limited risk

Areas where malaria transmission occurs

VANUATU

HONG KONG
MACAO
BRUNEI DARUSSALAM
SINGAPORE

MALDIVES

MAURITIUS

COMOROS

CAPE VERDE

- *Holoendemic.* Spleen rate in children constantly over 75%, but spleen rate in adults low.

In endemic areas the gametocyte rate is highest in the very young, but in epidemic malaria or areas where transmission has been considerably reduced, gametocytes occur at all ages.

16.5.2 Parasite

There are four human malaria parasites, *Plasmodium falciparum*, *P. vivax*, *P. malariae* and *P. ovale*. *P. falciparum* causes the most serious effects, but differs from *P. vivax* and *P. ovale* in having no persistent stage (the hypnozoite – Fig. 16.5) from which repeat blood-stage parasites can be produced. *P. vivax* has the widest geographical range, being found in

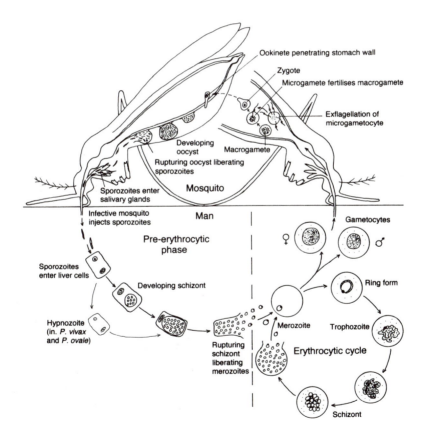

Fig. 16.5. Malaria life cycle.

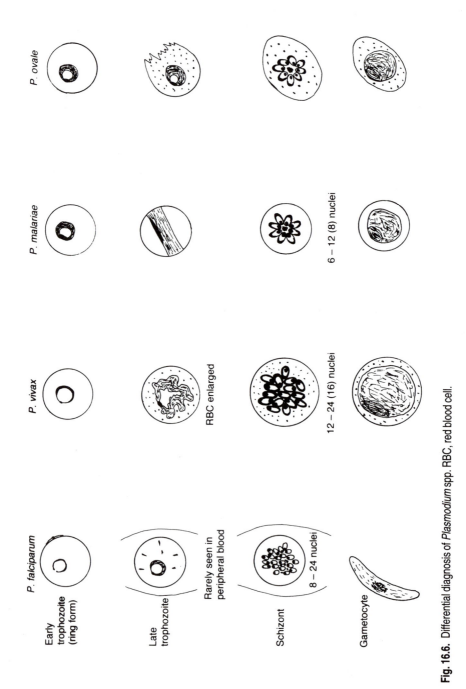

Fig. 16.6. Differential diagnosis of *Plasmodium* spp. RBC, red blood cell.

temperate and subtropical zones as well as the Tropics. *P. vivax* is predominant in some areas and becomes an opportunist parasite where *P. falciparum* is at the extremes of its range. During control campaigns *P. vivax* will replace *P. falciparum* initially. *P. vivax* infection will lead to relapses if a schizonticidal drug only is used for treatment. There are strain differences, e.g. the Chesson strain in Papua New Guinea, which requires a more prolonged radical treatment. *P. malariae* produces a milder infection but is distinguished from the other three by having paroxysms of fever every fourth day. There is an association between *P. malariae* in children and nephrosis. *P. ovale* is the rarest of the parasites and is suppressed by infections with other species.

Diagnosis is with a thick blood smear (to detect parasites) and a thin smear (to determine species), as shown in Fig. 16.6. A dipstick method for *P. falciparum* has recently been developed, which promises to make the diagnosis of malaria simpler.

The *incubation period* depends upon the species and strain.

- *P. falciparum* 9–14 days.
- *P. vivax* 12–17 days, but in temperate climates it can be 6–9 months.
- *P. malariae* 18–40 days.
- *P. ovale* 16–18 days.

The prolonged incubation period of *P. vivax* in temperate climates is due to the strain *P. v. hibernans*. It is probable that this prolonged incubation period allows the parasite to take opportunity of a very short duration of vector biting, which only occurs in summer months.

The duration of the developmental cycle in the mosquito (the extrinsic cycle) is determined by the temperature and species. *P. vivax* completes this more quickly than *P. falciparum*. At 19°C *P. falciparum* takes in excess of 30 days (beyond the life expectancy of the average mosquito), whereas *P. vivax* can still complete its cycle in less than 20 days. The absolute minimum temperature for *P. vivax* is 17°C but the extrinsic cycle is longer than the lifetime of the mosquito.

Species of parasite	Development time (days) at mean ambient temperatures		
	30°C	24°C	20°C
P. vivax	7	9	16
P. falciparum	9	11	20
P. malariae	15	21	30

Table 16.2 Principal anopheline vectors.

Geographical area	Species	Breeding place	Behaviour
Mexico, Central and S. America	A. pseudopunctipennis	Clear sunlit pools	Indoor human-biting
Mexico, Central and S. America	A. punctimacula	Shaded pools and streams	Outdoor biting
Central America and Caribbean	A. albimanus	Large sunlit waters with vegetation	Indoor human-biting
S. America	A. darlingi	Shaded fresh water	Lives in houses
Trinidad and Brazil	A. aquasalis	Brackish tidal swamps	Strong flyer
Trinidad and Brazil	A. bellator	Leaf bases of bromeliads in cocoa growing areas	Outdoor human-biting
Brazil and Argentina	A. albitarsis	Shaded large and small waters	Outdoor human-biting
Colombia and Venezuela	A. nuñeztovari	Sunlit muddy pools and lagoons	Outdoor biting
Mediterranean	A. sacharovi	Sunlit marshes	Prefers cattle
Egypt and Israel	A. sergenti	Irrigation channels, road construction pits	Indoor human-biting
S.W. Asia	A. superpictus	Sunlit freshwater pools and streams in hill country	Indoor human-biting
North Africa	A. pharoensis	Swamps and rice fields	Bites humans and animals
Africa and Arabia	A. arabiensis	Sunlit temporary pools	Indoor human-biting
Africa and Arabia	A. gambiae	Sunlit temporary pools	Indoor human-biting
Africa	A. funestus	Shaded clear water	Indoor human-biting
East Africa	A. merus	Brackish swamps	Indoor human-biting
West Africa	A. melas	Mangrove swamps	Lives indoors
Gulf to India	A. stephensi	Urban, in wells, gutters (shaded)	Lives indoors
Pakistan, India, Sri Lanka	A. culicifacies	Clear to brackish water	Prefers cattle
In foothills from Pakistan to Myanmar	A. fluviatilis	Shaded streams	Highland, lives indoors
India, Malaysia, Indonesia, S.E. Asia	A. sundaicus	Sunlit, salt-water lagoons	Lives in cowsheds
Malaysia	A. letifer	Stagnant drains and pools	Indoor human-biting
Malaysia	A. donaldi	Forest-shaded stagnant pools	Outdoor human- and monkey-biting
Malaysia	A. campestris	Forest-shaded stagnant pools	Outdoor human- and monkey-biting
Malaysia, Indonesia (China)	A. balabacensis	Shaded pools	Outdoor human- and monkey-biting
Nepal, Malaysia, Indonesia	A. maculatus	Rice paddies	Indoor human-biting
Indonesia	A. leucosphyrus	Forest-shaded pools	Bites and rests outdoors

Geographical area	Species	Breeding place	Behaviour
S.E. Asia	A. aconitus	Rice fields, swamps, ponds	Lives indoors
S.E. Asia	A. dirus	Shaded pools in forests	Outdoor biting
Philippines	A. flavirostris	Streams, rivers, irrigation ditches	Indoor human-biting
East Asia (China)	A. minimus	Sunlit rice fields and ditches	Lives indoors
China	A. sinensis	Rice fields and ditches	Outdoor human- and animal-biting
Melanesia	A. farauti	Sunlit temporary rainwater pools	Indoor human-biting
Melanesia	A. punctulatus	Sunlit temporary rainwater pools	Indoor human-biting
Melanesia	A. koliensis	Sunlit temporary rainwater pools	Indoor human-biting

16.5.3 Vector

The transmission potential will depend upon the species of *Anopheles* mosquito (Table 16.2), its feeding habits and the environmental conditions. This varies widely, with *A. gambiae* being the most efficient of all malaria vectors while a species such as *A. culicifacies* is comparatively inefficient. This depends upon a number of factors, such as the preferred food source (human or animal) or defensive action by the host (swatting mosquitoes that have a painful bite), but the most important is the length of survival. Only a few members of a population of *A. culicifacies* survive longer than 12 days, so members of this species have less opportunity to become infective and may die before completion of the extrinsic cycle, whereas 50% of a population of *A. gambiae* will live longer than 12 days. Longer-living mosquitoes are better vectors. Once a mosquito becomes infected, its potential for transmission (as well as its potential for acquiring infection) is determined by its feeding habits. If a mosquito takes all its meals on humans it has a higher transmission potential than if some of its meals are taken on animals. The degree of human feeding can be determined by precipitin tests on the blood meals of mosquitoes.

A mosquito must have a blood meal before it can complete its gonotrophic cycle and lay a batch of eggs. The gonotrophic cycle is normally about 2–3 days but varies with temperature, species and locality.

Biting patterns vary within species and from one mosquito species to another; human-biting preference may be indoors, outdoors or a mixture of the two. There is also a rhythm of mosquito activity, all anophelines being night-time feeders, with generally a maximum peak of biting

% total bites

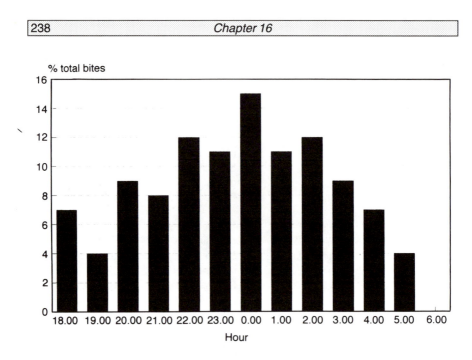

Fig. 16.7. Human-biting of *Anopheles farauti* under natural conditions: 80.8% of total catch biting indoors.

around midnight (Fig. 16.7). Indoor human–biting and night-time activity means that people are generally bitten when they are asleep and together in one place, giving the mosquito maximum opportunity for a successful feed.

The final component of vectorial capacity is mosquito density. Clearly a large number of mosquitoes have a far greater transmission potential than a small number. Some mosquitoes produce large numbers at certain favourable times of the year, while others maintain more constant populations. The environment largely determines mosquito density.

16.5.4 Environment

The most important environmental factors are temperature and water, with wind, phases of the moon and human activity having lesser effects. Temperature determines the length of development cycle of the parasite and the survival of the mosquito vector. This means that in temperate climates malaria can only be transmitted in brief periods of warm weather when the right conditions are available. In tropical regions, altitude alters the temperature, and highland areas will have less (although possibly epidemic) malaria.

Water is essential for the mosquito to breed. In arid desert countries the mosquito cannot survive, but wells and irrigation allow mosquitoes to breed and malaria appears. Rainfall generally increases the number of breeding places for mosquitoes, so there is more malaria in the wet season. However, the rain may be so great as to wash out breeding places, instead producing a decrease.

The mosquito, being a fragile flyer, is easily blown by the wind, sometimes to its advantage but generally to its disadvantage. On windy evenings mosquito biting may decrease considerably.

Nocturnal mosquitoes are sensitive to light so on a moonlit night there is a reduction in numbers. Measurements of mosquito density must be made on several nights, or ideally over a period of months.

Humans may alter their environment in many ways – by lighting fires, keeping lights burning or using insect repellents or insecticides. If these are persistent activities the mosquito will adapt to this change. An example is illustrated in Fig. 16.8 (compare with Fig. 16.7), where the vector altered from an indoor night biting pattern to an outdoor dusk and dawn one, due to prolonged residual house spraying with dichlorodiphenyltrichloroethane (DDT) (which has an irritant effect). Where the mosquito species is mainly zoophilic (feeds on animals), keeping domestic animals in proximity to the household will encourage mosquitoes to feed on them instead of on humans.

It is these environmental factors which determine whether malaria

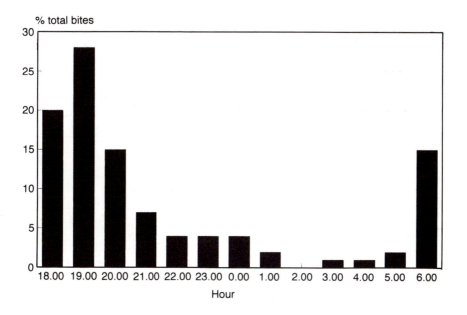

Fig. 16.8. Human-biting of *Anopheles farauti* after prolonged DDT spraying: 32.1% of total catch biting indoors. DDT, dichlorodiphenyltrichloroethane.

is *endemic* or *epidemic*. Where conditions of temperature and moisture permit all-year-round breeding of mosquitoes, endemic malaria occurs, but, if there is a marked dry season or reduction in temperature, conditions for transmission may only be suitable during part of the year, resulting in seasonal malaria. If conditions are marginal and only favourable every few years, epidemic malaria can result. Epidemic malaria is devastating, as large numbers of people who have no immunity are attacked. Endemic and epidemic malaria call for quite different strategies of control.

16.5.5 Control

Mathematical models can be helpful in determining the best strategy for the control of malaria and a schematic representation of one is shown in Fig. 16.9. This is based on the parasite life cycle (see Fig. 16.5), with which it should be compared. The stages at which the life cycle can be interrupted are as follows.

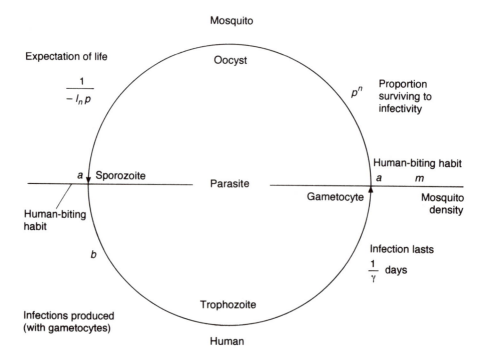

Fig. 16.9. Mathematical model of malaria based on the schematic life cycle of the parasite.

1. In *humans*.

- Reduction of the duration and intensity of infection by chemotherapy.
- Prevention of infection by chemoprophylaxis and vaccination.
- Reduction of the gametocyte load, the infective form for mosquitoes.

2. In *mosquitoes*.

- Prevention of human–biting (including deviating to other mammals).
- Reduction of expectation of life and proportion surviving to infectivity.
- Decreasing mosquito density.

16.5.6 Chemotherapy

Treatment of the uncomplicated case of malaria is with a 4-aminoquinoline, (chloroquine):

- 600 mg of chloroquine base as an initial dose;
- 6 hours later, 300 mg chloroquine base, followed by
- 300 mg chloroquine base for 2 or 3 more days.

Amodiaquine can also be used but serious side-effects have been reported.

Unfortunately, there are many areas of the world where chloroquine resistance is found and alternative drugs (Fansidar, quinine, Halofantrine, doxycycline, mefloquine, qinghaosu or its derivatives) need to be used. Chloroquine can still be used in areas of reduced sensitivity in the indigenous population (but not in non-immunes), especially where cost is the deciding factor. A possible regime is:

	Day 1 10 mg base kg^{-1}	Day 2 10 mg base kg^{-1}	Day 3 5 mg base kg^{-1}
70 kg adult	5 tablets	5 tablets	2 tablets

In *P. vivax*, chloroquine will only clear parasites from the blood, and to effect radical cure primaquine is administered in a dose of 15 mg base daily for 14 days, or given once a week at 30–45 mg base of primaquine for 8–12 weeks. People with deficiency of the enzyme glucose-6-phosphate dehydrogenase (G-6-PD) may have a haemolytic crisis with this drug. Primaquine can be used to reduce the reservoir of *P. vivax* in control programmes, but asymptomatic carriers may be reluctant to take the drug.

Case finding and treatment are an effective strategy only where there is a low level of malaria, so in general they need to be used in combination with other methods of malaria control. Mass drug administrations can be of value in rapidly reducing the parasite reservoir, but the effect is only temporary and is not an effective method of control on its own. From the mathematical model, treatment (r) alone, is unlikely to have much of an effect on the control of malaria.

16.5.7 Chemoprophylaxis

Chemoprophylaxis can be given to persons at particular risk, such as pregnant women, non-immune immigrants or migrant workers, but, if facilities allow, it would be preferable to give them priority in control programmes, such as with impregnated bed nets. Chloroquine 300 mg (two tablets) weekly can be used where chloroquine resistance is not a major problem, but local advice should be sought.

16.5.8 Vaccines

Attempts to produce a vaccine against malaria have been in progress since 1910. The first was a preparation of killed sporozoites, with merozoites and gametocytes also being tried. But none of these whole-parasite stages have produced lasting immunity. Greater response has been induced by separating the specific immunizing antigen. This has recently been achieved by isolating the deoxyribonucleic acid (DNA) fragments of the circumsporozoite antigen and cloning them through bacteria or yeasts. This has allowed large quantities of pure antigen to be produced and trials of a vaccine to take place. Unfortunately, initial results have not produced a sufficient level of protection in highly endemic areas, but there may be a place for combining vaccination with other control strategies. Even so, there will be all the other problems of vaccination programmes, such as preservation in a cold chain, response of the public and contraindications.

16.5.9 Reducing the Gametocyte Load

The gametocyte is the sexual form of the parasite that undergoes development within the mosquito. Preventing mosquitoes from taking up gametocytes could interrupt transmission. There are two ways this can be done.

● Administration of gametocidal drugs.
● Preventing mosquitoes from feeding on a malaria case.

Drugs which act on gametocytes are proguanil, pyrimethamine and primaquine. Quinine, chloroquine and amodiaquine are active against the gametocytes of *P. vivax* and *P. malariae*, but not against the more important *P. falciparum*. The action of proguanil and pyrimethamine is on the development of gametocytes within the mosquito, but they act on all four parasites. Primaquine has a highly active and rapid action on gametocytes of all species, whether in the blood or in the mosquito, and is used in combination with treatment in control programmes. It has also been proposed as a method of reducing the level of gametocytes within the population, but would require an almost perfect mass treatment, as well as the danger of toxicity (especially with G-6-PD-deficient individuals) and the development of resistance to the only medicament used for radical cure. For these reasons, the use of primaquine in this way is not considered a suitable method of malaria control.

Any person found to have malaria should, where possible, be protected by a mosquito net so as not to infect new mosquitoes. This is a particularly important measure during eradication and control campaigns, especially when endemicity is brought to a low level.

16.5.10 Personal Protection

Reducing the number of bites a mosquito can make on a person reduces the chance of contracting malaria. If effective, they should theoretically be quite successful, as human-biting adds a^2 to the mathematical model. Methods of personal protection have been covered in Section 5.3.1. They include clothing, mosquito nets and repellents. Items of clothing, such as socks and shawls, can be treated with repellents which retain activity for some time, or repellents can be applied directly to the skin. Some naturally occurring plants have repellent properties, such as *Tegetes minuta* in East Africa.

Mosquito nets are most effective if used properly. Providing subsidized mosquito nets can be used as a method of malaria control, especially for mothers and children, who are liable to go to bed early. This can be improved by *impregnating* the *nets* with synthetic pyrethroid insecticides (such as permethrin, deltamethrin or lambda–cyhalothrin). This repels mosquitoes and kills those which come into contact with the net, achieving a double effect of reducing biting and mosquito expectation of life. When used on a community scale the concentration of impregnated bed nets can produce a *mass effect*, reducing the mosquito population and the sporozoite rate. The method of impregnating bed nets will be found in Section 5.3.1.

As with residual spraying, it is preferable to impregnate nets all at one time, just before the main transmission season of malaria. Permethrin lasts for some 6 months, but deltamethrin and lambda–cyhalothrin retain activity for 9 months so in areas of seasonal malaria one application a year may be sufficient.

Bed nets are more effective and cheaper to maintain than screening the whole house, which is only recommended for people with a high standard of living. A small hole in the netting can render the rest ineffective. A knock-down spray can be used to kill mosquitoes that have entered a screened house.

The use of smoke from mosquito coils or vaporizing mats can be surprisingly effective and has the advantage that it is a cheap personal protection. Coils are easily manufactured locally, and naturally occurring substances, such as pyrethrum, can be incorporated. People often sit around fires in the evening and by the addition of certain plants a repellent smoke can be produced.

Mosquitoes can be diverted to bite other animals if they are the preferred blood meal. However, if the animals are taken away, such as to market, the mosquitoes may be forced to take their blood meals on humans. The habits of the malaria vectors will need to be known before encouraging this practice.

16.5.11 *Reduction of the Mosquitoes' Expectation of Life*

Mathematical models have shown the considerable advantage of reducing the mosquitoes' life expectancy to less than the parasite extrinsic cycle. In Fig. 16.9 it is seen that p^n, the maximum probability of a mosquito becoming infective, is related to the length of the extrinsic cycle n, by the nth power. This, then, is by far the most vulnerable part of the parasite life cycle.

Reduction of the mosquitoes' expectation of life is achieved by the use of residual insecticides (which has been covered in Section 5.3.2). These are applied to the inside surface of houses so that the resting mosquito (after it has taken its blood meal) absorbs a lethal dose of insecticide and dies before the parasites it has taken up in the blood can complete development.

This was the main method of the malaria eradication programmes used in many countries of the world. Unfortunately, insecticidal resistance, organizational breakdown and reluctance by people to have their houses sprayed resulted in an abandonment of the goal of eradication. Instead, residual house spraying is used for control. Trying to eradicate the last remaining cases becomes very difficult, but with just a control strategy malaria is reduced to within the ability and resources of the country. Synthetic pyrethroids impregnated into bed nets also have a residual action.

16.5.12 Decreasing Mosquito Density

The density of mosquitoes is determined by the number of larvae, so any method which reduces the larval numbers inadvertently reduces the potential number of adults. The larvae can be attacked by several different methods.

- Using insecticides and larvicidal substances.
- Modification of the environment.
- Biological control.

These have already been covered in Section 5.3.1. Larvicidal substances can be oils that spread over the surface and asphyxiate the larvae or have insecticidal properties. The size and flow of the body of water will determine which is the preferred method to use. Modification of the environment by drainage or filling in is the most permanent and effective, but is an expensive undertaking. It is worth spending money on engineering methods in areas of dense population such as towns, while in rural areas much can be achieved by using self-help schemes. The considerable advantage of this method is that, once done, it lasts for a long period of time, if not permanently, and in these days of resistant mosquitoes it is being seen more and more as an economical proposition. Reducing mosquitoes does not ensure a reduction in malaria and larviciding must be evaluated. From the mathematical model (m), it is likely to have a small effect only.

Biological control with fish or bacilli (*B. thuringiensis* or *B. sphaericus*) will reduce mosquito larvae to a certain extent, but a balance, as with much of nature, often results. Biological control can also be used directly against adults with the sterile-male technique. This has not been successful with mosquitoes because of the very large numbers involved and their short period of life. Another method that is being considered is species competition, whereby a non-malarial mosquito from another part of the world is introduced to compete with the resident vector. This has not met with any great success.

In epidemic malaria adult mosquito density can be rapidly reduced by using a fogging machine or ULV spray from aircraft. This will cut short the epidemic by killing off flying adults. But it needs to be repeated regularly as new adults will continually be produced from larvae which are not affected by the knock-down sprays.

16.5.13 Prospects for Malaria Control

Malaria attracts the wonder cure. First it was the eradication programme, now all hope is pinned on the vaccine, but it is more likely to be controlled by simple, non-dramatic methods, where care to detail is

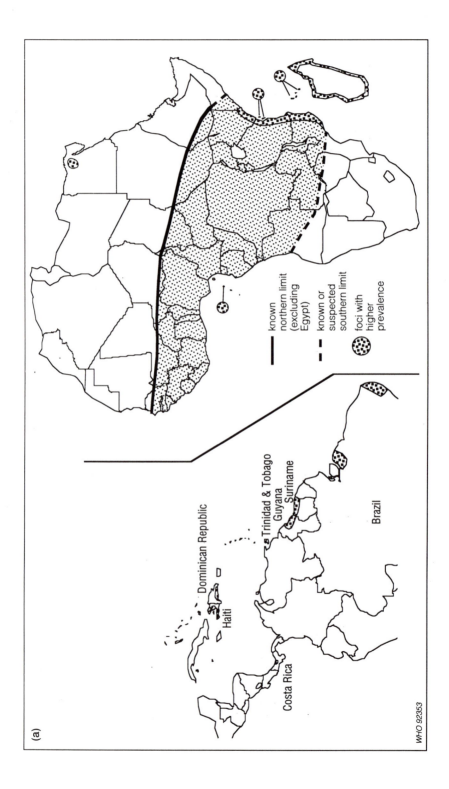

known
northern limit
(excluding
Egypt)

known or
suspected
southern limit

foci with
higher
prevalence

Dominican Republic

Haiti

Costa Rica

Trinidad & Tobago
Guyana
Suriname

Brazil

(a)

WHO 92353

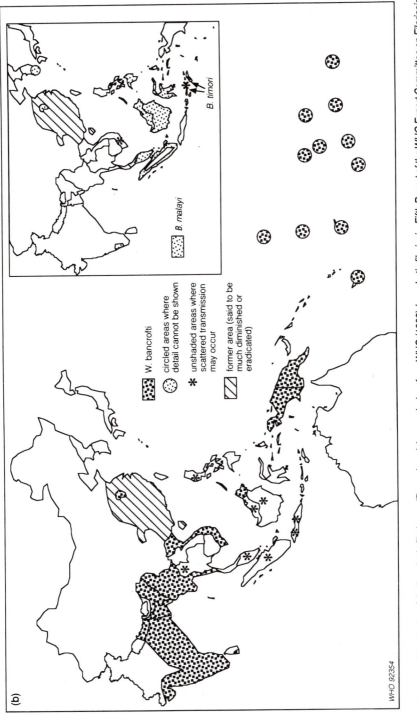
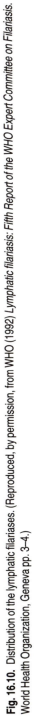

Fig. 16.10. Distribution of the lymphatic filariases. (Reproduced, by permission, from WHO (1992) *Lymphatic filariasis: Fifth Report of the WHO Expert Committee on Filariasis*. World Health Organization, Geneva pp. 3–4.)

Table 16.3. The vectors of lymphatic filariasis.

Filaria species and type	Endemic area	Principal vector
Wuchereria bancrofti – periodic		
	Tropical America	*Culex quinquefasciatus* *Anopheles darlingi*
	Tropical Africa	*Culex quinquefasciatus* *Anopheles arabiensis* *Anopheles funestus* *Anopheles gambiae* *Anopheles melas* *Anopheles merus*
	South-west Asia	*Culex molestus* *Culex quinquefasciatus*
	South and east Asia	*Culex quinquefasciatus* *Aedes poicilius* *Anopheles balabacensis* *Anopheles dirus* *Anopheles donaldi* *Anopheles flavirostris* *Anopheles candidiensis* *Anopheles anthropophagus* *Anopheles letifer* *Anopheles leucosphyrus* *Anopheles maculatus* *Anopheles minimus* *Anopheles sinensis* *Anopheles subpictus* *Anopheles vagus* *Anopheles whartoni*
	Micronesia	*Culex pipiens pallens* *Culex quinquefasciatus*
	Melanesia	*Anopheles farauti* *Anopheles koliensis* *Anopheles punctulatus* *Culex quinquefasciatus*
Wuchereria bancrofti – aperiodic		
	South Asia	*Aedes harinasutai* *Aedes niveus*
	Polynesia	*Aedes cooki* *Aedes fijiensis* *Aedes kesseli* *Aedes oceanicus* *Aedes polynesiensis*

Filaria species and type	Endemic area	Principal vector
		Aedes pseudoscutellaris
		Aedes samoanus
		Aedes tutuilae
		Aedes upolensis
		Aedes vigilax
Brugia malayi – periodic	South-East Asia	*Anopheles anthropophagus*
		Anopheles barbirostris
		Anopheles campestris
		Anopheles donaldi
		Anopheles kweiyangensis
		Anopheles sinensis
		Mansonia annulata
		Mansonia annulifera
		Mansonia uniformis
Brugia malayi – periodic	South Asia	*Mansonia annulata*
		Mansonia bonneae
		Mansonia dives
		Mansonia uniformis
Brugia timori – periodic	Flores, Timor	*Anopheles barbirostris*

(Reproduced, by permission, from WHO (1984) *Lymphatic Filariasis: Fourth Report of the WHO Expert Committee on Filariasis*, World Health Organization, Geneva, p. 111–112.)

applied. It is the encouragement of simple protective methods that everybody can follow, like impregnated mosquito nets, or of community-action environmental modification. A multiplicity of simple methods, carried out by many responsible people, is likely to be more successful in the long term than more complex methods. It will be people who will finally control malaria, but the health authorities must advise and assist them in the ways of achieving it.

16.6 FILARIASIS

The filarial infections are caused by nematode worms that use vector insects for their transmission. The most important are *Wuchereria bancrofti* and *Brugia malayi* (Fig. 16.10 and Table 16.3), which are mosquito-transmitted, and *Onchocerca volvulus*, which utilizes *Simulium* flies.

16.7 WUCHERERIA BANCROFTI

16.7.1 Parasitology

The most prolific parasites of humans, the nematodes have taken advantage of every possible system to extend their phylum, including insect vectors. Despite their size, the microfilariae of *Wuchereria bancrofti* are able to use various species of mosquitoes to complete their life cycle (Fig. 16.11). So successful are they that over 250 million people in the world are infected. Microfilariae, the larval form, are present in the peripheral blood and are taken into the mosquito's stomach when it feeds on humans. The larva loses its sheath inside the mosquito, migrates through the stomach wall and burrows into the muscles of the thorax. It becomes shorter and fatter, commonly described as sausage-shaped. Developmental changes take place and it elongates to a third stage, infective larva, leaving the thoracic muscles. It migrates to the proboscis, where it waits for the mosquito to feed and then breaks out on to the skin. The larva has to find its way into the tissues, generally through the wound made by the mosquito. (It is important to realize that the infective larva is *not* injected like the malaria parasite directly into the bloodstream.) This developmental stage in the mosquito, from the time of the blood meal until reinfection, takes 10 or more days, depending on the temperature, a very similar length of time to the development of *Plasmodium*.

Once in the body, the larva reaches the lymphatics and settles down in a lymphatic node to develop into an adult. It is the obstruction of the lymphatic drainage system by the adults, especially the fibrotic reaction when they die, that causes the serious disease manifestations of elephantiasis and chyluria. No multiplication took place in the mosquito, so one larva that was taken up in the blood meal becomes one adult in the human (if it survives all the stages). Since there are male and female worms, it is necessary for the two sexes to meet if the female is to be fertilized and produce microfilariae. These microfilariae are liberated into the lymphatic stream, reaching blood vessels via the thoracic duct. *W. bancrofti* has adapted to its vector by exhibiting microfilarial *periodicity* which normally corresponds with the mosquito biting time.

Diagnosis is by finding microfilariae in a measured sample of blood (for differential features of microfilariae, see Fig. 16.12). This is by thick blood smear, counting chamber or filtration of venepuncture blood, taken during the peak microfilarial output, which generally means collecting samples at night-time. The diethylcarbamazine (DEC) provocation test allows blood from nocturnally periodic filariasis to be taken during the daytime, but the results are not consistent so are unsuitable for monitoring control programmes. Monoclonal antibody immunoassay methods are useful in detecting positives, but do not measure

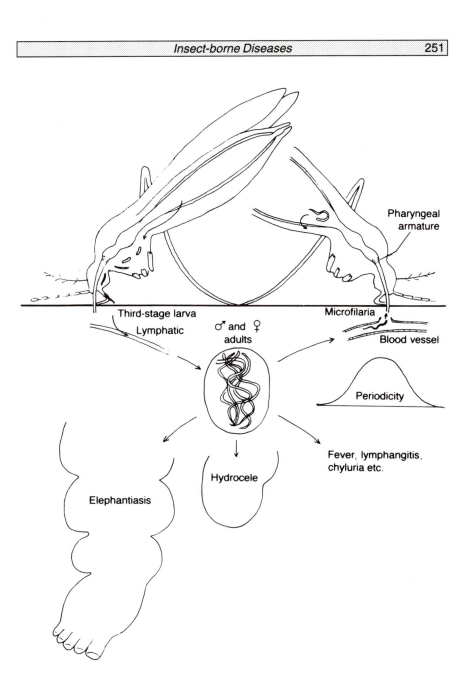

Fig. 16.11. Life cycle of *Wuchereria bancrofti.*

density. Effectiveness of control can only be determined from measured blood samples, as decrease in density occurs before conversion to negativity.

Clinical assessment methods, such as hydrocele or lymph-node

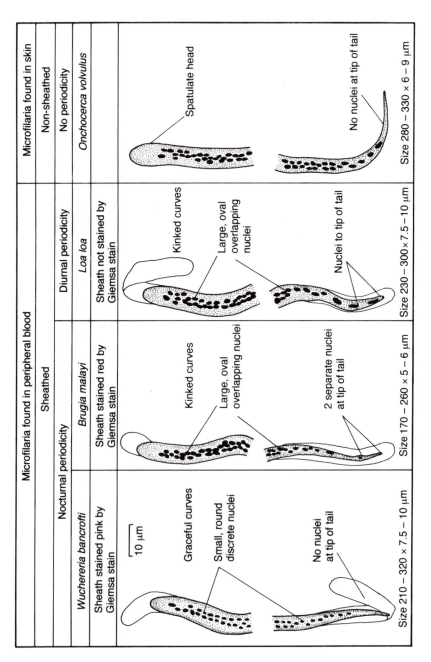

Fig. 16.12. Differential features of microfilariae of medical importance. (Courtesy of the Department of Medical Parasitology, London School of Hygiene and Tropical Medicine).

surveys, can be of value in rapidly defining the area in which blood surveys are to be made.

16.7.2 Epidemiology

Relevant *parasite* characteristics are as follows.

* Microfilarial longevity: 6 months.
* Periodicity of microfilariae: nocturnal, diurnal or aperiodic.
* Microfilarial density.
* Developmental cycle in mosquito takes 11–21 days (average 15) at an optimum temperature of 26–27°C. Extremes are 17°C to 32°C.
* Microfilarial loss when mosquito bites: only 20–40% enter skin.
* Probability of a larva reaching maturity is extremely low: one estimate is 1 in 700 (takes approximately 1 year).
* Probability of a mature worm finding a mate of the opposite sex is related to the intensity of infection. Many are unsuccessful.
* Longevity of adult worm is 7–12 years (mean 10), but period of microfilarial production is only 2–2.5 years.

Vector characteristics related to the parasite life cycle are as follows.

* Mosquito density. Peak biting time in relation to microfilarial periodicity.
* Microfilarial density. Above 50 per 20 mm^3 of blood in *Aedes* and *Culex* leads to mosquito mortality.
* Species of mosquito. Anopheline mosquitoes with pharyngeal armatures damage microfilariae, so large numbers of microfilariae are required to produce infection. In culicine mosquitoes very low levels of microfilariae can produce infection.
* Expectation of life of mosquito must exceed duration of developmental cycle of parasite.

There is no reservoir other than humans in *W. bancrofti*. There are no specific host factors; all races, both sexes and all ages of persons are equally susceptible to infection. (There are marked differences between individuals developing elephantiasis, but these are immunological rather than ethnic.)

Filarial infection is determined by the number of infected bites, which can either be the result of a high intensity over a short period of time or constant bites over a long period of time. Mosquito mortality occurs when density of microfilariae is excessive, so the chronic, long-term pattern is more common.

Three types of filariasis are seen: *rural* filariasis transmitted by nocturnal *Anopheles* mosquitoes with a generalized distribution similar to that of malaria; *urban* filariasis transmitted by *Culex* with a tendency

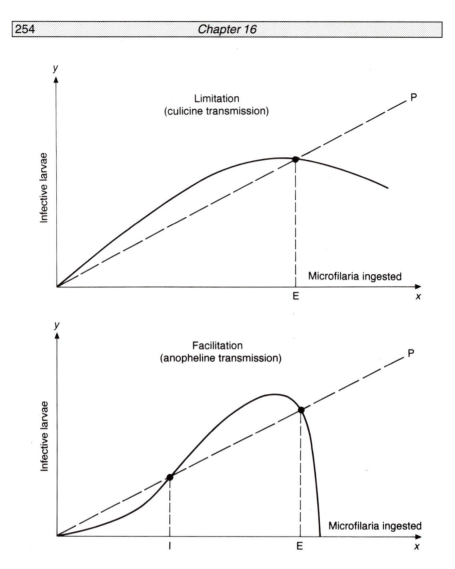

Fig. 16.13. Limitation and facilitation in filariasis. (Reproduced, by permission, from Pichon, G., Perrault, G. and Laigret, J. (1975) *Rendement parasitaire chez les vecteurs de filarioses.* (WHO/FIL/75.132), World Health Organization, Geneva.)

to invade new areas; and the Pacific Island variety which has a homogeneous (rural) distribution but is transmitted by day- and night-biting *Aedes* mosquitoes.

The type of vector determines the pattern of infection and control strategy. Culicine mosquitoes exhibit limitation and anophelines exhibit facilitation (Fig. 16.13). The broken line (P) represents proportionality, whereby the number of microfilariae ingested is sufficient to produce enough infective larvae to maintain infection. With limitation (culicines) it will be seen that this is always greater than proportionality until a point (E) is reached, where the number of microfilariae ingested is so large that damage occurs to the mosquito and mortality occurs. There is a similar pattern in facilitation (anophelines), except at low levels, when the number of microfilariae ingested is unable to produce sufficient infective larvae and infection is not maintained. This threshold level (I) is probably due to the pharyngeal armature in anopheline mosquitoes, which damages microfilariae. When there are many microfilariae ingested by the mosquito, sufficient will remain undamaged to produce infection, but at low microfilarial levels every microfilaria will be damaged. This applies to both W. *bancrofti* and B. *malayi*, so for control the type of mosquito is more important than the species of parasite.

16.7.3 Control

There are various places at which control can be implemented.

- Reduction of the number of bites by infected mosquitoes.
- Decreasing the number of microfilariae in the human host.
- Reduction of the mosquito expectation of life.
- Decrease the mosquito density.
- Alteration of the mosquito biting time.
- Reduction of the number of adult worms.

Reducing the number of infective bites

Multiplication does not take place when the organism enters the host, so the disease process and its severity depend upon repeated entry of the body by the parasites, many of which will be unsuccessful. The transmission process is surprisingly inefficient, requiring some 15,500 infective bites to produce a reproducing adult. This means that, for *Anopheles* mosquitoes, approximately eight infective bites per person per day can take place without the disease being transmitted.

Number of bites can be reduced by taking simple precautions of personal protection: mosquito nets, repellents, protective clothing, etc. Impregnated mosquito nets should be effective in nocturnally periodic filariasis, transmitted by anopheline mosquitoes. This would be an additional benefit of a malaria control programme.

Decreasing the number of microfilariae (mass chemotherapy)

The microfilaria is the stage of the parasite taken up by the mosquito to commence the transmission cycle. Reducing the number of microfilariae will decrease the chance of infecting mosquitoes. Diethylcarbamazine

(DEC) has a marked action on microfilariae and may also reduce micro-filarial production by adults. Many adult worms are also killed by DEC.

With infection transmitted by culicine mosquitoes, diagnostic tests (even filtration techniques) miss a large number of positive cases, so it is preferable to give mass drug therapy. Two approaches have been used, either a full course of therapy over a limited period of time or inter-mittent single-dose therapy over a long period of time. With the full course therapy, 6 mg kg^{-1} DEC is given weekly, monthly or a combination of both, up to a total dosage of 72 mg kg^{-1} DEC. Extending the period of administration appears to improve the effectiveness. With the inter-mittent approach, 6 mg kg^{-1} DEC is given to each person once a year but continued for at least 10 years. The full-course therapy produces the greatest reduction in microfilariae with a gradual return over subsequent years, whereas the intermittent course maintains a low level. It might be easier to mobilize the population for a limited period through the use of village organizations (e.g. women's groups, as used in Samoa) or to give an annual dosage using medical workers. The annual regime is now gen-erally preferred.

Ivermectin also has a microfilaricidal action, but does not kill adult worms. Its main advantage is in reduced side-effects and it can be safely used where onchocerciasis is also present. At a dose of 100 μg kg^{-1} every 6 months, satisfactory control is achieved, but 400 μg kg^{-1} is required for persistent cases. Combinations of DEC (6 mg kg^{-1}) and ivermectin (160 μg kg^{-1}), given at annual intervals, have been shown to give better control than either DEC or ivermectin on its own.

Before mounting a mass drug treatment control programme, a com-plete survey is needed. Follow-up surveys of samples of the population are made at annual or biannual intervals. Thirty per cent of the treated population should be sampled. Children less than 1 year old, pregnant and nursing mothers, the sick and the very old should be excluded from mass treatment. Side-effects, especially itching, can be most unpleasant and a pilot control study should precede the main campaign. Consider-able care should be taken in areas where both filariasis and onchocercia-sis coexist.

In areas where the vector is an anopheline, reducing the number of microfilariae in the individual and community below the threshold level should be sufficient to interrupt transmission. Case detection and treat-ment, conscientiously carried out over several years, could lead to eradication of the disease.

Reduction of the mosquito's expectation of life (vector control)

By reducing the lifespan of the mosquito to below that of the devel-opmental period of the parasite within the mosquito (range 10–15 days), transmission of infective larvae will be halted. The expectation of life of the mosquito is reduced by using residual insecticides, which are absorbed when the mosquito rests on an internal surface after taking a blood meal or touches an impregnated mosquito net. This is the classic method used in malaria control.

Insecticides are expensive and normally not justified for filariasis control. However, in the rural type of filariasis where the vector is an *Anopheles* mosquito, probably the same vector as for malaria, it may be cost-effective to try and control both diseases by residual spraying or impregnating bed nets. The degree of mosquito reduction required is much less for filariasis than it is for malaria, however, mosquito control needs to be for a prolonged period, at least 7 and preferably 10 years. This is more likely to occur by encouraging individuals to purchase their own mosquito nets, which are then impregnated with insecticides.

Decrease in mosquito density (larval reduction)

The number of mosquitoes able to bite humans is dependent upon the number of larvae that develop into them. By reducing the number of larvae, mosquito density is also diminished. This is a supplementary method of malaria control and has also been covered under vector control (Section 5.3.1). Various methods can be used: larvicides, genetic modification, environmental or biological control. These methods are particularly appropriate to culicine-transmitted urban filariasis, although the degree of larval reduction required is often difficult to achieve. In enclosed areas of water, such as latrines and septic tanks, expanded polystyrene beads are very effective. As with the other control methods of filariasis, a reduction in microfilarial levels will take a long time to achieve and larval control must be maintained for at least 10 years.

Alteration of mosquito biting pattern

The parasite of *W. bancrofti* has developed a periodicity of its micro-filariae which coincides with the biting pattern of the vector mosquitoes. It can either be nocturnal, diurnal or aperiodic. If it is possible to alter the time when mosquitoes bite, the chance of them taking up microfilariae will also be reduced. This has been noticed as an additional effect of residual house spraying (see Fig. 16.8) where DDT was used. The *Anopheles* mosquitoes were affected by the repellent action of DDT and changed their feeding time to dawn and dusk, rather than increasing to a maximum peak at midnight. It is probably not possible to utilize this as a main control method, but it is a subsidiary benefit where insecticides are being used.

Reduction of the number of adult worms

Unfortunately, there is no specific drug which acts on the adult worms, although DEC causes substantial mortality. The worms lie embedded in the lymphatics so cannot be removed surgically without damage, as practised in onchocerciasis control. Adults live for approximately 10 years (range 7–12 years), so, if reinfection can be prevented for this period, adult worms will die off and there will be no reservoir of infection. It is maintaining control methods for this period of time that is crucial with filariasis.

General points with filariasis control

The need for control methods to continue for many years has been constantly stressed above. If vector control methods are implemented, no microfilarial reduction will be seen for the first 2 or 3 years but then a steady decline will take place. The control method does not have to be very rigorous, but duration is essential.

In *Anopheles*-transmitted filariasis, there is a threshold microfilarial density and, if density can be maintained below the threshold, either by vector control for about 10 years or drug therapy for at least 5, the disease can be expected to die out. With culicine mosquitoes, the absence of a pharyngeal armature permits infection to occur with very low densities and it is also possible they may be able to concentrate microfilariae. Eradication is therefore more difficult and the disease can be expected to return once control methods have been removed.

Drug therapy is the main method of control, but vector control may be a feasible alternative, especially if the disease is transmitted by *Anopheles* mosquitoes and malaria is also a problem. Larval reduction can be used as an ancillary method. Personal protection can be surprisingly effective if followed diligently and methods such as impregnated mosquito nets could be effective on a large scale.

Due to the prolonged period of control required, intermittent mass chemotherapy at annual intervals is more cost-effective than limited intensive treatment for culicine-transmitted filariasis. Case finding and treatment are satisfactory in anopheline-borne infection.

16.8 *BRUGIA MALAYI*

This parasite has many similarities with *W. bancrofti*, with which it was originally grouped, but, since an animal reservoir has also been found, it is now considered to be a different genus. Rodents, monkeys and a large number of other animals harbour the parasite. There are two periodic rhythms, an aperiodic one in the animal reservoir and a nocturnally periodic one in humans.

B. malayi is transmitted mainly by *Mansonia* and *Anopheles* mosquitoes. The *Mansonia* mosquitoes are particularly difficult to control because the larvae attach themselves to the underside of water plants, where they are immune to surface oils and larvicides. Removal of these water plants by hand or with herbicides has produced some effect. No attempts have been made to diminish the animal reservoir. All the control methods used for *W. bancrofti* are also applicable, except that, with an animal reservoir, eradication is unlikely to be achieved. Reducing the number of infective bites will be effective where there is an animal reservoir. Eradication has been achieved in parts of China, where the vector is *A. sinensis* and there is no animal reservoir, using case finding and treatment.

Lymphoedema and, to an extent, elephantiasis lesions have decreased following repeated doses of DEC in the related species *B. timori*. Prolonged administration of DEC might also have some effect on the gross pathology of *W. bancrofti* and *B. malayi*.

16.9 ONCHOCERCIASIS

Differing from lymphatic filariasis, the microfilariae of onchocerciasis (*Onchocercus volvulus*) have a predilection for the skin and eye, leading in time to blindness. The vector, *Simulium*, breeds in fast-flowing streams, so the disease is associated with riverine areas, giving it its other name of river blindness. The distribution of the disease, principally in Africa and tropical America, is shown in Fig. 16.14.

It is convenient to consider onchocerciasis in four separate components: microfilaria, adult worm, vector and host.

16.9.1 Microfilariae

- Are found in the skin. Measured skin snips estimate density.
- Survive for up to 2.5 years.
- Density is important for infecting flies and in clinical effects.
- Periodicity, peak at 4. p.m. to 6 p.m., but relatively unimportant.
- Developmental cycle 6–13 days, depending on temperature.

16.9.2 Adults

- Live in skin, many of them in palpable nodules.
- Have greater chance of meeting and mating than *W. bancrofti*.
- Survive for 16–17 years, producing microfilariae into old age.

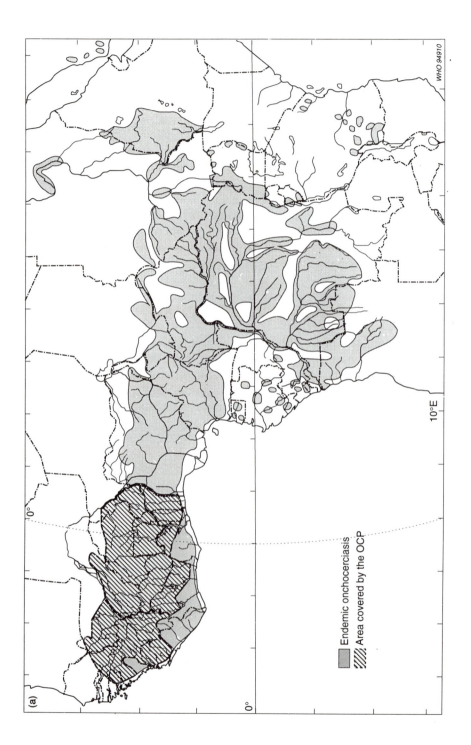

(a)

Endemic onchocerciasis

Area covered by the OCP

WHO 94910

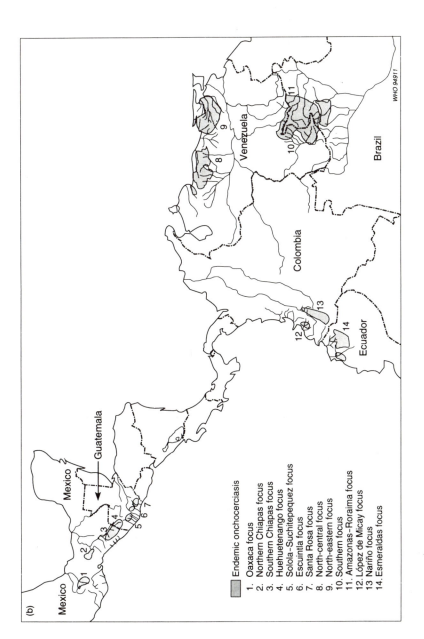

Fig. 16.14. Distribution of onchocerciasis. (a) Africa and the Arabian peninsula. (b) The Americas. OCP, Onchocerciasis Control Project. (From World Health Organization Technical Report Series (1995), *Onchocerciasis and its Control*, No. 852. Reproduced with permission of the World Health Organization, Geneva.)

The following labels appear on the map:

Mexico
Mexico
Guatemala
Colombia
Venezuela
Brazil
Ecuador

WHO 94911

Endemic onchocerciasis

1. Oaxaca focus
2. Northern Chiapas focus
3. Southern Chiapas focus
4. Huehuetenango focus
5. Solola–Suchitepequez focus
6. Escuintla focus
7. Santa Rosa focus
8. North-central focus
9. North-eastern focus
10. Southern focus
11. Amazonas–Roraima focus
12. López de Micay focus
13. Nariño focus
14. Esmeraldas focus

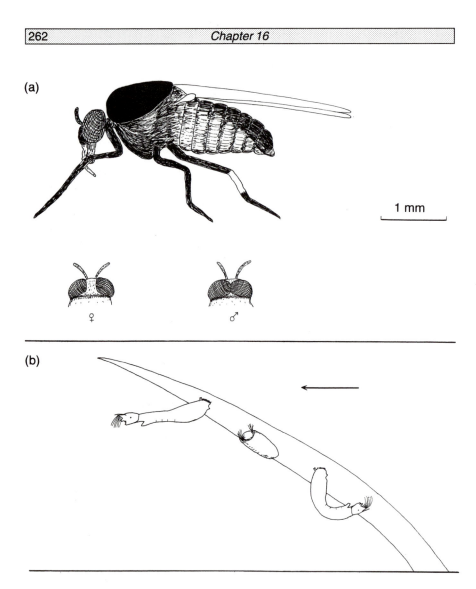

Fig. 16.15. *Simulium*, the vector of onchocerciasis. (a) Adult. (b) Larvae and pupa attached to a plant in a stream flowing in the direction of the arrow.

16.9.3 Vectors

- Various species of *Simulium* flies (Fig. 16.15 and Table 16.4).
- Strong flyer, carried by wind, can travel more than 100 km.
- Maximum density at breeding place. Focal infection.
- Daytime biting, but different species prefer different times of day.
- Outdoor biting.
- Biting preference for lower body in Africa, upper in South America.

Table 16.4. *Simulium* vectors of onchocerciasis.

Geographical area	Species	Breeding place	Habitat
West Africa, Central African Republic (CAR), Sudan, Uganda, Ethiopia (Yemen?)	S. damnosum species complex	Large rivers	Savannah, but sometimes forest
West Africa, CAR, Sudan	S. sirbanum	large rivers	Savannah
West Africa, CAR, Zaire	S. squamosum	Small to medium-sized rivers in hilly areas	Forest, savannah, mosaic
West Africa	S. soubrense	Large rivers	Forest, savannah
West Africa	S. sanctipauli	Large rivers	Forest
West Africa	S. yahense	Small watercourses	Forest
Cameroon, CAR, Tanzania	S. mengense	Large rivers	Forest
Zaire, Burundi, Uganda, Tanzania, Malawi	S. kilibanum	Large rivers	Forest
Zaire, Burundi, Rwanda, Uganda, Sudan	S. naevi species complex	Heavily shaded small permanent rivers in forest	Forest
Ethiopia	S. ethiopiense	Heavily shaded small permanent rivers in forest	Forest
Tanzania	S. woodi	Heavily shaded small permanent rivers in forest	Forest
Guatemala, Mexico	S. ochraceum	Small mountain streams	Highlands
Guatemala, Mexico, Venezuela	S. metallicum	Small streams	Highlands
Colombia, Ecuador, Venezuela	S. exiguum	Large rivers	Lowlands
Brazil, Venezuela	S. guianense	Large, fast-flowing rivers	Highlands
Brazil, Venezuela	S. oyapockense	Large rivers	Lowlands

- Most South American *Simulium* have pharyngeal armatures, African *Simulium* do not. Mortality due to superinfection not important in transmission.
- Many *Simulium* bite animals as well as humans.
- Longevity 2–3 weeks (maximum 3 months).

16.9.4 Host

- *O. volvulus* only infects humans (and epidemiologically insignificant chimpanzees and gorillas).
- Eye and skin pathology related to proximity of nodules.

- In Africa, savannah infection produces more blindness than forest infection.

16.9.5 Control

There are various approaches to control.

- Reduction of fly density.
- Avoidance of fly breeding places.
- Decrease in microfilarial density.
- Reduction of the number of adult worms.
- Reduction in the number of *Simulium* bites.

Reducing the fly density (larval reduction)

The larvae breed in water, so insecticide is sprayed on streams and rivers. The larvae are relatively sensitive to insecticides, so low-dose applications – 0.05 to 0.1 mg l^{-1} – are effective. Temephos (Abate) is suitable, as it is effective in a very low dose, is relatively non-toxic to fish and retains some residual action. It exerts its effect for some 20–40 km downstream in the wet season. The main difficulty is to ensure that every watercourse is treated. Owing to the flies' ability to cover large distances, recolonization soon takes place when insecticidal applications are discontinued. Although expensive, the extra cost of using aircraft and helicopters can be justified if many watercourses, spread over large areas of countryside, have to be covered.

Unfortunately, insecticidal resistance has occurred in a number of areas, so biological control with *Bacillus thuringiensis* is an alternative. This does not have the spreading power of insecticides and greater concentrations need to be used (in the order of 0.9 mg l^{-1}); it has to be mixed with water before it can be applied.

Avoidance of fly breeding places

Maximum contact between humans and flies occurs near *Simulium* breeding places, at rivers, when water needs to be collected. An association between rivers and the symptoms of the disease, particularly blindness, is known to the local people, which has led to depopulation of areas. Alternative water sources, such as wells or a piped supply, remove the need to visit rivers.

Reducing the microfilarial density

Ivermectin immobilizes microfilariae, which are flushed out of the skin and eye and killed in the lymph nodes. As microfilarial death occurs away from the skin and eye, irritation is minimized and ocular reaction reduced. It can be given as a single dose with retreatment at 6- and 18-month intervals. This means that mass therapy for onchocerciasis can be used as an adjunct to vector control.

Reducing the number of adult worms

Since the adult worms live for a considerable period of time, during all of which they are producing microfilariae, specific attack on the adult parasites can reduce both the symptoms and the potential for transmitting infection. There are two ways of attacking the adults.

- Suramin has a specific action on the adult worm and, as a consequence, on the number of microfilariae. However, it can produce severe complications and should only be used in selected patients, under strict medical attention.
- Nodulectomy, or the surgical removal of adult worms from skin nodules, can be a relatively effective procedure. This is particularly practised in the Guatemala onchocercal areas, as nodules are more commonly found in the upper parts of the body, where they are likely to produce ocular lesions.

Reduction in the number of Simulium bites

Personal protection is less effective against *Simulium* than with mosquitoes, as bed nets and coils are inappropriate. The wearing of long-sleeved shirts and long trousers with hat and net can be used by individuals investigating the disease, but are not methods that can be developed for mass use. Repellents have some effect. Avoiding passage through breeding sites will reduce fly biting.

General points on onchocerciasis control

As adult O. volvulus can live to a considerable age (15–17 years), any control programme would need to be maintained for this length of time before eradication could take place. However, most programmes seek to reduce the intensity of infection to a level where symptoms are absent. Two criteria are used in the Onchocerciasis Control Project (OCP) in West Africa.

- Less than 100 infective larvae per human per year.
- Annual biting rates of less then 1000.

The main method of control is using larvicides which can be extremely effective if carried out thoroughly. Species eradication of *S. naevi* was achieved in Kenya by methodically treating every watercourse with DDT. Where the disease covers a limited area, a similarly intense programme may be considered. Where there is a more diffuse focus, the borders of control need to be extended sufficiently to prevent reinvasion by *Simulium*. While resistance is a serious problem, resistant *Simulium* are less important in transmission.

With the advent of ivermectin, mass drug therapy or selective therapy for persons with heavy infections can be given right from the start of the programme. This will rapidly reduce the microfilarial level and the potential for infecting flies. Preventing blindness (with ivermectin) has been particularly valuable in obtaining the cooperation of people. Nodulectomy is a simple additional technique.

16.10 *LOA LOA*

Loiasis is a filarial infection found in West and Central African rain forests. The life cycle of the parasite is essentially the same as that of *W. bancrofti* except that the vectors are tabanid flies, *Chrysops*. These large, powerful flies inflict a painful bite, attacking either within the forest or on the forest fringe.

The disease is characterized by Calabar swellings (named after a town in eastern Nigeria), which are transient, itchy swellings. Fever and eosinophilia suggest they have an allergic aetiology. *L. loa* is often confusingly called the eye worm (to be differentiated from *O. volvulus*) as it is sometimes seen migrating across the conjunctiva, but it produces no pathology in the eye.

It is diurnally periodic and diagnosis is made by examining daytime blood. Both adults and microfilariae are killed by DEC, but caution needs to be exercised as allergic reactions can be profound. Low dosages of 0.1 mg kg^{-1} can be used to initiate treatment, gradually building up over 8 days to 8.6 mg kg^{-1}, which is continued for 3 weeks. Steroid cover may be required in those with more than 30 microfilariae mm^{-3}.

Extensive control measures are generally not warranted, the main preventive action being against the bites of *Chrysops*. Clearing the forest canopy, oiling of pools and mass treatment (with considerable caution) are methods that have been practised in areas of high transmission.

16.11 *MANSONELLA OZZARDI, M. PERSTANS* AND *M. STREPTOCERCA*

These three filarial parasites of humans are found commonly in blood and skin smears, but they produce little or no pathology. They are of minimal significance except to be differentiated from *W. bancrofti, O. volvulus* and *L. loa* (see Fig. 16.12).

16.12 TRYPANOSOMIASIS

There are two forms of trypanosomiasis, well defined by geographical limits – sleeping sickness, found in Africa, and Chagas' disease, found in Central and South America. They are caused by species of *Trypanosoma*.

16.13 SLEEPING SICKNESS

There are two forms of sleeping sickness in Africa, that due to *Trypanosoma brucei gambiense*, which produces a chronic disease, and that due to *T. b. rhodesiense*, an acute and fatal infection if not treated (Fig. 16.16). When seen in human blood, trypanosomes are either long slender, intermediate or short stumpy forms, probably representing a cycle of antigenic variation. They are introduced into the blood by the bite of the tsetse fly and multiply locally. After being disseminated round the body, they continue to multiply, rapidly in *T. b. rhodesiense*, less so in *T. b. gambiense*.

The forms produced in human blood are infective to any tsetse fly. They are taken up into the midgut, where they multiply, migrate into the space between the peritrophic membrane and the gut wall and pass forward to the salivary glands. The epimastigote (Fig. 16.17) becomes a trypomastigote, which is the infective form, introduced when the fly takes another blood meal. Mechanical transfer can occasionally happen if a contaminated fly bites another person within a short space of time.

The bite of the tsetse fly generally causes a local reaction, but 7–10 days after it has subsided it becomes red and inflamed, the first sign of infection. Trypanosomes multiply at the bite site and aspirated fluid will contain the dividing forms. In *T. b. gambiense* an enlargement of the lymph glands takes place, especially those in the cervical region. This rarely occurs in *T. b. rhodesiense*, the disease progressing rapidly to involve the central nervous system (CNS). The main clinical signs are a fever and protracted headaches. In *T. b. gambiense* infection the course is much more prolonged and personality changes can occur, but inevitably the disease leads to progressive lethargy, emaciation, coma and death.

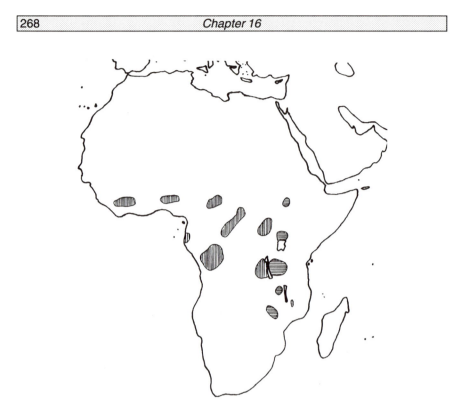

Fig. 16.16. Sleeping sickness foci in Africa. ⊞, *T. b. gambiense*; 昌, *T. b. rhodesiense*.

T. b. *gambiense* mostly occurs to the west of the central rift valley of Africa containing the lakes of Tanganyika, Kivu, etc., and *T. b. rhodesiense* to the east (Fig. 16.16). *T. b. gambiense* infection is particularly prevalent in Zaire and *T. b. rhodesiense* in Tanzania. These two types of diseases differ markedly in their epidemiology and control.

16.13.1 Glossina *(Tsetse Fly)*

The tsetse fly is easily recognized by its characteristic stance and behaviour. A large powerful fly, it rests on a surface with wings folded like a pair of scissors. Within the venation of these wings, a characteristic hatchet cell (Fig. 16.18) is defined. There is normally no doubt about identification when passing through 'fly' country, as they attack any moving object in large numbers, rendering a most painful bite. They are attracted by movement and will cling to the side of a vehicle travelling at 30–40 k.p.h. without being dislodged. They prefer dark colours and if there is a large object they will fly to that in preference. They are more

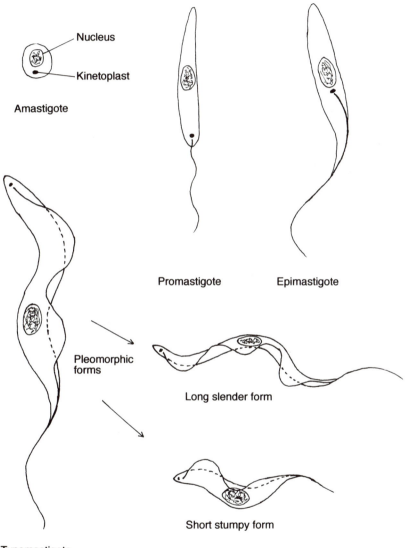

Nucleus

Kinetoplast

Amastigote

Promastigote

Epimastigote

Pleomorphic forms

Long slender form

Short stumpy form

Typomastigote

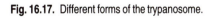

Fig. 16.17. Different forms of the trypanosome.

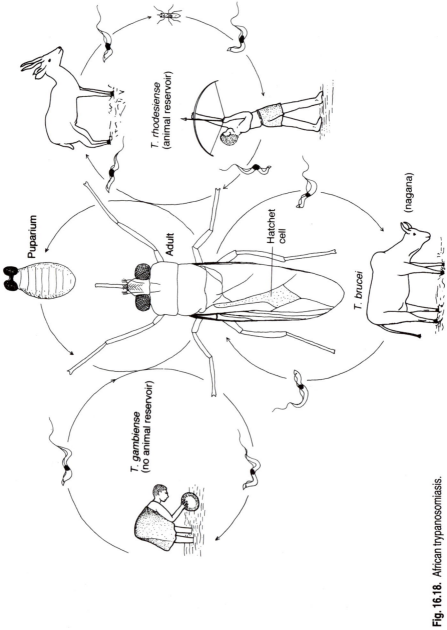

Puparium

Adult

Hatchet
cell

T. rhodesiense
(animal reservoir)

T. gambiense
(no animal reservoir)

T. brucei

(nagana)

Fig. 16.18. African trypanosomiasis.

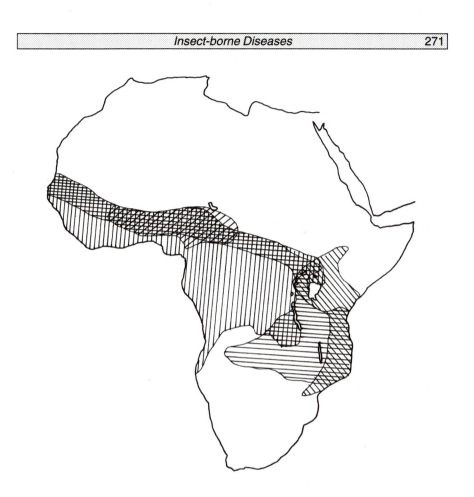

Fig. 16.19. Tsetse fly distribution. ▤, *Glossina morsitans*; ▥, *G. palpalis* and *G. fuscipes*; ▨, *G. tachinoides*; ▧, *G. pallidipes*.

abundant near their breeding place in the sandy soil beside rivers.

Distribution of tsetse flies is shown in Figure 16.19 where it will be noticed that distinct species are often related to particular sleeping sickness areas (compare with Fig. 16.16). Table 16.5 is a simplified guide to identifying the species of *Glossina*, but professional confirmation should always be obtained.

16.13.2 Gambiense Sleeping Sickness

Sleeping sickness, as with other vector-borne diseases is determined by the habits of the vector. In the gambiense type, the tsetse fly breeds in the tunnel of forest along the course of rivers (Fig. 16.20). Although powerful flyers, they do not range far from this shaded protection but

Table 16.5. A simplified key to *Glossina* of medical importance and their favoured habitats.

Hind tarsi	all segments dark above	*G. palpalis* group (1)
	only two distal segments dark above	*G. morsitans* group (2)
1.	Abdomen obviously banded dorsally	*G. tachinoides*
	Abdomen dark, unbanded dorsally	*G. palpalis* (W. Africa)
		G. fuscipes (E. Africa)
2.	Distal two segments of front and middle tarsi *without* dark tip	*G. pallidipes*
	Last two segments of front and middle tarsi *with* dark tips	(3)
3.	Bands of abdomen very distinct and sharply rectangular	*G. swynnertoni*
	Bands on abdomen rounded medially and less distinct	*G. morsitans*
In summary the vectors of *T. gambiense* are		*G. palpalis*
		G. tachinoides
		G. morsitans
and of *T. rhodesiense*		*G. morsitans*
		G. pallidipes
		G. fuscipes
		G. swynnertoni
		G. tachinoides (in S.W. Ethiopia)
Favoured habitats		
a.	Lake and riverside fringing forest	*G. palpalis*
		G. tachinoides
		G. fuscipes (near Lake Victoria)
b.	Fringing forest without permanent water	*G. pallidipes*
c.	Miombo woodland, thickets and game savannah woodland	*G. morsitans*
d.	Restricted to northern Tanzania game savannah woodland	*G. swynnertoni*

travel extensively through this tunnel of forest in search of blood meals. Any mammals, including humans that come to the river to drink or cross are attacked and fed upon.

The important reservoir of *T. b. gambiense* infection is humans (although the domestic pig may be involved), and those whose occupation brings them into contact with the infected fly are more likely to succumb to infection. Since women are involved in the collection of water, the preparation of food and the washing of clothes, they are more commonly infected in gambiense sleeping sickness.

The disease can occur in endemic and epidemic form. There are well-known foci from which people become infected at a constant rate, but movements of infected flies or, especially, people into new areas can

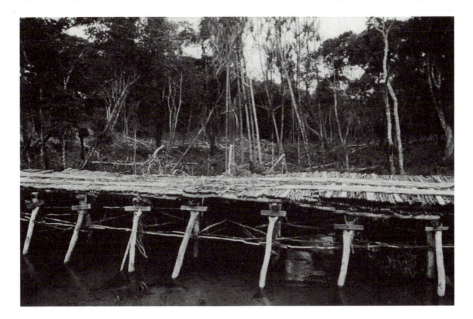

Fig. 16.20. Tunnel of forest along the banks of a river with selective clearance (leaving the big trees).

initiate epidemics. Generally, infected flies are comparatively few in number, so that a large number of bites are required before a person becomes infected. Where the community that is fed upon is small and stable (less than 10 persons km^{-2}), there are only a few cases, who are either cured or die. When this community is much larger (above 10 persons km^{-2}), as when an infected person travels to a more densely populated area, the infection can be transmitted to other people, who in turn form a reservoir to infect more flies, and an increasing number of cases occur. Epidemic sleeping sickness is more likely in *T. b. gambiense* infection, as it is a more chronic disease and cases provide a reservoir (to infect flies) before symptoms cause them to seek medical attention. While endemic foci are difficult to eradicate, control measures should prevent epidemics from occurring. In mass examination of the population or ongoing surveillance, examination for enlarged cervical nodes and gland puncture can be used. Immunobiological methods are being increasingly used. A cheap and accurate method is the Card agglutination test (CATT), in which a drop of finger-prick blood is mixed with a suspension of trypanosomes and the result read directly.

16.13.3 Rhodesiense Sleeping Sickness

The principal vector of *T. b. rhodesiense* is *G. morsitans*, which breeds along watercourses, but then travels widely throughout the extensive shade cover provided by the forest belt. This open type of forest, commonly called *Miombo* (mainly *Brachystegia* and *Julbemardi* spp.), is found in large areas of East Africa. It is inhabited by smaller wild animals, especially the bushbuck, which form a reservoir of infection. Towards the margins of this forest belt, it breaks up into thickets separated by savannah grassland in which large numbers of wild animals are found. The tsetse fly ranges widely over these areas, feeding on animals and using the thickets for cover and shade.

Rhodesiense sleeping sickness is mainly an occupational disease of the hunter, the honey collector and the woodcutter, who travel through the forest and fringing savannah. Adult males are therefore the main sufferers.

Rhodesiense infection is not a focal disease and, because of its short clinical course, epidemics are uncommon. However, movements of people, such as the development of new settlements in forest areas, can encourage the flies to establish a more regular feeding pattern on the human population so that, if an infected person enters this community, serial transmission and an epidemic will occur. The first signs that this is happening is where women and, especially, children become infected.

Various species of *Glossina* are able to transmit *T. b. rhodesiense* and, although *G. morsitans* is the commonest, riverine tsetse that transmit *T. b. gambiense* sleeping sickness can also be involved.

16.13.4 Control

Methods of control are most easily understood by considering the vector, parasite and host.

Vector control

A knowledge of the habits and behaviour of the local vector is necessary before embarking on methods of vector control. The environment is modified so that it is unsuitable for the fly, but not so damaged that the water-table is affected or soil eroded.

With the riverine type of habitat, areas of the forest tunnel are cleared. Total clearance is not required, as this leads to erosion of river banks, so a selective form of clearance can be performed, as illustrated in Fig. 16.20. The big trees are left with their extensive root systems, but all dense undergrowth is removed. Clearance should be continued for half a kilometre on either side of a river crossing, water collection place or inhabited area.

In East Africa, where extensive forest provides a habitat for the fly, the forest margin is pushed back from any place of habitation. A band of at least 1 km, preferably 2 or 3, should be left between the area of habitation and the forest. This must also include any cultivated area, and regulations are required to prevent people from moving into the cleared part to start new cultivation. Ringbarking is a more economical method of forest clearance than cutting down every tree.

Where forest clearance is impractical, insecticides can be used. This is easiest along the course of substantial rivers, using a boat and spraying the forest on either side. In the savannah-type habitat, isolated thickets can be treated. Extensive insecticidal application to *miombo* forest is inappropriate. Insecticides have to be repeated whereas forest clearance is permanent, and the relative costs of these two techniques need to be considered.

The vector can also be controlled by trapping. A well-designed trap will collect enough flies to considerably reduce the biting risk. An effective trap has a fine metal mesh treated with insecticides; it is shaded to attract tsetse flies, which are rapidly killed when they touch the screen. These must be regularly maintained.

Parasite reduction

Finding the parasite is often quite difficult. For *T. b. gambiense*, the organism is aspirated by needle puncture from enlarged glands. In *T. b. rhodesiense*, blood smears are satisfactory, although several may need to be taken before a positive is found. Blood-concentration techniques are valuable where the facilities are available.

In a sleeping sickness area a *surveillance* service should be set up. Sleeping sickness workers are recruited more on their knowledge of the local community than on their medical skills, as the simple techniques of gland puncture or making a blood slide can easily be taught. The workers cover a set area and take slides from people with symptoms of persistent fever and headache, or from those who pursue a particular occupation, such as hunters, honey collectors or woodcutters. In *T. b. gambiense* infection, palpation for neck glands can provide a useful estimate of prevalence.

Finding cases in the early stages of the disease not only increases the chance of successful treatment, but also removes a potential source of infection of tsetse flies. In an epidemic of *T. b. rhodesiense*, a mass blood-slide examination can be performed in the worst-affected areas to detect asymptomatic cases.

Treatment of cases requires hospitalization as the drugs are highly toxic. Suramin is effective in early and intermediate cases of both *T. b.*

rhodesiense and *T. b. gambiense*. When the central nervous system (CNS) is involved, melarsoprol is the drug of choice. Eflornithine is very effective in all stages of *T. b. gambiense* infection (including cerebral), but is not effective in *T. b. rhodesiense*. Pentamidine has been used as a prophylactic against *T. b. gambiense* for people at special risk. There is no prophylactic against *T. b. rhodesiense* infection.

Another approach to reducing the parasite reservoir in *T. b. rhodesiense* is to destroy the animal population. This used to be practised on a wide scale, but animal conservation has now questioned the wanton slaughter of animals. In most cases it will be found that the human reservoir is more important than the animal, but where there is evidence that flies are becoming infected from this alternative source then game can be killed or driven off.

Alteration of the human habitat

Sleeping sickness has been responsible for large movements of people from their traditional homelands, either by self-choice, or by government action, to avoid an epidemic. Moving people away from the sleeping-sickness areas is the ultimate method of control, but one to be taken only when all else fails.

The preferable alternative to moving populations is to modify the habitat so that it is unsuitable for transmission. Methods of forest clearance have already been described, while providing water supplies will remove the reliance on obtaining water from rivers.

The density of population largely determines the endemicity, as mentioned above. Two different approaches can be taken.

- Keep the population close together and clear an area of forest around them.
- Encourage the people to spread out very widely so that they partially clear a large area of forest.

In the first method the people are safe as long as they remain within the village, but once they pass through the forest they are subjected to a considerable number of bites. In the second alternative, people will become infected in the initial stages of forest clearance, but once this has been done protection will be much greater and more use can be made of the land. In the initial period of forest clearance, a surveillance service will be required to find these pioneer cases. The most unsatisfactory solution is a moderately large population spread evenly over the area, this is the potential situation for an epidemic.

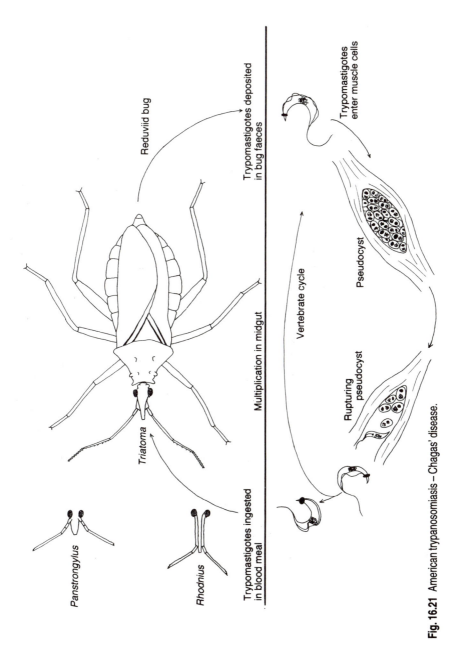

Reduviid bug

Trypomastigotes deposited in bug faeces

Trypomastigotes enter muscle cells

Multiplication in midgut

Vertebrate cycle

Pseudocyst

Rupturing pseudocyst

Triatoma

Trypomastigotes ingested in blood meal

Panstrongylus

Rhodnius

Fig. 16.21 American trypanosomiasis – Chagas' disease.

16.14 CHAGAS' DISEASE

American trypanosomiasis or Chagas' disease presents as an acute infection, generally in children, with fever, local swelling at the site of inoculation and enlargement of the regional lymph nodes. After the acute phase has subsided, chronic symptoms occur from enlarged heart, colon and other parts of the body. Heart failure and cardiac irregularities are common, leading to disability and death.

16.14.1 Epidemiology

Chagas' disease is caused by *Trypanosoma cruzi* and transmitted by Reduviidae bugs. The parasite life cycle is illustrated in Fig. 16.21.

Occurring throughout South and Central America (Fig. 16.22), the epidemiology of this disease differs from area to area according to the species of the Reduviidae and the reservoirs of infection. Essentially, though, there are two cycles, *wild* and *domestic*, which are illustrated in Fig. 16.23.

In the wild cycle, armadillos, opossums, raccoons and a number of other animals have been found infected, living in close proximity to their burrow-inhabiting bugs. This infection remains as a zoonosis until disturbed by a domestic animal, commonly a dog, that ferrets around the burrows of these wild animals. It is attacked by the bugs and acquires the infection. On returning to the house, the dog becomes a reservoir for the domestic bugs. After 8–10 days, the bugs become infective and transmit the disease to man.

In Central America the cycle is semidomestic, with the reservoir maintained in the domestic rat (*Rattus rattus*), from which house-haunting bugs pass on the infection to people in the house. Although the bugs feed on humans it is the passage of trypanosomes in the bug faeces, which are rubbed into the wound or conjunctiva, that produces the infection.

The bugs live in cracks in the walls and floors and within the thatch in the roof. The mud-and-wattle type of structure is particularly suited to the conditions required. The number of bugs hiding within the cracks and crevices can be several hundred.

Infection can also be transmitted by blood transfusion. Small epidemics in a group of people sharing the same food suggest that bug faecal contamination of food could lead to transmission by the oral route.

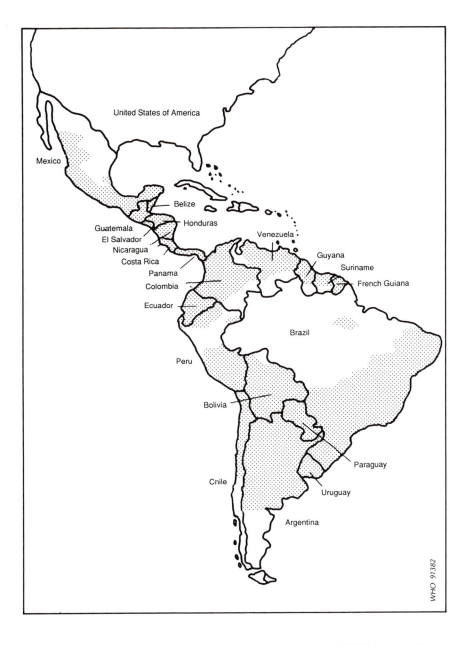

Fig. 16.22. Distribution of Chagas' disease. (Reproduced, by permission from WHO Expert Committee (1991) *Control of Chagas' Disease: Report of a WHO Expert Committee*, World Health Organization, Geneva.)

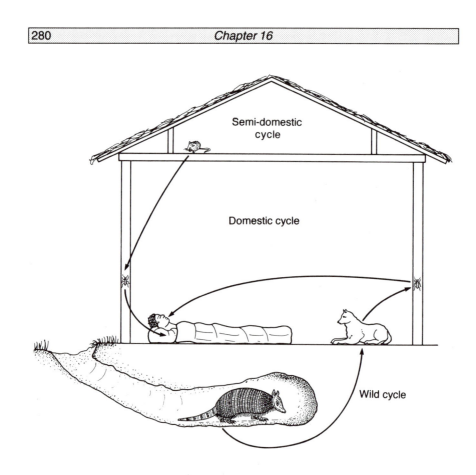

Fig. 16.23. Epidemiology of American trypanosomiasis.

16.14.2 Control

The methods of control are to reduce the number of bugs that can come into close proximity with humans and the reservoir of disease. These requirements are both satisfied by improvements to housing. Unfortunately, trypanosomiasis is a disease of poverty and building new and better houses is rather impractical in this segment of the population. If assistance can be given, proper foundations and cement walls will not only deny a place for the bugs to live, but also prevent rats and armadillos from making their burrows underneath them. Even with existing houses much can be done by applying a layer of mud plaster to walls and erecting a simple ceiling. Where cost prohibits any of these methods, residual insecticides can be sprayed on the walls and ceilings. This can be effectively carried out as a control programme, using a similar methodology to malaria. Firstly, a pyrethrum spray is administered, which draws the bugs out of their hiding places and marks the infected houses. In the attack phase, a residual insecticide is sprayed on all houses in an infected locality (not just infested houses). A second spraying is made 90 days after the first to houses where bugs have been found in either the preliminary or the attack phase. Spraying continues at this time interval until the number of infested houses falls below 5%. Maintenance is achieved by regular house searches, instituting focal spraying when reinfestation is discovered.

An alternative is to protect the individual from being bitten by the use of mosquito nets. If the net is impregnated with an insecticide (e.g. permethrin), this will prevent the bug from feeding through the net if it is touching the body.

The dog is probably the most important domestic reservoir and householders should question the value of maintaining such animals if they are proving a threat to the health of the family. Good hygiene, trapping and poison will keep down rats. Control of the wild reservoir is unlikely to be successful.

In areas of high endemicity screening of blood donors is required and crystal violet (1:4000) can be added to the blood.

16.15 LEISHMANIASIS

Leishmaniasis is a group of diseases due to infection with *Leishmania*, present in a number of different forms. They are defined more by geographical boundaries (Fig. 16.24) than by climate or socio-economic factors, which largely determine the distribution of other diseases. Transmitted by the minute and fragile phlebotomine sandflies, they have a complex parasitology.

There are three main clinical forms of the disease, cutaneous, mucocutaneous and visceral (kala-azar). The cutaneous infection starts with a papule and enlarges to become an indolent ulcer, which either heals or lasts for many years. In the New World infections, a more aggressive form of mucocutaneous leishmaniasis (espundia, chiclero ulcer) results in nasopharyngeal destruction and hideous deformities. The visceral form is a chronic infection, with fever, hepatosplenomegaly, lymphadenopathy and anaemia. There is progressive emaciation and weakness, with generally a fatal outcome if not treated. Post-kala-azar dermal leishmaniasis can occur after apparent cure of the visceral case.

Treatment is with sodium stibogluconate or meglumine antimonate, but pentamidine or amphotericin B may be required in cases that do not respond, especially in mucocutaneous leishmaniasis. Because of the toxicity of the preparations, treatment should be undertaken in hospital.

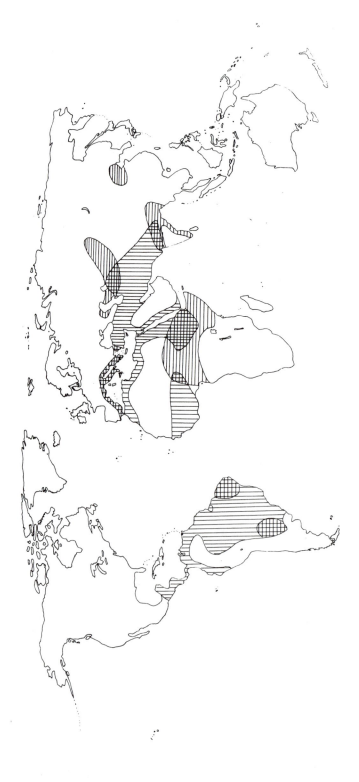

Fig. 16.24. The global distribution of cutaneous and visceral leishmaniasis. ▥, Cutaneous; ▤ visceral.

16.5.1 Parasitology

There are seven species of *Leishmania* and a number of subspecies.

• Visceral leishmaniasis	*L. donovani* (*donovani, infantum, chagasi, archibaldi*)
• Mucocutaneous	*L. braziliensis* (*braziliensis, peruviana*)
	L. guyanensis (*guyanensis, panamensis*)
• New World cutaneous	*L. mexicana* (*mexicana, amazonensis, pifanoi, garnhami, venezuelensis*)
• Old World cutaneous	*L. major*
• Old World cutaneous	*L. tropica* (*killicki, tropica*)
• Old World cutaneous	*L. aethiopica*

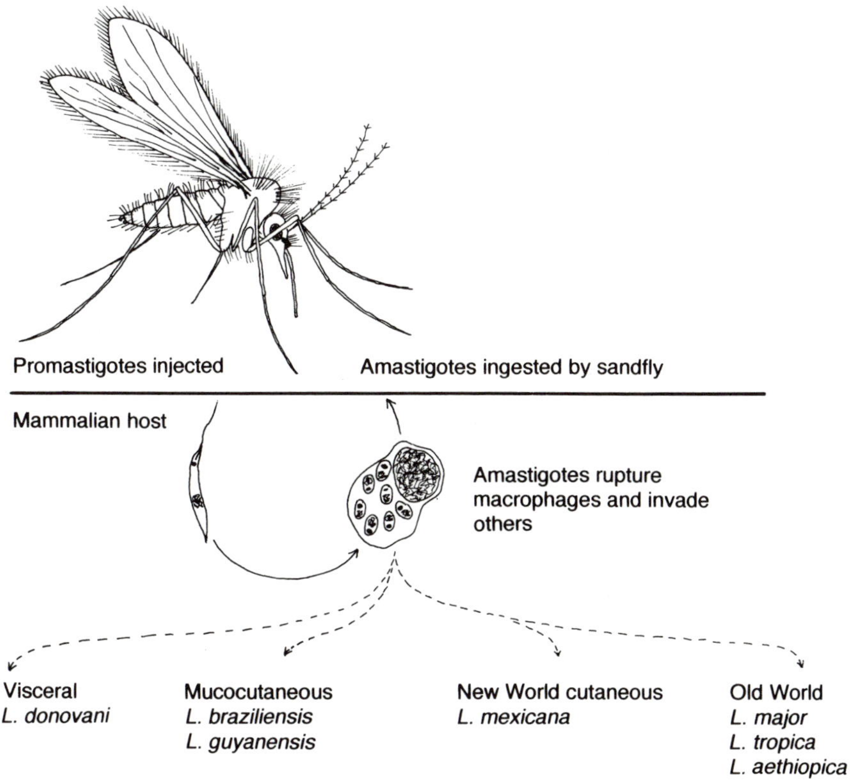

Promastigotes injected   Amastigotes ingested by sandfly

Mammalian host

Amastigotes rupture
macrophages and invade
others

Visceral	Mucocutaneous	New World cutaneous	Old World
L. donovani	*L. braziliensis*	*L. mexicana*	*L. major*
	L. guyanensis		*L. tropica*
			L. aethiopica

Fig. 16.25. Leishmaniasis.

They are all transmitted by the bite of the sandfly and undergo the same simple life cycle. Promastigotes enter humans with the bite of the sandfly, change into amastigotes (see Fig. 16.17), and are engulfed by macrophages. They multiply and finally rupture the cell, invading other macrophages. When the sandfly takes a blood meal, they change into promastigotes. These multiply continuously so that the number produced can be so large as to block the foregut. When the insect next bites, it is forced to regurgitate promastigotes into the host before it can take a blood meal (Fig. 16.25).

In cutaneous leishmaniasis the amastigotes remain at the site of introduction, contained by the macrophages of the skin. In visceral leishmaniasis, large mononuclear cells and polymorphonuclear leucocytes become invaded and subsequently carry the parasites to the viscera, especially the liver, spleen and bone marrow. The mucocutaneous form is intermediate, the parasite restricting its attack to the reticuloendothelial system of the mucous membranes of the mouth, nose and throat.

The epidemiology is due to the intimate relationship between the vector and humans and the non-human reservoirs that maintain the disease.

16.5.2 Vectors

Phlebotomus and *Lutzomyia* are weak flyers, utilizing a hopping flight that carries them only a short distance from the habitat. They require conditions of high humidity, found in animal burrows in arid areas as well as in moist tropical forests. Typical habitats are tree holes, animal burrows, termite hills, rock crevices, foliage clumps and fissures that develop in the ground during the dry season.

The life cycle, from oviposition to emergence of the adult, can take 30–100 days, depending on species and temperature, while the adult lives for approximately 2 weeks. Only the female sucks blood and lizards, birds and mammals are satisfactory alternatives to humans.

Most species feed out of doors during the evening and night, or in the day when there is shade or the weather is overcast. If it is windy, they are unable to fly. They are not able to bite through clothing and mainly attack the lower parts of the body. The main vectors are summarized in Table 16.6.

16.5.3 Reservoir

A range of reservoirs are found in this complex of diseases. In central Asia, cutaneous leishmaniasis is a zoonosis, the gerbil the reservoir and

Table 16.6. The vectors and reservoirs of leishmaniasis.

Type and parasite	Geographical area	Main vector	Reservoir
Visceral			
L. donovani (including infantile)	Mediterranean, S.W. Asia	*Phlebotomus peniciosus, P. ariasi, P. major syriacus, P. longicuspis*	Dogs, foxes
	Central Asia	*P. major syriacus, P. smirnovi, P. longiductus*	Dogs, jackals, foxes
	China	*P. chinensis*	Dogs
	India, Bangladesh	*P. argentipes, P. papatasi*	Humans
	Sudan, Chad	*P. orientalis, P. martini*	Wild rodents and carnivores
	Kenya	*P. martini*	Dogs
	Central and South America	*Lutzomyia longipalpis*	Dogs, foxes
Mucocutaneous			
L. braziliensis	Central and South	*L. wellcomi, L. umbratilis,*	Rodents and forest
L. guyanensis	America	*L. trapidoi*	animals
Cutaneous (New World)			
L. mexicana	Mexico, Belize, Guatemala	*L. olmeca*	Forest rodents
	Amazon basin	*L. flaviscutellata*	Forest rodents
	Peru	*L. peruensis, L. verrucarum*	Dogs
Cutaneous (Old World)			
L. major	Mediterranean	*P. papatasi*	Rodents, dogs, gerbils
	S.W. Asia	*P. papatasi, P. sergenti*	Dogs, rodents
L. tropica	Central Asia	*P. papatasi*	Rodents, gerbils
	India	*P. sergenti*	Dogs
	West Africa	*P. duboscqi*	Dogs, rodents
L. aethiopica	Ethiopia	*P. longpipes*	Hyrax
	Kenya	*P. pedifer*	Rodents

humans accidentally entering the focus become infected. In India there
is a domestic reservoir, mainly dogs, but direct human-to-human transmission also occurs. These are summarized in Table 16.6.

16.5.4 Host

An immunity develops following an infection with the parasite, but
there is little cross-immunity. *L. tropica* has been used for a long time as
an inoculum, inducing a sore on a hidden part of the body so as to prevent
a more disfiguring lesion developing on the face. *L. major* will protect

against L. *tropica* as well as L. *major* lesions and suspensions of living organisms have been prepared for this purpose. There is no cross-immunity with kala-azar and the other species of *Leishmania*, but an attack of kala-azar will protect against developing kala-azar in any other part of the world.

16.5.5 Control

Cases of the disease are normally sporadic and control measures inappropriate, but where an outbreak of the disease occurs specific action can be taken. Because of the fragile nature of the vector, it is easily attacked with insecticides, either as a residual house spray where the vector comes indoors, or by DDT powder blown into mammal burrows, ant hills and similar microhabitats. A longer-term solution is to alter the micro-environment such as by the destruction of termite hills and killing of rodents. Proper control of domestic animals, especially dogs, can be effective where they are important reservoirs. Repellents and personal protection adequately protect the individual from being bitten. Sandfly nets can be used, but the fine mesh required often makes them hot and impractical. Low-dose inocula and attenuated vaccines have been developed to minimize the severity of the disease in some endemic areas.

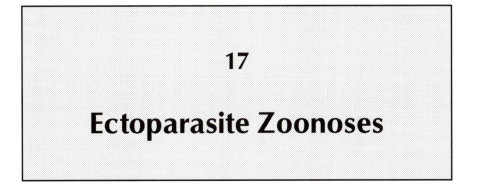

17

Ectoparasite Zoonoses

Ectoparasite zoonoses cover a group of infections that are either vector-borne (by ectoparasites), zoonoses or both. They are sustained within an animal reservoir by ectoparasites which feed on their blood. When humans accidentally become involved in this cycle, infection can occur. Control is of either the ectoparasite, the animal or both.

17.1 PLAGUE

A classic example of an ectoparasite zoonosis is plague, essentially an infection of rodents, in which it is maintained by their flea vectors. The greatest of all epidemic diseases, plague has ravaged Asia and Europe, altering the course of history. Today it is confined to established foci (Fig. 17.1), from which it erupts from time to time, but, fortunately, effective control now prevents the uncontrollable pandemics of the past.

17.1.1 Organism

The fragile organism that causes plague is *Yersinia pestis*, a small oval-shaped bacillus that stains negative with Gram stain. Fresh aspirate from a gland if stained with Giemsa gives a bipolar staining, which can be diagnostic in preliminary field investigations. The organism is sensitive to heat above 55°C, to 0.5% phenol for 15 min and to sunlight. Culture on to blood agar or desoxycholate can be made from blood, throat swabs, sputa and material aspirated from buboes. *Y. pestis* occurs in three varieties, *orientalis*, *antigua* and *mediaevalis*, separated by their ability to ferment glycerol and reduce nitrates. These can be useful in elucidating the oganism in epidemics.

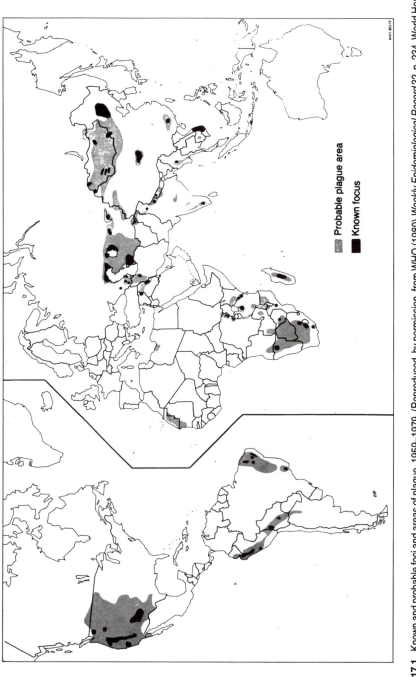
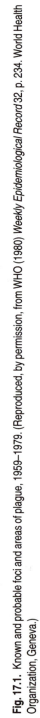

Fig. 17.1. Known and probable foci and areas of plague, 1959–1979. (Reproduced, by permission, from WHO (1980) *Weekly Epidemiological Record* 32, p. 234. World Health Organization, Geneva.)

Probable plague area

Known focus

17.1.2 Reservoir

The reservoirs of infection are mammals, and over 340 species have been found susceptible to plague. These are classically rodents, rats and mice, but many others, including rabbits, monkeys, dogs and camels, have been incriminated.

Rodents differ in their susceptibility, so that a focus will die out where there is a highly susceptible colony but persist where resistance is high. While it is the resistant rodents that maintain a focus, it is the movement of susceptible animals which is responsible for extending plague. Where the speed of mortality is high and the pool of susceptible animals limited, the exacerbation will collapse and the focus return to its original boundary, but, when a coincidence of susceptible rodents abuts domestic rodents, the stage is set for an epidemic in the human population. Foci of infection have been delineated (Fig. 17.1), some of which have given rise to plague outbreaks, while others have all the potential but human disease has not occurred.

17.1.3 Vector

A focus of plague is determined by three factors: the organism, the reservoir host and the flea vector. Many fleas have been incriminated as possible vectors, but species of *Xenopsylla* are the most important (*X. cheopis*, *X. brasiliensis* and *X. astia*). In identifying fleas, they can either have a comb on the head or be combless, *Xenopsylla* being combless. This differentiates *Xenopsylla* from *Ctenocephalides*, which are the common dog and cat fleas. The human flea *Pulex* is also a combless flea, but lacks the other distinguishing feature of *Xenopsylla*, the presence of a meral rod (these important features are illustrated in Fig. 17.2).

Fleas are able to survive for considerable periods without taking a blood meal (6 months) and the larval and pupal stages are well adapted to changing fortune. If there is a limited food supply or low temperature, the larva may prolong this stage from 2 weeks to more than 200 days and the pupae remain cocooned. When vibrations in the habitat, the emission of carbon dioxide or a rise in humidity indicate that an inhabitant has returned, the larva rapidly develops and the emergent flea feeds on the new host. Fleas are not specific, but prefer their normal host species, and fertility may be reduced if they cannot feed on them. Fleas rapidly abandon a dead host and use their powerful hind legs to help them hop on to a new one. Once re-established they tend to crawl around and settle to a regular feeding pattern. If fleas take in *Y. pestis* with their blood meal, these multiply in the proventriculus and lead to a blockage of the feeding apparatus. When the flea tries to feed again, it regurgitates bacteria into the bloodstream while trying to take up blood. It is unsuccessful, so it

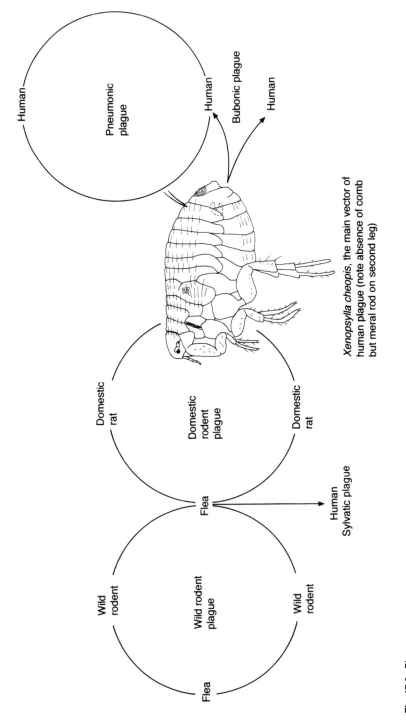

Human — Pneumonic plague

Human — Bubonic plague

Human

Xenopsylla cheopis, the main vector of human plague (note absence of comb but meral rod on second leg)

Domestic rat — Domestic rodent plague — Domestic rat

Human Sylvatic plague

Wild rodent — Wild rodent plague — Wild rodent

Flea

Flea

Fig. 17.2. Plague.

moves to a new host and tries again. Blocked fleas are important in rapidly infecting many people.

17.1.4 Transmission

Figure 17.2 illustrates the different transmission cycles of plague, the trio of bacillus, rodent and flea, into which humans can be fatally drawn. In the established focus of wild rodent plague, infection is maintained in a comparatively resistant colony of animals, who suffer little from the disease. If humans stray into this focus as hunters or trappers, fleas from wild rodents they have killed may bite them and cause plague. This is sylvatic plague and is generally an isolated case with little epidemiological significance. The more important event is when some change takes place in the wild rodent focus and domestic rodents become involved. Wars of nature are similar to wars of humans and a replacement of one group of plague-resistant rodents by another with no resistance could cause a change in the ecological balance. Or, from the opposite approach, an increased domestic rodent population may expand into the wild rodent one. Whichever of these alternative mechanisms takes place, the deprived flea seeks a new host and settles on a domestic rodent. The domestic rodent, being highly susceptible to plague, is rapidly killed, which brings the flea of the domestic rodent in search of a new host and, because of their proximity, humans are likely to become the next victims.

Plague is a disease of civil disturbance and war. In recent history the largest human focus has been in Vietnam. Persistent endemic foci in Madagascar and East Africa produce the most cases at this time. The multimammate rat (*Mastomys natalensis*) acts as an intermediary between the feral rodent reservoir and the domestic rat. Feeding on the remnants of the harvest, it is driven to alternative stores of food in the home when the rains start. This brings a seasonal pattern of plague. If drought occurs, the desperate multimammate rat is forced early into conflict with the domestic rat and an epidemic can occur with the drought.

17.1.5 Clinical

The disease in humans, due to the bite of an infected flea, is called *bubonic plague* after the bubo or swelling that develops at the regional lymph nodes which are draining the site of inoculation. It is commonest in the groin and secondly in the axilla, while it can also occur in the cervical lymph nodes. This latter site is more likely in the case of sylvatic plague, as infection can also occur from ingesting the organism directly from the reservoir rodent. (Some populations eat rodents as a normal item in the diet, while in drought conditions people may be driven to eat whatever they can find, including rats.)

The bubo appears on the first or second day after an *incubation period* of 2–6 days. It is painful and tender, becomes fluctuant and often breaks down to discharge pus. There is an associated high fever, confusion and irritability and signs of haemorrhage may develop. These may be subcutaneous, into the stomach or in the intestines. These symptoms lead to prostration and shock, with death soon after.

In a few cases the disease may be overwhelming from the start, with *septicaemic plague*. All the signs are more severe and develop so rapidly that a bubo is not formed and the patient is dead within a few days. In the generalized spread of the organism around the body, it can invade the lungs and, should a sufferer of bubonic or septicaemic plague start coughing out bacteria, transmission can occur via the respiratory route. This leads to *pneumonic plague*, where spread is from person to person and the flea is not involved. It is highly infectious and lethal, so stringent protective action must be taken. About 5% of bubonic patients develop terminal pneumonia and transmit infection via the respiratory route. The onset of pneumonic plague is very rapid with shallow, rapid breathing, watery blood-stained sputum, high temperature, pulmonary oedema and shock. Death occurs between the third and fifth day.

Asymptomatic cases of plague are common during epidemics and can be detected near foci by antibody testing. A mild form of the disease, with swollen glands and a slight rise in temperature, can occur as *pestis minor*, but many cases go undiagnosed. They tend to occur towards the latter part of an epidemic. During an epidemic, routine throat swabs may detect Y. *pestis*, but there is no good evidence that transmission can occur from these cases.

17.1.6 Treatment

Effective treatment depends upon the speed of making a diagnosis and treating early. If plague has already been diagnosed in the area, a confirmatory test should not be awaited. The clinical presentation of fever and bubo in a severely ill patient can be rapidly confirmed by the finding of bipolar organisms (with Giemsa stain) in an exudate or gland puncture. Otherwise a specimen is sent to a laboratory (Carey–Blair transport medium will preserve the organism) and treatment started immediately. This is by one of the following.

- Tetracycline 3 g orally immediately, followed by 1 g three times a day, up to a total of 40 g.
- Streptomycin 1 g intramuscularly, followed by 0.5 g every 4 hours, up to a total of 20 g.

Chloramphenicol and co-trimoxazole have also been used.

Streptomycin can cause a Herxheimer reaction so tetracycline is preferable in the critically ill. Resistant strains have occurred and the sensitivity of the organism should be monitored.

Isolation of cases is mandatory and the terminal bubonic case with pneumonia or pneumonic plague is highly infectious and extreme precautions should be taken. Gowns and full face masks should be worn, while goggles are required to protect the eyes, as *Y. pestis* can be absorbed through the conjunctiva.

17.1.7 Control

The methods of control depend upon the transmission cycle (Fig. 17.2).

Wild rodent plague foci are often extensive and harmless, and to try and destroy them is a considerable task. If they are localized and close to habitation, it might be feasible to alter the environment by cultivation or in a way that discourages rodents. Precautions need to be taken that a plague epidemic is not generated by such activity. Where hunters or soldiers have to pass through a plague focus, personal protection can be obtained by long trousers tucked into socks, treated with repellents or impregnated with insecticides. Warnings should be given about the danger of touching or eating any animals killed.

Domestic rodent plague depends upon the two components of the rat and the flea, but the order in which they are attacked is crucial according to the stage of the disease. To kill rats during a plague epidemic only makes the infected fleas search for a human host and increases spread. In the presence of plague, *the fleas must be controlled first.* Using insecticide powder (dichlorodiphenyltrichloroethane (DDT), bendiocarb, carbaryl or fenitrothione), burrows can be insufflated and rat runs liberally dusted. Rats pick up insecticide on their fur and take it into their nests with them. Fleas do not like cleanliness and people should be encouraged to wash with soap and warm water. Clothes can be searched and fleas picked off, but it is preferable to boil clothing in order to kill off any larvae or missed adults.

The control of rats can be by cats, traps or poisoning. Rat protection with shields and guards should be used after rats have been removed. A well-trained cat can be most efficient. Trapping is an effective means of rat control if carried out properly. Traps can be made out of scrap pieces of metal and are therefore simply manufactured in Third World countries. A knowledge of the rat runs is gained and the trap left baited but unsprung. Once the bait has been taken, the trap is set. Traps must be visited regularly, all dead rats disposed of (by burning) and the traps set again.

Poisoning can be with either acute or chronic poisons. The number of poisons is considerable and where available it is preferable to solicit professional advice. Poisons strong enough to kill rats are also able to kill other animals that may consume them. They are also dangerous to humans, especially children, so proper safety precautions must be observed. *Zinc phosphate* is a useful acute poison. A good bait should be used, such as broken maize or rice, and the poison is mixed with the bait in a proportion of 1:10, using cooking oil to dissolve the poison. Alternatively, the poison can be mixed with water and bait and then dried out before applying to the traps. There is a danger from the dust and gases produced when preparing baits, so a mask and gloves should be used. Copper sulphate is an antidote and can be administered in 0.25 g portions every 10 minutes until vomiting is induced. The most commonly used chronic poison is *warfarin*, which is mixed with bait in a ratio of 1:19. With chronic poisons, the bait should be placed first and only if it is taken should it be mixed with poison on subsequent applications.

Gassing is very effective, as it kills both rats and fleas at the same time, but strict precautions must be observed. Rodents living in burrows can be gassed, blocking all exits; hydrogen cyanide gas is most commonly used.

Plague vaccine will protect persons at risk for several months, but should not be relied upon. *Chemoprophylaxis*, using 250 mg tetracycline four times a day for a week or doxycycline 100 mg a day for a week should be given to close contacts of cases and to medical workers at risk.

Quarantine of all cases is required by international health regulations for a period of 6 days. All persons should be dusted with insecticides to remove fleas and precautions taken to prevent aerosol spread from pneumonic cases. Any patients dying of plague should be buried or burnt with aseptic precautions.

Surveillance of foci should be maintained, with regular trapping of rodents to examine them for infection and their flea populations.

17.2 TYPHUS

Like plague, typhus is a disease of history, particularly associated with the conflicts of humans. When the anger of humans causes war, disruption of civilizations, famine and refugees, the disease of war, typhus, enters into the attack.

Typhus was confused with typhoid for a considerable period of time because they both produced fever, prostration and a rash. Indeed, typhoid obtained its name when it was finally separated from typhus, as being a less infectious disease, with markedly abdominal symptoms and a milder rash.

There are many similarities between the epidemiology of typhus and that of plague, and it is convenient to approach the disease in the

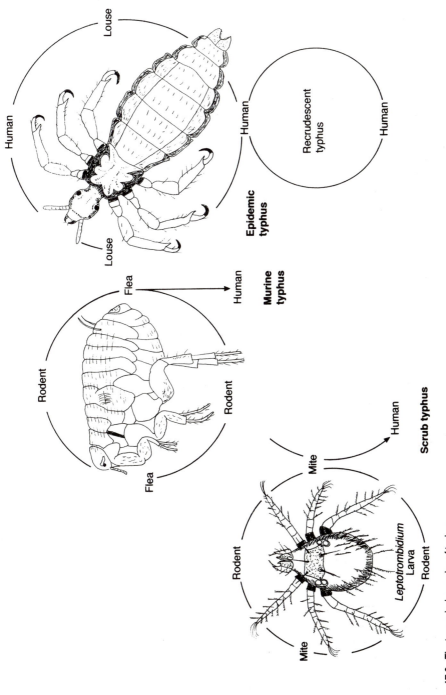

Fig. 17.3. The transmission cycles of typhus.

reverse order to which it is normally described in order to assist in its description. While plague is a composite disease of three different cycles utilizing the same organism and vector, there are three different forms of typhus, each with its own organism and vector (Fig. 17.3).

17.2.1 Organism

The causative organism of typhus is a *Rickettsia*, an intracellular bacteria. Rickettsiae require cellular tissue of humans or the ectoparasite in which to develop and reproduce, but can survive in the environment if suitable conditions prevail (e.g. in louse faeces). Otherwise, they are sensitive to heat, being killed by a temperature of 60°C for 30 min, and they are easily killed by antiseptics.

The typhus-producing rickettsiae and their ectoparasites are as follows.

● Scrub typhus	*R. tsutsugamushi* (*R. orientalis*)	Trombiculid mites
● Murine typhus	*R. mooseri*	Flea, *X. cheopis*
● Epidemic typhus	*R. prowazeki*	Human louse

To differentiate between flea-borne and louse-borne typhus, serological tests are required. Various tests have been developed.

● Labelled antibody techniques using fluorescence or labelled enzyme with enzyme-linked immunosorbent assay (ELISA).
● Haemagglutination tests using red cells coated with specific antigen. In the presence of antibody, agglutination takes place, which can be measured by serial dilution.
● Complement fixation or radioimmune assay technique.

17.2.2 Scrub Typhus

Like wild rodent plague, scrub typhus is a zoonosis in which humans are not involved. Well-defined areas, *mite islands*, harbour rodents, mites and the *Rickettsia* which is transmitted between them. A large number of rodents have been incriminated, including rats, and it is their system of burrows and runs and their range of activity that determine the limits of the mite island. The rodents are fed upon by the larval stage of various leptotrombiculid mites. The nymphs and the adults live on other arthropods, finding all they require to eat among the surrounding vegetation. Only the larva needs to take blood, a necessary requirement for it to become a nymph and subsequently an adult. The larva climbs up on to grass or vegetation and awaits the passage of a rodent or any other passing mammal to which it attaches itself. Once it has fed, it drops off and continues its development in the soil. If during its feeding it sucks up *R. tsutsugamushi*, these develop in the nymph and adult stage so that they are passed transovarially and infect the next generation of bloodsucking larvae. The mites appear to be unaffected by this infection. The mites therefore act as a reservoir of infection, hardly requiring the mammalian host, except to provide a blood meal for their own continuity. Such is the balance of this arrangement that a mite island can persist undisturbed, causing harm to no one unless accidentally entered by humans. The larval mite will attack humans just as it will attack birds and other mammals that come crashing through its hunting ground, transmitting the infection to its unusual host.

The illness in humans commences after an *incubation period* of some 10–12 days (range of 7–21) with fever, headache, exhaustion and progressive prostration. A macular rash appears after a few days and the infective mite bite develops into an eschar. This is a red indurated area with a central vesicle that subsequently breaks down to leave a black scab. This feature is an aid to diagnosis. The severity of the disease varies markedly from area to area, being a severe and fatal illness, similar to epidemic typhus in some places, while in others it is so mild and innocuous that it passes as flu. I remember visiting a school near to a well-known mite island which expected all new students to have a minor illness for a day or two and then be immune for the rest of their academic stay.

As epidemic typhus is historically the disease of disruption and war, scrub typhus is the disease of travelling armies. Large groups of soldiers passing through or camping in mite islands quickly become subject to devastating epidemics. Control is by preventing the larval mite from attacking humans by wearing protective clothing impregnated with repellents or insecticides – long trousers tucked into boots with high lace-up sides or gaiters to cover the gap, impregnated with diethyltoluamide, dimethylphthalate or a synthetic pyrethroid. Repellents should also be smeared on to arms and necks, because it is these sites that are attacked when working in the undergrowth. If an area of scrub typhus is known and it is desired to clear it permanently, the undergrowth should be cut down and burnt, leaving the ground to dry out thoroughly before being safe to use. A less permanent method is to spray the area with insecticides. Tetracycline can be taken as a prophylactic by those at particular risk, but such methods are never reliable.

Mite islands can be very small and localized or can cover extensive areas, but generally they are associated with transitional vegetation or fringe habitats. These are areas separating different vegetation zones, such as forest and grassland. Mite islands are nearly always the result of human activity, where forest is destroyed either for timber or in slash-and-burn agriculture. The land regenerates as secondary growth and rats and other rodents move in and provide suitable conditions for the leptotrombiculid mites.

17.2.3 Murine Typhus

Scrub typhus has been given the alternative name of rural typhus, which adequately distinguishes it from urban typhus, which is the main characteristic of the flea-borne disease. Murine typhus, then, is a disease of towns and habitation, maintained there by domestic rodents, *Rattus rattus* and *R. norvegicus*. In contrast to scrub typhus, the mammal in murine typhus is the reservoir of the disease and the common rat flea, *X. cheopis*, acts only as a transmitter. Many other mammals have been found infected – mice, cats, opossums, shrews and skunks – but the key in all these alternative sites is always the domestic rat.

The flea becomes infected by biting the host, the infection appearing not to have any effect on the flea or shorten its lifespan. *R. mooseri* is not transmitted by the bite of the flea but is passed in its faeces. If infected faeces are rubbed into an abrasion or inhaled as an aerosol, other rats become infected. The body of the flea is also highly contagious and, if crushed, the organism is liberated. While *X. cheopis* is the main vector, the organism has been isolated from *Pulex irritans*, the common human flea, and from lice, mites and ticks. These probably do not form an important means of transmission, but could explain epidemics where *X. cheopis* is not found.

Humans are infected by their close association with domestic rodents. *R. mooseri* can be transmitted directly when the flea is squashed or scratched into an abrasion and its tissue juices or faeces contaminate the wound. The habit of some people when catching fleas of crushing them between their teeth is also a potential method of infection. However, it would seem that the direct attack on humans by the essentially healthy rat flea is uncommon and the more important method of transmission is from an aerosol of organisms in the flea faeces. These are carried on the rats' fur or sent into the air when disturbed. *R. mooseri* can be inhaled or swallowed or enter through other mucous membranes such as the conjunctiva. Murine typhus is common where rats live in constant contact with humans. It is endemic in Pakistan, India and the Malaysian peninsula, but may become epidemic in any part of the world where rats are found, such as in ports.

The illness presents as a gradual increase in fever, followed by a rash. It is milder than the epidemic form of typhus. Mortality is low and complications are rare, so that most people fully recover in a week to 10 days. Treatment is with tetracycline or chloramphenicol if the diagnosis is made early.

Control is the same as for plague (see Section 17.1), where the subject is covered in more detail. Essentially it is the control of fleas and rats, with the use of insecticide powders to kill the fleas first, followed by measures against rats. Buildings should be protected against reinfestation and new structures built with rat-proofing.

17.2.4 Epidemic Typhus

While scrub typhus and murine typhus are zoonoses, epidemic typhus is an infection where only humans and the louse are involved. The body louse *Pediculus humanus corporis* is the main vector, but *Phthirus pubis* and *Pediculus humanus capitis* may be involved. The body louse can spend its entire life cycle on the same host, laying its eggs in the seams of his/her clothing and finding all the food and shelter it requires. Female lice lay some 5–10 eggs per day, which hatch in 6–9 days, depending on temperature. If the clothes are kept on the body, the temperature is maintained and hatching takes place rapidly, but, if they are removed and cool down, development may take 2–3 weeks. One month is the maximum period they can survive, so clothes that are not worn for this length of time will be free of lice.

The egg hatches into a nymph, which in all respects resembles a small adult, and sucks blood. Three nymphal stages are passed through before it becomes an adult louse. Lice, both males and females, can survive only by taking blood meals and if deprived can last no longer than 10 days. They are sensitive to temperature and will abandon a dead person as well as one with a high fever. The lifespan of an adult louse is about 1 month and during this time a female may lay some 200–300 eggs.

The organism of epidemic typhus is R. *prowazeki*, which is ingested in the blood meal and can infect both males, females and all nymphal stages. The rickettsiae develop in the epithelial lining cells of the stomach, which they distend to such an extent that rupture takes place, liberating them back into the damaged gut lumen. These are then passed into the louse faeces, in which they can survive for 100 days or more. The damage caused to the louse can be sufficiently severe to kill it within 10 days and this helps to explain why few lice are found on a person suffering from typhus.

Humans become infected by scratching the louse faeces into abrasions or the puncture wound left by the feeding parasite, or if the lice are crushed on the skin or in the mouth. Dried lice faeces can remain viable for a considerable period of time and fine particles that are inhaled or enter the conjunctiva can be a potential hazard to those not infested with lice.

Lice thrive in conditions of deprivation and poverty, where clothing is worn without changing and people live in close proximity to each other. Lice cannot travel far or survive for long without a blood meal, so it is the crowding together of people that allows lice to crawl across and infest a new host. Where clothing is changed or washed or the ambient temperature is high, body lice do not occur and typhus is not found. But, in times of human disruption brought about by war, famine or social upheaval, the crowding together of people in conditions of poor sanitation provides the stage for an outbreak of typhus. A similar situation can occur in the highland areas of tropical countries, so that outbreaks of typhus have been reported from Rwanda, Burundi, Guatemala, Bolivia and Peru.

Various claims have been made for non-human reservoirs of *R. prowazeki*, but humans appear to be an adequate reservoir and their lice an ideal vector. The difficult question is what happens to the organism when an epidemic has subsided. The probable answer is found in *Brill–Zinsser disease*, more suitably called *recurrent typhus*. In this condition, people are found to have *R. prowazeki* in their bodies long after they had the disease. The organism remains dormant until some event causes a breakdown in host resistance and overt disease reappears. Cases have been found 20 and 40 years after the person was in a typhus area and where lice have been absent for this length of time. But, if lice feed on these cases, they become infected and can transmit epidemic typhus.

The *incubation period* is 10–14 days, but can be shorter if the infecting dose is large. There is a sudden onset, with headache, pains, rigors and malaise as the temperature rapidly rises to 40°C or more, where it remains for the duration of the illness. The characteristic rash appears between the fourth and seventh day and consists of petechial haemorrhages on the trunk and limbs but sparing the face, palms and soles. As the disease progresses, the patient becomes semistuporous, with confusion, anxiety and considerable dullness. He/she appears unable to hear, talks nonsense and has to be fed. By the third week, if treatment has not been given, the patient will progressively recover or else sink further into heart failure, bronchopneumonia and death.

Treatment should be commenced as soon as possible, even before the diagnosis is confirmed, as speed is of the essence if treatment is to be effective. Tetracycline is the drug of choice, at a dose of 500 mg four times a day. Longer-acting tetracyclines can be given at a lower dose and, where all of these are unavailable, chloramphenicol can be used. Careful nursing is of the utmost importance.

Control of epidemic typhus is control of the louse. In an epidemic this is most effectively done by insufflating an insecticide powder into people's clothing. This can be by a blower with a long nozzle that is pushed up the arms of clothing, down through necks and up trousers and skirts. The clothing should be thoroughly treated remembering that the lice live between the underclothing and body. DDT is the cheapest and most suitable insecticide, but, where resistance has developed, benzene hexachloride (BHC), malathion or newer preparations such as temephos, propoxur or synthetic pyrethroids can be used. Samples of lice should be tested for insecticidal resistance before and during mass treatments. Since it is conditions of overcrowding that generate epidemics, it is often not too difficult to disinfect large numbers of people in a comparatively short time. Dead bodies should be dusted with insecticides before burial.

Prophylactic antibiotics, generally tetracycline, can be given to contacts to reduce the extent of the reservoir. Treatment centres should be set up to discover cases early and antibiotics given.

Vaccines have been successful in controlling epidemics, but they suffer from various disadvantages. A killed vaccine (Cox) is painful when injected and does not give complete immunity, whereas a live attenuated vaccine appears to give solid immunity for over 5 years, but must be prepared carefully, as virulence can increase. Vaccines can either be used for mass administration in the face of epidemics or be given to persons at increased risk.

In the long term, typhus will only disappear when all lice are removed. People should be encouraged to wash themselves and their clothes. Clothes must be boiled or washed at over 60°C, which is a higher temperature than most washing machines achieve. Ironing clothes kills both adults and eggs.

Surveillance is the cornerstone of epidemic control.

- Human cases: notify disease and make urgent reports of suspicious cases.
- Louse surveys at clinics, prisons and similar collections of people.

7.3 DISEASES TRANSMITTED BY HARD TICKS

17.3.1 Hard Ticks

Hard ticks are responsible for transmission of rickettsiae and arboviruses. Those of medical importance are *Dermacentor*, *Amblyomma*, *Haemaphysalis* and *Rhipicephalus*. A female *Dermacentor*, to characterize the group of hard ticks, is illustrated in Fig. 17.4. The feature that distinguishes hard from soft ticks is the presence of a scutum (shield) and protruding mouth-parts. Care has to be taken in identifying the engorged specimen, for the body is so greatly distended as to obscure the head and mouth-parts (Fig. 17.4). The female has a smaller scutum than the male, but, since both males and females take blood meals, there is no real need to distinguish between them.

Eggs are laid in a large mass on the ground, hatching after weeks or months into six-legged larvae. These larvae resemble mites, but are differentiated from them by the prominent mouth-parts and the scutum

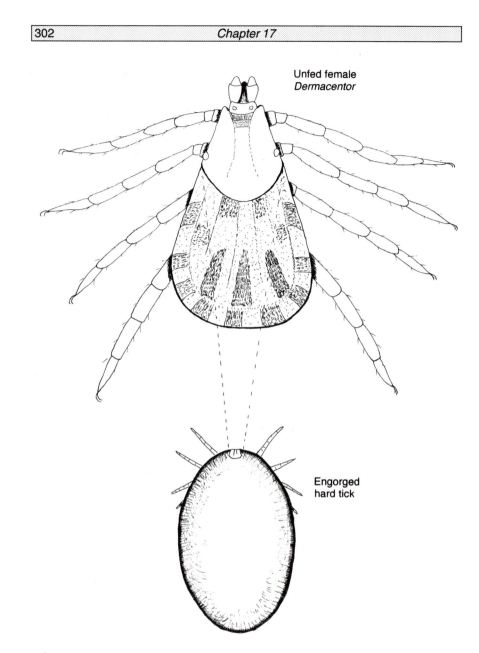

Fig. 17.4. Hard ticks.

originating from just behind the head. Larvae climb on to grass or prominent vegetation to await a passing mammal on to which they crawl and make their way to an area of soft skin, such as in the ears, on the eyelids or below the belly. In humans they may surreptitiously climb up the leg and attach themselves to the scrotum or between the buttocks.

Once in a favourable site they pierce the skin with their powerful mouth-parts, inject saliva and feed on the host's blood. Larvae will remain attached for from 3 days to a week, after which they drop to the ground and seek a place to moult. Developing into an eight-legged nymph, it repeats a similar feeding pattern, being attached for 5–10 days and then falling to the ground once more for the final moult. From the nymph develops a male or female adult, which subsequently quests for a new host, on which it remains for a considerable period of time (up to a month), becoming greatly engorged with blood. Finally dropping off, the female digests her blood meal and begins egg laying. After egg laying the female dies.

The life cycle of ticks is modified by temperature and humidity. If it becomes too cold, the cycle of development will be delayed until more favourable conditions return. Larvae and nymphs tend to feed on small mammals and humans, whereas adults prefer larger animals, such as cattle and game animals.

Control of ticks is mainly through the use of insecticides and repel-lents. DDT, malathion and propoxur are suitable insecticides, admin-istered as dusting powders or solutions to infested animals. Cattle are commonly treated by making them swim through an insecticidal bath or dip. This should be carried out on a regular basis, with monitoring of ticks for insecticidal resistance. Dogs are important carriers of ticks and should be similarly treated by insecticidal baths, making sure that they are totally immersed as the ears are a common site for ticks to attach.

Repellents, such as diethyltoluamide or dimethylphthalate, smeared on skin or as a solution to impregnate clothing, are effective in preventing ticks from becoming attached.

Ticks take some 2 hours to attach themselves and start feeding, so a careful search of the body, paying particular attention to the groin, should be made after passing through tick-infested country. Larval and nymph stages can be very small. Ticks should not be pulled off directly as the mouth-parts may be left behind, which will continue to cause irritation. Applying methylated spirit, ether, benzene or similar solution will kill the tick and sterilize the wound.

17.4 ROCKY MOUNTAIN SPOTTED FEVER

First described in the Rocky Mountains of North America, the disease caused by *Rickettsia rickettsi* is also found in Mexico, Brazil and other countries of South and Central America.

The illness commences suddenly, with onset of high fever, headache, malaise, muscle pains and the characteristic rash. Appearing about the third day, it is maculopapular from numerous petechial haemorrhages and covers the whole body, including the palms and soles. *Diagnosis is* made clinically, with the additional help of serological tests, described under typhus (see Section 17.2), taking care to differentiate it from measles and meningococcal meningitis. *Treatment* is with tetracycline or chloramphenicol.

Humans are infected by the bite of a tick, although they can also acquire infection by scratching in tick faeces or crushing it on their skin or mucous membranes. Larval and nymphal stages, as well as adult ticks, can transmit the infection. Rickettsiae can be maintained by transovarial transmission, so the tick is the reservoir.

Prevention is by avoiding any known tick country or wearing protective clothing, impregnated with repellents or insecticides. The common vector is the dog tick, and the control of dogs and their ectoparasites is effective.

17.5 TICK TYPHUS

Going under a host of names – boutonneuse fever, African tick typhus, Kenya tick typhus, Indian tick typhus, to give but a few – infection with *Rickettsia conorii* has been reported from a number of different parts of the world.

Generally a mild illness of a few days, characterized by an eschar at the site of the tick bite, it has a fever and rash similar to those of other rickettsial diseases. The reservoir of infection is the tick, but as with Rocky Mountain spotted fever, it is the dog tick, brought into close proximity by its canine host, that is responsible for most infections. Alternatively, humans acquire the infection from passing through scrub forest which rodents and their ticks are inhabiting. Rodents serve as a secondary reservoir.

Diagnosis and *treatment* are the same as for other rickettsial diseases. As well as the precautions outlined above, a regular search routine should be instituted to pick off ticks from the body when passing through any area of scrub and bush. At night, people should sleep off the ground, e.g. on camp-beds, and dogs should be kept away.

17.6 ARBOVIRUSES

Kyasanur forest disease, named after the part of India from which it was first described, is transmitted by *Haemaphysalis* ticks. Clinical features are similar to the other haemorrhagic fevers described in Section 16.2. Reservoirs are ticks and the rodents on which they feed. Control is the same as for the other tick-borne diseases.

Crimean/Congo haemorrhagic fever found in West, Central, East and South Africa, as well as Asia, is transmitted by *Hyalomma* ticks.

(Person-to-person infection can also occur.) It presents as a haemor-rhagic fever after an incubation period of 7–12 days. Domestic animals serve as reservoirs and people working in high-risk areas can be vaccinated.

Hard ticks can also be responsible for spreading other arbovirus diseases normally transmitted by mosquitoes, such as Japanese, St Louis, Eastern and Western equine encephalitis (see Section 16.2).

17.7 INFECTIONS TRANSMITTED BY SOFT TICKS

Soft ticks differ from hard ticks in having a retracted head and no scutum. As their name implies, soft ticks do not have a rigid structure but a leathery body that looks like a collapsed bag. This hangs over the body structures, so that viewed from the top, only the legs can be seen protruding from it (Fig. 17.5). When the tick takes a blood meal, its collapsed body fills and becomes greatly distended. The tick digests the blood meal, utilizing a structure called a coxal gland, which is like a filter, to remove excess fluid. This is important in relapsing fever, as the spirochaete of *Borrelia duttoni* is passed out in the coxal fluid.

The life cycle is similar to that of hard ticks except that there are several nymphal stages (four in *Ornithodorus moubata*). Each stage needs to take a blood meal before passing on to the next nymphal stage. Finally, the fourth instar changes into an adult and egg laying commences after the female has become engorged with blood. Ticks can live for several years, so that many eggs can be laid in her lifetime. In contrast to hard ticks, the female does not die after egg laying but is able to continue taking blood meals, laying eggs after each.

O. moubata is the main soft tick of medical importance, living close to humans and feeding on them and their domestic animals. Ticks rest in cracks and crevices of poorly built houses, emerging at night to feed on sleeping occupants. Ticks can remain alive for over 5 years after a single blood meal, and are able to attack humans again after they reoccupy a house following a prolonged absence. Also, the eggs are coated with a waxy protective layer, so allowing them to remain viable for several months. They are laid in walls, floors and furniture and will hatch in 1–4 weeks if conditions are suitable. Once established, soft ticks are very persistent occupants.

17.8 RELAPSING FEVER (TICK-BORNE)

Two different patterns of tick-borne relapsing fever are found, *endemic in Africa* and *epidemic in other parts of the world*, due entirely to the habits of the tick vector.

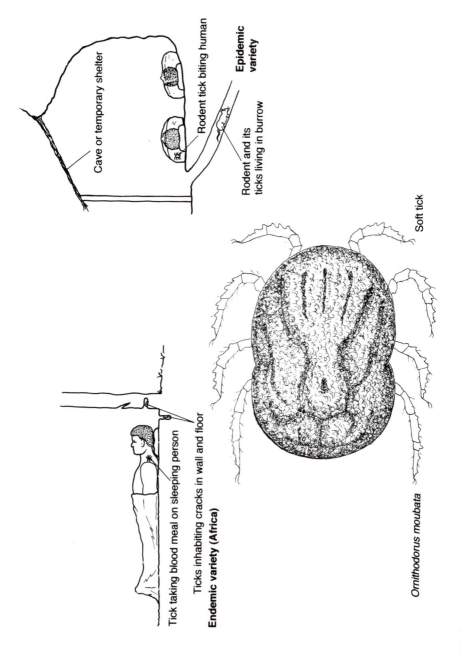

Cave or temporary shelter

Rodent tick biting human

**Epidemic
variety**

Rodent and its
ticks living in burrow

Tick taking blood meal on sleeping person

Ticks inhabiting cracks in wall and floor

Endemic variety (Africa)

Ornithodorus moubata

Soft tick

Fig. 17.5. Epidemiology of the tick-borne relapsing fevers.

In Africa the vector *O. moubata* is domestic in habit (as described above) living in and around the homes of humans, transmitting the disease from person to person. The reservoir is the tick, but humans act as a secondary reservoir. When a tick feeds on an infected person, the spirochaetes of *B. duttoni* are ingested with the blood meal. They multiply in the gut and enter the haemocoele, where they increase to enormous proportions. The spirochaetes pierce all organs of the tick's body, including the salivary gland, the coxal organ and the reproductive system, leading to *transovarial infection*. Nymphal stages may already be infected when they take blood meals or can become so from their hosts. In relapsing fever the spirochaete is transferred by the bite of the tick and from the coxal fluid, not from the faeces. In *O. moubata* adults, the coxal fluid is the main source of spirochaetes, but, in the nymphs and other species of *Ornithodorus*, it is the salivary glands.

The *incubation period* in humans is 3–10 days, after which fever develops, with a recurring or relapsing pattern, as the name of the disease indicates. The period of fever lasts for a few days and then recurs after 7–10 days, with up to ten or more relapses occurring in the untreated case. The onset of fever is sudden with headache, myalgia and vertigo. A transitory petechial rash can occur and a variety of other systems may be involved. There can be bronchitis, nerve palsies, hepatosplenomegaly and signs of renal damage.

Diagnosis is made from spirochaetes, found in the blood during febrile periods. Mass screening of blood slides can be used in surveillance. Blood slides can be either stained or viewed by dark-ground illumination. An improvement on this technique is the direct centrifugal method originally developed for malaria.

Treatment is with a single dose of 300,000 units of procaine penicillin immediately, followed next day by tetracycline 500 mg four times daily for 10 days. This regime provides adequate treatment while at the same time minimizing reaction.

Babies and young children are particularly susceptible to infection in endemic areas, with adults exhibiting immunity. However, immunity is lost by pregnancy and congenital infection can occur. It is a cause of abortion, stillbirth and premature delivery. This is particularly the pattern in Central and East Africa.

In other parts of the world, the infection is a zoonosis, with a transmission cycle maintained between rodents and their parasitic ticks. Humans enter this cycle as an intruder or by accident, much as they do in sylvatic plague or scrub typhus. Rodent-inhabited caves or camp-sites near rodent burrows are areas where sporadic infection can occur. When temporary shelters or log cabins are erected near a zoonotic focus, rats invade these buildings and their ticks begin to feed regularly on humans. An endemic pattern, similar to that in Africa, may then develop. Ticks responsible for transmitting relapsing fever in other parts of the world are *O. tholozani* in Asia, *O. erraticus* in North Africa and *O. rudis* in Central and South America.

Control of soft ticks is by the use of insecticides, such as malathion, diazinon or propoxur, sprayed around houses. Special attention needs to be paid to any cracks and crevices where ticks may hide. In addition, insecticides can be mixed with the floor or wall plaster during construction or repair work. BHC as 140 mg base m^{-2} is a suitable preparation. Infants (and adults) can be protected from house-invading ticks by sleeping under a mosquito net. Ticks are also deterred from entering rooms in which a night-light is glowing.

The rodent reservoir is of major importance in bringing ticks close to human habitations. Every effort should be made to prevent rodents invading houses or burrowing underneath them, using suitable methods of house construction.

17.9 RELAPSING FEVER (LOUSE-BORNE)

Louse-borne relapsing fever is an epidemic disease occurring in the same situations or even at the same time as epidemic typhus. The organism, *Borrelia recurrentis*, is a spirochaete, indistinguishable from *B. duttoni* in stained preparations and with some cross-immunity between the two. Distribution is similar to that of epidemic typhus, being found in the highland areas of Africa, India and South America.

The disease is associated with poor personal hygiene and overcrowding, in which lice flourish. Lice become infected by feeding on humans during the pyrexial period. The spirochaete invades the haemocoele of the louse, much in the same way as with ticks. Humans are infected only by *crushed* lice, the liberated spirochaete entering the bite wound or any abrasion. Crushing lice between the fingernails or teeth is a possible way of acquiring infection. The spirochaete can enter through mucous membranes and possibly even unbroken skin. Because the lice have a short lifespan and are killed during transmission, humans are the only reservoir. There is an endemic focus in Ethiopia, from which epidemics appear to originate. All the conditions favourable for an epidemic seem to occur about once every 20 years.

The disease is very similar to tick-borne relapsing fever, but the number of relapses is generally less. It is also more responsive to treatment, with a single dose of 300 thousand units of procaine penicillin on the first day, followed by tetracycline 250 mg the next. Severe reactions to antibiotic therapy are commoner in louse-borne than in tick-borne relapsing fever.

Control and further details about the louse *P. h. corporis* will be found under epidemic typhus (see Section 17.2.4). Essentially, delousing is the main control method.

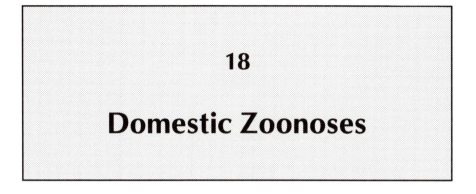

18

Domestic Zoonoses

Domestic zoonoses are diseases due to domestic animals and pets.

18.1 PARASITES FROM DOGS AND CATS

The most important source of disease from which humans suffer is humans themselves, but the animals on which they depend for their livelihood and companionship are responsible for many others. Paramount among these is the dog; a list of infections that it transmits or in which it is a reservoir will be found in Table 18.1. Some have been mentioned in previous chapters, while others will be covered here.

18.2 HYDATID DISEASE

Echinococcus granulosus is a cyclophyllidean tapeworm of canines, in which the adult worm is found. Eggs passed in the faeces contaminate pasture land and, when eaten by herbivorous domestic and wild animals, particularly sheep, pigs and goats (also found in cattle, camels and horses), develop into hydatid cysts. The hydatid cyst is a fluid-filled sack containing enormous numbers of scolices, any of which can become an adult worm in the dog. The common means of infection is for dogs to be fed the offal of domestic animals (Fig. 18.1). In the wild, jackals, wolves and wild dogs become infected by killing and eating infected herbivores.

Humans enter this cycle accidentally when they swallow the eggs and hydatid cysts develop inside them. There are several ways infection can occur.

- Through food items, e.g. fruit or vegetables contaminated by dog faeces.

Table 18.1 Some infections transmitted to humans from dogs.

Viruses	Rabies
	Lymphocytic choriomeningitis (LCM)
	Arboviruses
Rickettsiae	*Rickettsia rickettsiae*
	R. conori
Bacteria	*Salmonella*
	Escherichia coli
	Leptospirosis
	Mycobacteria
	Tularaemia
Fungi	Ringworm
Protozoa	*Leishmania* spp.
	Chagas' disease
Helminths	*Echinococcus*
	Multiceps
	Larva migrans (*Toxocara, Ancylostoma*)
	Echinostoma
	Fasciolopsis
	Heterophyes
	Opisthorchis
	Paragonimus
	Dracunculus
	Dirofilaria
	Strongyloides
	Schistosoma japonicum
	Dipylidium
Arthropods	Ticks
	Fleas
	Pentastomids (*Linguatula*)

- Drinking water contaminated by dog faeces.
- Close contact with dogs, e.g. by touching their fur or being licked by them. (When a dog licks itself it can spread eggs all over its body as well as them sticking to its tongue.)

Hydatid cysts have been recorded from all parts of the body and can cause serious disease. The commonest site is the liver, with lung, abdomen, kidney and brain in descending order of frequency. The main pathological effect is produced by the cyst increasing in size, which in a vital organ can rapidly lead to serious and often fatal effects. Also the cyst contents are infective so, if the cyst is ruptured either accidentally or at operation, then numerous new cysts are formed. The liberation of so much foreign protein in the body can result in a severe anaphylactic reaction.

Diagnosis of the disease is clinically, e.g. chest X-ray or enlargement

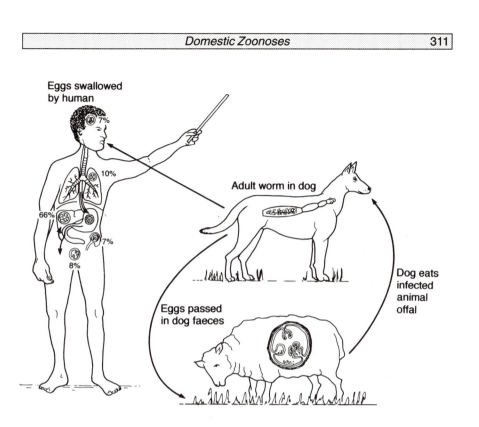

Fig. 18.1. Hydatid disease – *Echinococcus granulosus.*

of the liver, while immunological methods are also useful. A diagnostic aspiration of the cyst must never be made. Treatment is by surgical removal; either this must be complete or the contents must first be sterilized by formalin, if there is a risk of rupture.

The disease is widespread, but occurs in concentrated pockets, such as sheep-rearing areas or where dogs live in very close proximity to humans. A unique example is in the Turkana people of northern Kenya, where dogs are trained to care for young children, so the rate of infection is very high.

A rare species is *Echinococcus multilocularis*, which, as its name suggests, forms multiloculated lesions, which invade the body much in the same way as a neoplastic growth. It is a parasite of the Arctic and colder regions of the world.

Control can be implemented at several points in the life cycle. Infected material should not be fed to dogs or, if this cannot be avoided, it must be well cooked. Dogs can be treated to remove any adult worms. Measures to reduce faecal contamination, such as fencing water sources and food gardens or the general training of dogs, can be taken. Ultimately, though, this will depend on humans' relations with their animals, by keeping them in their proper place, destroying unwanted animals and observing personal hygiene.

18.3 TOXOCARIASIS

The larvae of the ascarid roundworms of dogs (*Toxocara canis*) and less commonly cats (*T. catis*) can invade humans, wandering in the body unable to complete their development. If eggs are accidentally swallowed, the larvae penetrate the tissues and wander until they die. An unfortunate site of predilection is the eye, and the young child playing with the puppy is in danger of contracting blindness. The body responds to this invasion by the production of eosinophils. Diethylcarbamazine or thiabendazole can be used in treatment. The method of control is to reduce stray dogs and prevent others from contaminating playgrounds, streets and public places with dog faeces.

18.4 LARVA MIGRANS

The larval forms of several animal parasites wander aimlessly in the human body, if they enter it by mistake. Examples are the cat and dog hookworms, *Ancylostoma brasiliense*, *A. stenocephala* and *A. canium*. The signs are a serpiginous track of wandering larvae, which is painful and red at the advancing end, causing intense pruritus. It lasts for some time, advancing a little more each day.

The *Toxocara* larvae, mentioned above, and the cat and dog filariae *Dirofilaria immitis*, *Brugia pahangi* and *B. patei*, can cause a more serious visceral larva migrans. The body reacts to these parasites, especially when they pass through the lungs, with a profound eosinophilia (tropical eosinophilia). Symptoms are cough, especially paroxysmal, not unlike asthma, with the production of large quantities of sputum, sometimes streaked with blood. A diagnosis of tuberculosis can mistakenly be made. Diagnosis is largely made on clinical grounds but the filaria antigen of *D. immitis* can be used as a skin test. The condition responds dramatically to diethylcarbamazine and control is similar to that of the other filarial infections.

A localized form of larva migrans occurring in Thailand and China results from *Gnathostoma spinigerum*, an intestinal parasite of cats and dogs. Humans are infected by the larval stage through eating raw fish. The disease presents as a single migratory swelling, either superficially or in the deeper tissues, cerebral lesions being not uncommon. It causes intense itching and eosinophilia. If the larva comes near the surface of the body, its surgical removal can result in cure; otherwise diethylcarbamazine has been reported to have some effect. Ensuring that fish are properly cooked is the easiest method of control.

18.5 TOXOPLASMOSIS

The coccidial parasite *Toxoplasma gondii* is found in the cat. Oocysts are passed in cat faeces and, if these are accidentally swallowed by humans, they become infected. Alternatively, pseudocysts can be swallowed in undercooked meat (generally mutton). The *Toxoplasma* parasites that develop from the oocysts disperse to many parts of the body, including the central nervous system (CNS), where they form small inflammatory foci (pseudocysts). They result in surprisingly little pathology to their host, occasionally producing lymphadenopathy and a low-grade fever.

The serious results occur in congenital infections passed on by an acutely infected mother, where CNS involvement of the infant leads to death or mental defects. Disseminated toxoplasmosis can also occur in the immunodepressed, e.g. those with acquired immune deficiency syndrome (AIDS).

Diagnosis can be made by immunological tests or by lymph-node biopsy. Pyrimethamine, with or without sulphonamides, can be used for treatment. Control is by personal hygiene, especially hand washing after touching cats. Cats should be banished at mealtimes and when food is being prepared. The habit of giving cats scraps of food during the course of a meal should be strongly discouraged. All meat should be properly cooked.

18.6 RABIES

A disease that strikes terror into the hearts of humans because of its invariable fatality, rabies is widely spread throughout the world. As important in temperate as tropical countries, its control is aimed principally at managing the dog population.

Rabies is caused by a rhabdovirus. The virus withstands freezing temperatures for considerable periods of time, but is killed by boiling, sunlight and drying. It is not easily destroyed by disinfectants. Monoclonal antibody techniques have allowed the differentiation of four related viruses, including Mokola and Duvenhage which produce rabies-like illness.

The virus has a special affinity for brain and mucus-secreting tissue, especially the salivary glands. Large quantities of virus particles are present in the saliva from 1–10 days before the development of symptoms in the animal, right up until it dies.

The virus has an affinity for nervous tissue and, once in the body, it travels along peripheral nerves to the CNS. From the central area it can also travel peripherally and this is how the salivary glands become infected. Cases have occurred in caves, where the only possible means of transmission is an aerosol of bat faeces, so the respiratory route is a possible, but less important, means of entry.

Rabies is common in Europe, Russia, Africa, India, the Philippines, China and Japan. It is mainly transmitted by members of the dog family, including wolves, foxes, jackals and hyenas, but domestic animals such as the cat and cow have also been responsible. Other infected wild animals are mongooses, skunks and racoons. In South America the vampire bat transmits rabies, particularly to cattle, but insectivorous bats have also been found infected.

Virus enters the body through a bite or abrasion of the skin. Classically it is a dog bite, but, if the abraded skin is licked by a dog, cat or cow that has infective saliva, infection can occur. Humans are rarely infected by the bite of the vampire bat, it being responsible mainly for infecting cattle. Humans have occasionally been infected by entering caves, where fine particles of bat faeces contaminate the conjunctiva or enter the respiratory mucosa.

The disease in the dog occurs in two forms, the furious and dumb. In *furious* rabies the animal becomes restless, wanders away from home and bites anybody or anything that comes in its way. It is unable to bark and may attempt to eat sticks and stones but is foiled in the attempt by a difficulty in swallowing. It foams at the mouth, suffers from the progressive paralysis of *dumb* rabies and is dead within a few days. Sometimes the furious course is not followed and only dumb rabies is manifest.

While the disease is invariably fatal in domestic dogs, cats and cows, it would appear to have a more variable effect in wild dogs, such as foxes and wolves. Certainly rabies reduces fox populations, but individuals do recover from the disease. There is little evidence to support the finding of a reservoir in such canines, but this may not be the case in rodents and bats. Rabies virus has been found in mongooses and the multimammate rat, *Mastomys natalensis*. These animals suffer from rabies, but subclinical infections may occur. When canines feed on small mammals, they can acquire rabies. Vampire bats have been shown to recover from the disease and rabies virus has also been isolated from insectivorous bats, which do not take blood meals. This suggests that rabies may exist in a mild and asymptomatic form for most of the time in these mammals. However, when humans are bitten or when they enter the virus-contaminated habitat, they are at risk of losing their lives.

The *incubation* period depends upon the proximity of the point of introduction of the virus (generally a bite) to the brain. It is usually 2–8 weeks, but 2 years has been recorded. The disease starts quietly with malaise, fever, sore throat and lack of appetite. Paraesthesia develops and abnormal muscle movements occur. The patient then enters the excitable stage, when he/she becomes anxious, there is difficulty in swallowing and frank hydrophobia, and generalized convulsions may take place. The patient either dies in the convulsive stage or enters progressive paralysis as the terminal symptom. In the bat form of the disease there is no excitable stage and the patient dies from respiratory paralysis.

The clinical picture following a history of an animal bite is usually sufficient to make the diagnosis, but the virus may be isolated from saliva, tears, cerebrospinal fluid (CSF), urine and many other tissues if facilities exist to culture it. Treatment is hopeless, although two cases have survived with intensive care on life-support systems.

18.6.1 Prevention

Fortunately rabies virus can be inactivated on its passage along the peripheral nerves and this is the main method of protecting the individual bitten by a rabid dog. The first procedure is to wash out the wound thoroughly with 20% soap solution, followed by water and a quaternary ammonium compound or 0.1% iodine. If there is a high suspicion of infection, rabies antiserum should also be injected locally around the wound. Tetanus toxoid and penicillin should be administered, as tetanus is often a greater danger than rabies.

If the biting animal can be caught, it should be tied up and observed for 10 days. After this time, it will either have died from the disease or remained well. If it has died or was killed, then the head is severed with aseptic precautions (as the saliva is highly infectious), packed in ice and sent to a laboratory for culture and histological studies. Section of the brain will show characteristic Negri bodies. Monoclonal antibodies can also be used.

Vaccines

The three recommended vaccines are human diploid-cell vaccine (HDCV), rabies vaccine adsorbed (RVA) and the duck embryo vaccine (DEV). HDCV is preferable, but the most expensive. The schedules for the full course are as follows.

- HDCV 1 ml i.m. immediately and on days 3, 7, 14, 28 and 90.
- RVA 1 ml i.m. immediately and on days 3, 7, 14, 28 and 90.
- DEV 1 ml subcutaneously daily for 21 days and then at 10 and 20 days after completion of the course.

If pre-exposure immunization has been given, then proceed as follows.

- HDCV: give one dose immediately and a second in 5 days.
- RVA: give one dose immediately and a second in 5 days.
- DEV: give five daily doses of DEV and one 20 days after the last dose.

Table 18.2 Post-exposure and antirabies guide. This is only a guide and should be used in conjunction with local knowledge of rabies endemicity and the animal involved.

Type of animal	Status of animal	Type of exposure	Treatment
Domestic Dog Cat Cow	Healthy and remains so for 10 days	Any	None
	Signs suggestive of rabies, animal retained for 10 days	Mild, scratch or lick, bite	Rabies vaccine (discontinue if animal not rabid by day 5)
	Rabid or becomes so during retention	Mild, scratch or lick Bite	Rabies vaccine Antirabies serum plus vaccine (discontinue if animal not rabid by day 5)
	Escaped, killed or unknown	Mild, scratch or lick Bite	Rabies vaccine Antirabies serum, plus vaccine
Wild Fox Wolf Racoon Mongoose Bat, etc.	Regard as rabid if unprovoked attack	Bite	Serum immediately followed by course of vaccine

Hyperimmune antirabies serum

Hyperimmune antirabies serum is given as soon as possible, half around the wound and the rest intramuscularly. Human immune globulin is preferable; if only horse serum is available, a test dose must first be given. The dose is as follows.

- Human immune globulin 20 iu kg^{-1} body weight.
- Animal immune globulin 40 iu kg^{-1} body weight.

Table 18.2 summarizes the procedure to be followed in treating a person who has been attacked by a rabid animal.

18.6.2 Control

Control measures can be aimed at the domestic dog, the reservoir of wild animals and the protection of humans.

- Control of domestic dogs. These can be licensed and all strays destroyed; preferably combine licensing with vaccination.
- Vaccination of all domestic animals with an approved vaccine at bi-annual intervals should be mandatory in all endemic areas. All dogs not vaccinated should be destroyed.

- Control of the wild animal reservoir is a massive undertaking but alteration of habitat and local destruction around a dwelling or place of work can be practised.

As rabies follows a natural cycle in many wild animals, their total destruction over large areas may upset this balance and produce a rebound increase. It is preferable to try and maintain a balance of nature. Immunization of wild animals can be achieved by leaving vaccine baits. This has been effectively used in Europe. With bat rabies, control of bats is largely unsuccessful and it is preferable to immunize cattle, which are the main victims.

Protection of humans who are at special risk can be by HDCV, RVA or DEV. This is not without some danger, but is minimal with HDCV.

- HDCV and RVA are given in three injections of 1 ml, the second after a month interval, and the third after a year, followed by annual boosters. An alternative shorter course is 1 ml on days 0, 7 and 21.
- DEV is given in two injections 1 month apart, followed by a third after 6–7 months.

18.7 LEPTOSPIROSIS

Leptospirosis is a very widespread zoonotic infection of animals, being endemic in many rodents, especially rats. The organism *Leptospira interrogans*, has been found in a variety of other animals – opossums, mongooses, skunks, hedgehogs, squirrels, rabbits and dogs, to name but a few – but the two domestic rats, *Rattus rattus* and *R. norvegicus*, are far and away the most important reservoirs.

L. interrogans has a large number of serovars, the most important of which is *icterohaemorrhagiae*. It is passed in rats' urine and can contaminate any area that they frequent. For the survival of the organism there must be moisture, such as a canal, sewer, damp soil, the washings of abattoirs or similar conditions. The pH of the soil or water is important and the spirochaete cannot survive in an acid environment. Leptospirosis is therefore commoner in places where the soil is alkaline. Salt water and chlorine solutions rapidly kill the organism.

Leptospira enters the skin of humans through minor abrasions, although it does appear to be able to enter unbroken skin or through mucous membranes. It is therefore the exposure of humans to contaminated moist areas, such as swimming in canals or walking barefoot over damp rat-infested soil, that invites infection. A direct rat bite can also transmit the disease.

A double infection cycle also occurs utilizing domestic animals. Cattle, dogs, pigs and water buffaloes are infected by coming into contact with rats' urine and these domestic animals subsequently excrete leptospires in their urine, close to where humans may come in contact with it.

Where rats are common and conditions are favourable, the infection is widespread. In many areas surveyed, it has been found in a large percentage of the population, endemic in the community with the occasional severe case. It is common in the Tropics, particularly where the soil is alkaline or irrigation is used for agriculture. Infection is therefore common in rice-paddy areas and sugar-cane estates, the latter because rats are common in the cane fields and abrasions readily occur during harvesting. This association of the disease with certain occupations is helpful in making the diagnosis. Such occupations as mine workers, farmers, canal cleaners, sewer workers and people employed in the cleaning and preparation of fish or in abattoirs are at greater risk.

The *incubation period* is between 4 and 18 days, usually about 10. *Clinical features* are many and variable, with jaundice and haemorrhages in the skin, mucous membranes and many internal organs, after a preliminary illness of fever, headache, malaise, vomiting and myalgia. The disease may progress to a more serious form, with liver failure, renal failure or meningitis. However, many others have mild infections and the vast majority do not exhibit any symptoms at all. In endemic areas children are probably most commonly infected.

A milder form of the disease is transmitted by dogs' urine, containing serovar *canicola* and is given the separate name of *canicola fever*.

Diagnosis is by finding the motile organism in a wet blood film during the first week of the disease. After this time, serological tests or animal inoculation can be used, while leptospires may be found in the urine from the third week onwards. Culture of the organism can take up to a month.

Treatment is with penicillin 1 mega unit every six hours for one week, but this must be given within the first 7 days of the illness or else it has no effect on the clinical course. In the late case, life-saving measures to combat renal and liver failure will be required.

Control is the avoidance of areas contaminated with rat urine, often a difficult thing to achieve. Various measures can be taken.

- The reduction of rats by extermination and protection of buildings, especially those used for preparing meat or fish and those housing domestic animals. (See under plague (Section 17.1).)
- Burning of sugar-cane fields after harvest.
- Wearing of protective clothing to reduce abrasions and contamination with moisture.
- Avoiding canals, lakes and bodies of water known to be infected.

Secondary infection and canicola fever can be prevented by the following.

- Controlling the number of dogs and their unsanitary habits.
- Providing proper pens for domestic animals so that urine does not collect and make the surroundings sodden.

  An attack can also be made against the spirochaete.

- Where water is used for washing down food premises, a solution of chlorine can be added or alternatively salt water used.

  Vaccination of humans is generally unsuccessful, but vaccination of animals may be worthwhile.

18.8 BRUCELLOSIS

Brucellosis is a widespread disease in the world, varying markedly in prevalence and severity from place to place. It produces an acute or chronic fever (undulant fever). Its control is through the proper management of domestic animals and pasteurization of milk.

The organism is a Gram-negative bacillus, with three species important to humans – *Brucella melitensis*, *B. abortus* and *B. suis*. *B. melitensis* causes the disease in goats, which was first investigated in Malta (Melita was the Roman name for the island). *B. abortus* as its name implies, causes abortion in cattle. *B. suis* is an infection of pigs. Both pigs and sheep are often infected with *B. melitensis* and *B. abortus*.

The organism is killed by heating at 60°C for 10 min and by 1% phenol for 15 min. It survives well in milk and cream cheeses that have not fermented or gone hard. In places contaminated by the faeces and urine of infected animals, survival can be for months and even years, especially at lower temperatures. With temperatures above 25°C, survival time is reduced.

The disease is mainly of animals, resulting in economic loss to the society and ill health to those involved in looking after animals. It is often not recognized, although it is found in a large number of animals if looked for. In Sudan and Nigeria, 60% of cattle have been found to be infected. Cattle become infected by eating placentae, licking a dead fetus or close contact with contaminated surroundings, such as occur in cattle paddocks (barns) or shelters. The young can obtain infection through the milk of their mothers.

Humans are infected by consuming raw milk or milk produce. *B. melitensis* is mainly spread by unpasteurized goat's milk or the consumption of cream cheeses prepared from it. *B. abortus* has less invasive power and virulence when consumed in cow's milk and so asymptomatic infection from drinking cow's milk can occur. In those whose occupations bring them in close proximity to animals, infection can occur through the skin, probably via an abrasion, the mucous membrane or the conjunctiva or as an aerosol through the respiratory tract. Such people as farmers, shepherds, goatherds, vets and abattoir workers are at greater risk.

The *incubation period* is from 5 days to 5 weeks but may be up to 7 months. The severity and duration of the disease is very variable and may go undiagnosed for a considerable period of time. Characteristically there are intermittent or irregular fevers (undulant fever) with generalized aches and pains. The patient is unduly weak and tired, often retiring in the second half of the day. There may be depression, a cough and lymphosplenomegaly. Recovery may occur spontaneously, or the disease become chronic, with the undulant pattern of fever and fatigue more pronounced. If not treated, this can continue for 6 months to a year, after which 80% of patients fully recover. Abortion is more frequent in women with the disease.

Diagnosis is difficult but isolation of the organism from blood, bone marrow or urine should be attempted. Serum agglutination tests can be used, but a rise in titre is required. A useful screening test is the rose bengal plate test; it may give false positives, but its speed and simplicity readily commend it.

Treatment is with tetracycline 3 g daily for 21 days. In severe infections streptomycin 1 g daily can also be given for 3 weeks. Co-trimoxazole (Bactrim, Septrin) have also been found effective.

Control is by pasteurization or boiling of cow's and goat's milk. Where pasteurization is not a legal requirement, people should be told of the risks of drinking raw milk and advised to boil it.

Anybody working with animals, especially those concerned with slaughter of animals or coming into contact with products of abortion, should wear overalls and gloves that are frequently washed and sterilized. Proper animal husbandry reduces areas of highly contaminated pasture land that perpetuate infection.

Where facilities permit, herds or flocks can be rendered *Brucella*-free by diagnosis and slaughter of infected animals. A useful test for this purpose is the milk ring test on cow's milk. Haematoxylin-stained *Brucella* antigen is added to a sample of cow's milk and, if positive, a blue ring appears at the interface. By removing infected animals from a herd and preventing them from coming into contact with others, whole areas of land and even complete countries have been made *Brucella*-free. This is a large and expensive undertaking and beyond the means of many Third World countries. An alternative is to vaccinate herds. The live attenuated vaccine S19 gives protection for 7 years or more. Calves should ideally be vaccinated at 6–8 months. Vaccination can also be given to adult animals, but should not be administered if an eradication programme is envisaged, as it then becomes impossible to tell whether an animal is infected or not.

18.9 ANTHRAX

Essentially an infection of cattle, anthrax ranks with rabies and plague as a much feared and fatal disease. It derives its name from the Greek for coal (anthrax), the colour of the fully developed skin lesion. It is the systemic effects that follow this that lead to the more serious manifestations, but with antibiotics it now carries a low mortality. Widespread in the bovine populations of the world, its persistence in the environment and in the produce of cattle makes it an ever-present threat in both the developing and the developed world.

Bacillus anthracis is a rod-shaped organism occurring in pairs or chains and staining positively with Gram stain. In the vegetative state in the animal or where there is a low oxygen content, the bacilli are surrounded by a capsule. If the dead animal's flesh and blood becomes exposed to the air or the organism is cultured in an atmosphere containing oxygen, spores develop. These appear as round filling defects in the stained rods, which they do not distend. Because of the characteristic appearance and staining properties of the organism, a rapid diagnosis can be made from the exudate of lesions.

The vegetative form is killed by heat at 55°C for 1 hour, which has its importance in the survival of the organism in the dead animal. If the carcass is not opened, the outside temperature is sufficient to encourage putrefaction, raising the internal temperature enough to kill off anthrax bacilli. A temperature of 30°C for 80 hours is sufficient to render the carcass free of organisms. However, if it is butchered or a post-mortem is performed, exposure to the air encourages the development of highly resistant spores, which are one of the most persistent forms of life yet known to humans. They have survived 160°C for 1 hour and −78°C despite thawing and refreezing, while in pastures they have been found viable after 12 years and possibly for up to 60 years. When warm, moist conditions prevail, the spore changes into the vegetative form. This has to compete with other soil bacteria, to which it is a poor rival.

The disease commonly affects cattle, sheep, goats and horses, but has occurred in dogs and cats. It is probably widespread in the wild and has been found in elephants and hippopotamuses and on the claws and beaks of vultures and other scavenger birds.

Anthrax spores are ingested or become accidentally inoculated through the skin, e.g. thistle scratches around the muzzle or legs of an animal close-grazing in an infected pasture. Biting flies have also been incriminated. The spores germinate into the vegetative form, which rapidly invades, increasing in virulence. A local lesion grows at the point of inoculation and extensive oedema develops around it. The capsulated bacilli produce a lethal factor, which causes widespread symptoms, anoxic hypertension or cardiac collapse, which can result in the sudden death of the animal. After death, the animal appears black from tarry blood that is slow to clot.

Humans are infected by contact with the deceased animal, either in butchering and handling of the infected meat, or at a place far removed from the death of the animal from spores in its hide, hair or bones. The *incubation period* is less than 7 days, and as short as 2 days in the rapidly fatal pulmonary form. But the commonest presentation is the cutaneous form of the disease. This commences with a small papule at the site of inoculation. By the second day a ring of vesicles surround it, which are at first clear but then become bloodstained. The central papule then ulcerates and enlarges to form a depressed dark eschar. This increases in size and darkens to the black coal colour that gives the disease its name. Pus is never present despite the development of oedema around the lesion. The oedema is extensive and may cause respiratory embarrassment if around the neck. The associated lymph nodes are often enlarged, but must be left to resolve spontaneously. The primary lesion commonly occurs on the head or face, while the neck and forearm are also often affected. Surprisingly the fingers are rarely involved.

As well as the primary lesion and its surrounding oedema, there are systemic symptoms of varying severity. The patient feels unwell, with nausea and lack of appetite, chills and rigors, although the temperature is normal or only slightly raised. A high temperature or weak pulse is a serious sign. The most severe form of anthrax is the pulmonary disease, which results from the inhalation of a very large dose of spores. Illness sets in rapidly, with cough, dyspnoea, cyanosis and a high temperature. Lymph nodes enlarge and there is splenomegaly. This passes into a stage of cardiovascular collapse and the patient is dead within 2 or 3 days.

Intestinal anthrax is another uncommon but severe form of the disease. The primary lesion occurs in the intestines and the massive oedema that results produces intestinal obstruction as well as the systemic symptoms described above. It results from people eating infected meat, which is a common cause of anthrax outbreaks in the Tropics, but surprisingly cutaneous disease still occurs much more frequently than the intestinal form.

Diagnosis is made by examination of the fluid from the vesicle in a person who gives a history of contact with an animal that recently died. A smear is made on to two slides, one being stained by Gram and the other fixed by heat and stained with methylene blue or Giemsa. The first shows Gram-positive rods and the second demonstrates the red capsule surrounding the blue bacilli. This finding can be confirmed by culture on selective media.

Treatment is with penicillin, to which the organism is very sensitive. One megaunit of procaine penicillin daily for 3 days or an equivalent combination of benzathine and benzylpenicillin should be adequate. No local treatment is required and surgical removal of the eschar or incision

of oedema only leads to unpleasant scarring and development of intract-
able sinuses. The local lesion resolves completely if left alone. Anti-
anthrax serum is rarely, if ever, used these days and early and large doses
of penicillin are the only hope for respiratory and intestinal cases.
Supportive measures need to be given for shock and tracheostomy may
be required when there is severe oedema of the neck.

Control is difficult due to the persistence of the organism in the
environment, but once an outbreak starts it should be possible to bring it
to an end by vigorous control of animals and their slaughter. No animal
that dies from anthrax should be allowed to be butchered and sold for
meat. Its hide and bones are also infectious, so should be buried deep with
lime or burnt. Anthrax is a common disease in pastoralists, who often
conserve cow dung as a fuel. This makes an ideal material for incinerat-
ing the carcass, as it burns slowly but continuously, so reducing the
whole animal to ash.

The animal should not be cut open to obtain specimens or perform
autopsy, but cutting off an ear is quite sufficient for diagnostic purposes.

Once anthrax is recognized, all animals should be vaccinated with a
live attenuated vaccine. Due to the persistence of the organism in the soil,
especially at a site where an infected animal has been buried, anthrax is
likely to recur year after year at the same site, so-called anthrax districts.
Hot, moist areas are particularly liable to offer the right conditions for
continuous sporulation and germination, leading to a steady infectious
state throughout the year. In contrast, hot arid areas encourage spore
formation and, when the vegetation dries out, close grazing brings the
animal into proximity with the spores in the dust, so a dry-season
outbreak is more common. This can be anticipated and cattle vaccinated
prior to the anthrax season.

Anthrax is an occupational disease in those persons who deal with
hides, hair (including wool) and bones of animals. The spores can persist
almost indefinitely in these animal remains and when tested are found
to be present in a large proportion. Pastoralists particularly will not
waste an animal that dies and taking off its skin and leaving the bones to
dry in the sun encourages formation of spores, which remain with these
products when they are shipped all over the world. It is an impossible
task to identify these infected animal products and, because of the high
proportion involved, an uneconomic process to destroy them. Quite
surprisingly people who handle infected hides and products only rarely
develop anthrax but they should of course be warned and provided with
facilities to be examined and treated. Protective clothing should be
provided and there should be a ventilation system to remove spores from
the air when unpacking, beating or a similar process occurs. Many
industrial processes disinfect the animal products, but where this does
not occur sterilization can be introduced. With persons at increased risk
of developing anthrax, vaccination can be offered. The vaccine is from a

sterile filtrate of B. *anthracis* and is given in 0.5 ml doses at 6 weeks after the initial dose, then 6 months and thereafter at annual intervals. Modified anthrax can occur in the vaccinated.

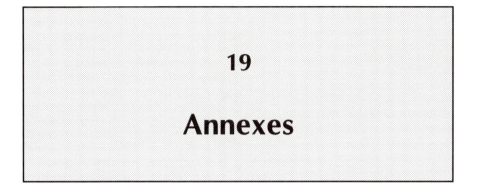

19

Annexes

19.1 COMMUNICABLE DISEASES: AGENT, TRANSMISSION AND INCUBATION PERIODS

Communicable diseases are listed in alphabetical order by the most commonly used name. Other names will be found in the index. Those diseases printed in **bold** are covered in the text.

Incubation periods are the usual range, but exceptions to these limits do occur. Agents are arboviruses (A), bacteria (B), ectoparasites (C), enteroviruses (E), fungi (F), helminths (but not nematodes) (H), nematodes (N), protozoa (P), rickettsiae (R), spirochaetes (S), toxins (T) and other viruses (V).

Disease	Clinical features (agent)	Transmission	Incubation period
Absettarov	Fever (A)	Vector (*Ixodid* ticks)	–
Actinomycosis	Systemic induration and fibrosis (B)	Person-to-person; swallowed, inhaled or through skin lesions	Months–years
Acute respiratory infections	(B, V)	Respiratory (droplet), also oral contact with contaminated articles (hands, utensils, material)	1–10 days
Aeromonas	Diarrhoea, vomiting (B)	Water and contaminated food	–
AIDS	Immune deficiency (V)	Sexual contact; via blood, tissues; perinatal transmission	2 months–10 years
Alenquer	Fever (A)	Vector (unknown)	3–6 days
Amoebiasis	Diarrhoea and systemic lesions (P)	Faecal-contaminated water and food; flies; sexual contact	2–4 weeks

325

Disease	Clinical features (agent)	Transmission	Incubation period
Amoebic meningoencephalitis	(P)	Nasal contact with contaminated water	3–20 days
Angiostrongylus	Meningitis (N)	Food (uncooked snails, slugs, seafood and vegetables)	1–3 weeks
Anisakiasis	Intestinal abscesses (N)	Food (uncooked fish)	Hours
Anthrax	Skin, intestinal or respiratory lesions (B)	Contact with infected animal tissues via skin, oral or respiratory route. Possibly also biting flies	2–7 days
Apeu	Fever (A)	Vector (culicine mosquito). Reservoir in rodents	3–12 days
Apoi	Encephalitis (A)	Vector (unknown)	5–15 days
Argentine haemorrhagic fever	(V)	Respiratory (rodent contaminated dust). Through broken skin (rodent contamination)	7–15 days
Armillifer	Calcified nodules (arthropod)	Eating raw snakes or drinking water contaminated by snakes	–
Ascaris	Malnutrition and intestinal symptoms (N)	Ingestion of soil or food contaminated by soil	10–20 days
Aspergillosis	Bronchial obstruction and eosinophilia (F)	Respiratory (from compost, hay and stored grain)	Days–weeks
Babesiosis	Fever and haemolytic anaemia (P)	Vector (*Ixodes* ticks). Blood transfusion	1 week–1 year
Bacillary dysentery (shigellosis)	(B)	Faecal–oral, direct or contaminated water and milk. Flies	1–7 days
Balantidiasis	Diarrhoea (P)	Faecal–oral or contaminated food and water (association with pigs)	Days
Bangui	Fever and rash (A)	Vector (unknown)	4–5 days
Banzi	Fever (A)	Vector (mosquito)	5–15 days
Bartonellosis	Fever, rash (B)	Vector (*Lutzomyia* sandflies)	16–22 days
Bhanja	Fever and encephalitis (A)	Vector (tick)	4–5 days
Blastomycosis	Pneumonia, rash (F)	Respiratory (dust-borne spores)	Weeks–months
Bluetongue	Fever (A)	Vector (*Culicoides*)	3–12 days
Bolivian haemorrhagic fever	(V)	Respiratory (rodent-contaminated dust). Through broken skin (rodent contamination)	7–15 days
Botulism	Paralysis (B, T)	Food (preserved). Skin (through wounds contaminated by soil)	12–36 hours

Disease	Clinical features (agent)	Transmission	Incubation period
Brazilian purpuric fever	Conjunctivitis (B)	Contact with conjunctival secretions. Respiratory	1–3 days
Brucellosis	Irregular fever (B)	Food (milk and dairy produce). Contact with or inhalation of animal tissues and excretions	5 days–5 weeks
Bunyamwera	Fever (A)	Vector (*Aedes* mosquito)	3–12 days
Buruli	Ulcer (B)	Inoculation of organism, possibly by insect	–
Bussuquara	Fever (A)	Vector (mosquito)	5–15 days
Bwamba	Fever and rash (A)	Vector (mosquito)	3–12 days
California encephalitis	(A)	Vector (mosquito)	5–15 days
Campylobacter	Diarrhoea (B)	Food or unpasteurized milk. Water. Contact with infected animals	1–10 days
Candidiasis	Thrush (F)	Contact with lesions or secretions. Faecal contact	2–5 days
Candiru	Fever (A)	Vector (unknown)	3–6 days
Capillariasis, hepatic	Hepatitis and eosinophilia (N)	Food (uncooked liver)	3–4 weeks
Capillariasis, intestinal	Malabsorption syndrome (N)	Food (uncooked fish)	Months
Capillariasis, pulmonary	Pneumonitis (N)	Ingestion of foods contaminated by soil	3–4 weeks
Capnocytophaga	Fever, meningitis (B)	Dog bite, scratch or lick	1–5 days
Caraparu	Fever (A)	Vector (culicine mosquitoes). Rodent reservoir	3–12 days
Cat-scratch	Fever, lymphadenitis (B)	Cat scratch, bite or lick	3–14 days
Catu	Fever (A)	Vector (mosquito)	5–15 days
Central European encephalitis	(A)	Vector (ticks). Consumption of unpasteurized goat's and sheep's milk	7–14 days
Chagas'	Carditis and megacolon (P)	Vector (Reduviidae). Blood transfusion. Congenital	5–15 days
Chagres	Fever (A)	Vector (phlebotomine sandflies)	3–6 days
Chancroid	Genital ulcer (B)	Sexual contact	3–5 days
Chandipura	Fever (A)	Vector (mosquito)	5–15 days
Changuinola	Fever (A)	Vector (phlebotomine sandflies)	3–6 days
Chickenpox	Rash (V)	Direct contact. Respiratory (aerosol of vesicular fluid)	2–3 weeks
Chikungunya	Fever, rash, arthritis (A)	Vector (*Aedes* mosquito). Reservoir in baboons and bats	3–12 days
Cholera	Diarrhoea (B)	Faecal contamination of food or water	1–5 days

Disease	Clinical features (agent)	Transmission	Incubation period
Chromoblasto-mycosis	Skin growths (F)	Inoculation through abrasion or via splinter	Months
Coccidioidomycosis	Respiratory infection, erythema nodosum (F)	Respiratory (dust-borne) organisms in soil	1–4 weeks
Cold, common	Respiratory infection (V)	Respiratory (droplet), also through mouth and conjunctiva	1–3 days
Colorado tick	Fever (A)	Vector (*Dermacentor*). Reservoir in small mammals	4–5 days
Condylomata acuminata	Genital warts (V)	Sexual contact	1–2 months
Congenital cytomegalovirus	CNS and liver abnormalities (V)	From genital secretions or breast milk. Adults infected by sexual contact or blood transfusion	3–12 weeks
Conjunctivitis	(B)	Contact with eye discharges. Respiratory. Flies	1–3 days
Creeping eruptions	Urticaria and eosinophilia (N)	Contact with soil contaminated by human, dog and cat faeces	–
Creutzfeldt–Jakob	Encephalopathy (V)	Unknown. Rarely from tissue transplant	Years
Crimean–Congo	Haemorrhagic fever (A)	Vector (*Hyalomma* ticks). Contact with blood and secretions of cases and animals (sheep, goats, cattle)	7–12 days
Cryptococcosis	Meningitis (F)	Respiratory	–
Cryptosporidium	Diarrhoea (P)	Faecal–oral, and from dogs and cats	1–12 days
Dakar bat	Fever (A)	Vector (unknown)	5–15 days
Dengue	(Haemorrhagic) fever (A)	Vector (*Aedes* mosquito)	3–15 days
Dhori	Fever (A)	Vector (tick)	3–12 days
Diphyllobothrium	Macrocytic anaemia (H)	Food (uncooked freshwater fish)	3–6 weeks
Diphtheria	Pharyngitis. Cutaneous lesions (B)	Direct contact with case or carrier. Respiratory	2–5 days
Dipylidium	Tapeworm (H)	Swallowing infected flea	–
Dirofilariasis	Pulmonary eosinophilia (N)	Vector (culicine mosquitoes)	–
Dugbe	Fever (A)	Vector (tick)	4–5 days
Duvenhage	Rabies-like illness (V)	Animal saliva via bite or abrasion	–
Eastern equine encephalitis	(A)	Vector (culicine mosquito). Bird and rodent reservoir	5–15 days
Ebola	Haemorrhagic fever (V)	Direct and indirect contact with blood, secretions or tissues. Sexual contact	2–21 days
Echinococcus	Hydatid cysts (H)	Dog to person via fur, licking or contaminated food and water	Months–years

Disease	Clinical features (agent)	Transmission	Incubation period
Echinostoma	Diarrhoea (H)	Food (raw snails, fish or freshwater plants)	–
Ehrlichiosis	Fever (R)	Vector? (possibly tick)	1–3 weeks
Enteritis necroticans	Gangrene of bowel (B)	Food (uncooked pork and beef). Potentiated by protease inhibitor in sweet potato	6–12 hours
Enterobius	Anal pruritis (N)	Faecal–oral, direct or indirect in dust	2–6 weeks
Enteroviral carditis	(E)	Faecal–oral or respiratory (mucus or faecal material)	3–5 days
Entomophthora-mycosis	Granuloma in skin or nasal passages (F)	Organism found in soil and rotting vegetation, but method of transmission is not known	–
Epidemic haemorrhagic conjunctivitis	(E)	Contact with eye discharges. Respiratory. Water	1–12 days
Epidemic myalgia	(V)	Faecal–oral or respiratory (mucus droplets)	3–5 days
Erysipelas	Cellulitis (B)	Contamination of abraded skin or wound	1–3 days
Erythema infectiosum	Rash (V)	Respiratory (droplet). Perinatal. Blood transfusion	4–20 days
Everglades	Encephalitis (A)	Vector (mosquito)	5–15 days
Fascioliasis	Liver damage (H)	Food (uncooked freshwater plants)	–
Fasciolopsis	Intestinal ulceration (H)	Food (uncooked fresh water plants)	3 months
Filariasis	Lymphoedema (N)	Vector (anopheline or culicine)	3–12 months
Fish poisoning	Vomiting and paraesthesia (T)	Food (toxic fish)	1–30 hours
Food poisoning	Diarrhoea and vomiting (B, T)	Contaminated food	
		staphylococci	1–6 hours
		Bacillus cereus	1–12 hours
		Clostridium perfringens	9–24 hours
		Uncooked seafood and contaminated seawater	
		Vibrio parahaemolyticus	12–48 hours
Gastrodiscoides	Diarrhoea (H)	Food (raw vegetables and water plants)	–
Gastroenteritis	Diarrhoea (B, V)	Faecal-contaminated food, water and milk	1–3 days
Germiston	Fever (A)	Vector (mosquito)	5–15 days
Giardia	Diarrhoea (P)	Faecal–oral or contaminated water and food	5–20 days
Gnathostoma	Systemic abscesses (N)	Food (uncooked fish or poultry)	–

Disease	Clinical features (agent)	Transmission	Incubation period
Gonorrhoea	Urethral discharge (B)	Sexual contact	2–7 days
Granuloma inguinale	Genital ulcers (B)	Sexual contact	Weeks–months
Guama	Fever (A)	Vector (mosquito)	5–15 days
Guaroa	Fever (A)	Vector (mosquito)	5–15 days
Guinea worm	Leg worm (N)	Water (swallowing infected copepods)	1 year
Haemorrhagic fever with renal syndrome	(V)	Respiratory (rodent excreta aerosol)	l0–20 days
Hand, foot and mouth disease	Stomatitis and skin lesions (E)	Direct contact with mouth lesions. Respiratory. Faecal–oral	3–5 days
Hanzalova	Fever (A)	Vector (*Ixodes* ticks)	–
Hepatitis A	Jaundice (E)	Faecal–oral. Contaminated water or food	15–50 days
Hepatitis B	Jaundice (V)	Inoculation. Sexual contact. Blood transfusion. Perinatal	7–26 weeks
Hepatitis C	Jaundice (V)	Inoculation. Blood transfusion. Sexual contact	3–10 weeks
Hepatitis delta	Jaundice (V)	Inoculation. Sexual contact	3–10 weeks
Hepatitis E	Jaundice (E)	Water-borne. Faecal–oral	3–7 weeks
Herpangina	Pharyngitis (E)	Contact with nose and throat discharges. Respiratory. Faecal–oral	3–5 days
Herpes genitalis	Genital lesions (V)	Sexual contact	2–12 days
Herpes simplex	Cold sores or systemic lesions in infants (V)	Contact with saliva or lesions. Perinatal	2–12 days
Heterophyes	Enteritis (H)	Food (uncooked fish)	–
Histoplasmosis	Pulmonary and other lesions (F)	Inhalation of spores (from soil)	5–18 days
Hookworm	Anaemia (N)	Larvae penetrate skin	Weeks–months
Hymenolepis	Enteritis (H)	Faecal–oral. Ingestion of insects	1–2 weeks
Ilesha	Fever and rash (A)	Vector (unknown)	3–12 days
Ilheus	Encephalitis (A)	Vector (mosquito)	5–15 days
Impetigo	Skin infection (B)	Direct contamination (mainly by hands)	4–10 days
Inclusion conjunctivitis	(B)	Infection of the newborn by genital contact of conjunctiva. Direct infection can occur from conjunctival secretions	6–19 days
Influenza	Respiratory infection (V)	Respiratory (droplet) or direct contact with mucus	1–3 days
Inkoo	Fever (A)	Vector (mosquito)	5–15 days
Isosporiasis	Diarrhoea (P)	Faecal–oral and from dogs and cats	–

Disease	Clinical features (agent)	Transmission	Incubation period
Issk-Kul	Fever (A)	Vector (tick)	4–5 days
Itaqui	Fever (A)	Vector (culicine mosquitoes). Rodent reservoir	3–12 days
Jamestown canyon	Encephalitis (A)	Vector (mosquito)	5–15 days
Japanese encephalitis	(A)	Vector (*Culex*). Reservoir in birds and pigs	5–15 days
Kamerovo	Fever (A)	Vector (tick)	4–5 days
Kasokero	Fever (A)	Vector (unknown)	5–15 days
Kerato-conjunctivitis	(V)	Direct or indirect contact with conjunctival secretions	5–12 days
Koutango	Fever and rash (A)	Vector (mosquito)	5–15 days
Kumlinge	Fever (A)	Vector (*Ixodes* ticks). Reservoir in rodents and birds	–
Kunjin	Encephalitis (A)	Vector (mosquito)	5–15 days
Kuru	Cerebellar ataxia (V)	Tribal practice of eating human brain (containing virus)	4–20 years
Kyasanur forest	Haemorrhagic fever and encephalitis (A)	Vector (*Haemaphysalis* ticks). Reservoir in rodents and monkeys	3–8 days
La Crosse	Encephalitis (A)	Vector (*Aedes*). Reservoir in *Aedes* eggs	5–15 days
Lassa fever	Haemorrhagic fever (V)	Contact with blood and secretions. Sexual contact. Endemic transmission by *Mastomys natalensis* excretions	5–15 days
Le Dantec	Encephalitis (A)	Vector (unknown)	3–12 days
Legionnaires'	Pneumonia (A)	Respiratory (water, aerosol)	1–6 days
Leishmaniasis	Cutaneous and systemic lesions (P)	Vector (phlebotomine sandflies). Mammalian reservoir specific to locality	Weeks–months
Leprosy	Skin and nerve lesions (B)	Close personal contact, possibly respiratory	1–20 years
Leptospirosis	Fever and renal failure (S)	Animal (rat, pig, cattle, dog) contamination of water in contact with abraded skin, swallowed or inhaled	4–18 days
Linguatula	Nasopharyngitis (arthropod)	Food (raw liver of sheep, goats and cattle)	–
Lipovnik	Meningitis (A)	Vector (tick)	4–5 days
Listeriosis	Meningoencephalitis (B)	Ingestion of milk and cheese. Sexual contact and perinatally	3–60 days
Loa loa	Calabar swelling (N)	Vector (*Chrysops* biting fly)	–
Louping ill	Encephalitis (A)	Vector (tick). Reservoir in sheep and deer	7–14 days

Disease	Clinical features (agent)	Transmission	Incubation period
Lyme	Rash, meningitis (A)	Vector (*Ixodes* ticks). Reservoir in ticks and mammals	3–30 days
Lymphocytic choriomeningitis	(V)	Swallowed or inhaled mouse excretions	8–15 days
Lymphogranuloma venereum	Rectovaginal lesions (B)	Sexual contact, or direct from lesions	3–30 days
Madrid	Fever (A)	Vector (culicine mosquitoes). Rodent reservoir	3–12 days
Malaria	Fever (P)	Vector (*Anopheles* mosquitoes). Blood transfusion (*Plasmodium malariae*	9–18 days 18–40 days)
Mansonellosis	(N)	Vector (*Culicoides* and *Simulium*)	–
Marburg	Haemorrhagic fever (V)	Direct and indirect contact with blood, secretions or tissues, sexual contact	2–21 days
Marituba	Fever (A)	Vector (culicine mosquitoes). Rodent reservoir	3–12 days
Mayaro	Arthritis, fever, rash (A)	Vector (culicine mosquitoes)	–
Measles	Fever and rash (V)	Respiratory (droplet). Contact with nasal or throat secretions	10–14 days
Melioidosis	Pulmonary consolidation (B)	Ingestion, inhalation or broken-skin contact with soil	Months–years
Meningitis	(B, V)	Respiratory (droplet)	2–10 days
Metagonimus	Diarrhoea (H)	Food (uncooked fish)	–
Microsporidiosis	Diarrhoea (P)	Ingestion, inhalation?	–
Mokola	Rabies-like illness (V)	Animal saliva via bite or abrasion	Weeks–months
Molluscum contagiosum	Skin lesions (V)	Direct contact with lesions. Sexual contact	10 days–6 months
Monkeypox	Pox rash (V)	Close contact with reservoir animals. Limited person-to-person	–
Mononucleosis, infectious	Glandular fever (V)	Swallowing or inhaling infected saliva. Blood transfusion	4–6 weeks
Mucambo	Fever (A)	Vector (mosquito)	–
Mucormycosis	Thrombosis and infarction (F)	Inhalation of spores. Inoculation by needles	–
Mumps	Parotitis (V)	Respiratory (droplet) contact with saliva	12–24 days
Murray Valley	Encephalitis (A)	Vector (*Culex*). Reservoir in birds	5–15 days
Murutucu	Fever (A)	Vector (culicine mosquitoes). Rodent reservoir	3–12 days
Mycetoma	Localized induration and sinuses (B, F)	Inoculation from soil or plants (e.g. thorns)	Months

Disease	Clinical features (agent)	Transmission	Incubation period
Mycoplasma	Pneumonia (V)	Respiratory (droplet)	5–20 days
Nairobi sheep	Fever (A)	Vector (tick)	4–5 days
Negishi	Encephalitis (A)	Vector (unknown)	5–15 days
Nepuyo	Fever (A)	Vector (culicine mosquitoes). Rodent reservoir	3–12 days
Nocardiosis	Systemic lesions (B)	Respiratory (dust-borne)	Days–weeks
Non-gonococcal urethritis (NGU)	(B)	Sexual contact	1–2 weeks
Non-venereal syphilis	Maculopapular skin rash (S)	Direct contact with lesions or indirect via eating and drinking utensils	3 weeks–3 months
Norwalk	Diarrhoea (E)	Faecal–oral, food-borne, water-borne or respiratory	1–2 days
Nyando	Fever (A)	Vector (mosquito)	3–12 days
Omsk haemorrhagic fever	(A)	Vector (*Dermacentor* ticks or contact with muskrat	3–8 days
Onchocerciasis	Blindness (N)	Vector (*Simulium* flies)	6 months–1 year
O'nyong-nyong	Arthralgia (A)	Vector (*Anopheles* mosquito)	3–12 days
Ophthalmia neonatorum	(B)	Genital secretions of mother to conjunctiva of infant	1–12 days
Opisthorchis	Liver damage (H)	Food (uncooked freshwater fish or crayfish)	Months
Orf	Maculopapular lesion (V)	Contact with mucous membranes of infected sheep and goats	3–6 days
Oriboca	Fever (A)	Vector (culicine mosquitoes). Rodent reservoir	3–12 days
Oropouche	Fever and meningitis (A)	Vector (mosquitoes and possibly *Culicoides*). Reservoir in monkeys, sloths and birds	3–12 days
Orungo	Fever (A)	Vector (*Aedes* and *Anopheles*)	3–12 days
Ossa	Fever (A)	Vector (culicine mosquitoes). Rodent reservoir	3–12 days
Paracoccidioido-mycosis	Mycosis of respiratory tract (F)	Respiratory (dust-borne)	Months–years
Paragonimus	Lung damage (H)	Food (freshwater crabs and crayfish)	Months
Paratyphoid	Diarrhoea (B)	Faecal contamination of food and water. Flies	1–10 days
Pasteurellosis	Cellulitis (B)	Cat scratch or dog bite	12–24 hours
Pediculosis	Urticaria (C)	Direct or indirect contact with infested person	8–10 days
Pertussis	Whooping cough (B)	Respiratory (droplet)	7–10 days
Pinta	Maculopapular rash (S)	Direct contact with lesions, facilitated by trauma	1–3 weeks
Piry	Fever (A)	Vector (mosquito)	3–12 days

Disease	Clinical features (agent)	Transmission	Incubation period
Plague	Bubo (B)	Vector (fleas)	2–6 days
	Pneumonia (B)	Respiratory	2–6 days
Pneumocystis	Pneumonia (P)	Presumably respiratory from animal or human source	Months
Pneumonia	(B, V)	Respiratory (droplet)	Depends on organism
Poliomyelitis	Paralysis (E)	Faecal–oral or respiratory	5–30 days
Pongola	Fever (A)	Vector (mosquito)	3–12 days
Powassan	Encephalitis (A)	Vector (tick)	7–14 days
Psittacosis	Pneumonitis (B)	Respiratory (inhaling bird droppings)	5–15 days
Puerperal fever	Genital-tract infection (B)	Contamination of genital tract during delivery by droplets, hands or faeces	1–3 days
Punta Toro	Fever (A)	Vector (phlebotomine sandflies)	3–6 days
Q	Fever (R)	Respiratory (animal tissues or excretions). Milk. Direct contact with infected animal	2–3 weeks
Quaranfil	Fever (A)	Vector (tick)	4–5 days
Rabies	Encephalomyelitis (V)	Animal saliva via bite or abrasion. Respiratory	2–8 weeks
Rat-bite fever	(B)	Rat bite or indirect contact with rats	3 days–3 weeks
Relapsing fever	(R)	Vector (louse or tick)	3–10 days
Restan	Fever (A)	Vector (culicine mosquitoes). Rodent reservoir	3–12 days
Rheumatic fever	Cardiac damage (B)	Respiratory (droplet). Ingestion of food and milk	1–3 days
Rickettsial pox	Fever and rash (R)	Vector (mites). Rodent reservoir	3–13 days
Rift Valley fever	Haemorrhagic (A)	Vector (culicine mosquitoes). Direct contact with animals	3–12 days
Rio Bravo	Encephalitis (A)	Vector (unknown)	5–15 days
Rocio	Encephalitis (A)	Vector (probably mosquitos)	5–15 days
Rocky mountain spotted fever	(R)	Vector (ticks). Reservoir in ticks	3–13 days
Ross River	Arthritis (A)	Vector (culicine mosquitoes). Rodent reservoir	3–12 days
Rotavirus	Diarrhoea (V)	Faecal–oral. Respiratory	1–3 days
Rubella	Maculopapular rash (V)	Respiratory. Congenital	15–20 days
Russian spring–summer encephalitis	(A)	Vector (tick)	7–14 days
St Louis encephalitis	(A)	Vector (*Culex* mosquito)	5–15 days

Disease	Clinical features (agent)	Transmission	Incubation period
Salmonellosis	Diarrhoea (B)	Food (generally contaminated by faecal or gut contents). Milk and eggs. Faecal–oral. Water-borne	12–36 hours
Sandfly fever	(A)	Vector (phlobotomine sandflies)	3–6 days
Sarcocystis	Diarrhoea (P)	Food (uncooked meat)	–
Scabies	Urticaria (C)	Direct skin contact	2–6 weeks
Scarlet fever	Rash (B)	Respiratory (droplet). Ingestion of food and milk	1–3 days
Schistosomiasis	Liver or bladder damage (A)	Water contact	–
Semliki	Encephalitis (A)	Vector (mosquito)	3–12 days
Sepik	Fever (A)	Vector (mosquito)	5–15 days
Shingles	Vesicular skin rash (V)	Direct contact. Inhalation of vesicular fluid	13–17 days
Shokwe	Fever (A)	Vector (mosquito)	3–12 days
Shuni	Fever (A)	Vector (mosquito or *Culicoides* midges)	3–12 days
Simian B	Meningoencephalitis (V)	Monkey saliva via bite or abrasion	3 days–3 weeks
Sindbis	Arthritis, rash (A)	Vector (culicine mosquitoes). Reservoir in birds	3–12 days
Sleeping sickness	Fever and headache (P)	Vector (*Glossina* tsetse fly). Mechanical. Congenital	Weeks–months
Smallpox	Pox rash (V)	Respiratory, skin contact	10–12 days
Snowshoe hare	Encephalitis (A)	Vector (mosquito)	3–12 days
Sparganosis	Subcutaneous nodules (H)	Eating frogs and other amphibians	–
Spondweni	Fever (A)	Vector (mosquito)	3–12 days
Sporotrichosis	Skin nodules (F)	Percutaneous from soil or vegetation. Respiratory	1 week–3 months
Staphylococcal	Skin and wound infections (B)	Autoinfection or contact with lesions	5–10 days
Streptococcal sore throat	(B)	Respiratory (droplet). Ingestion of food or milk	1–3 days
Strongyloides	Creeping eruption (N)	Larvae penetrate skin. Autoinfection. Oral	–
Syphilis	Skin, bone and heart lesions (S)	Sexual contact. Blood transfusion. Perinatal	9–90 days
Tacaiuma	Fever (A)	Vector (mosquito)	3–12 days
Taenia saginata	Tapeworm (H)	Food (uncooked beef)	10–14 weeks
Taenia solium	Tapeworm and cysticercosis (H)	Food (uncooked pork). Autoinfection. Swallowing eggs	8–12 weeks
Tahyna	Fever (A)	Vector (mosquito)	–
Tamdy	Fever (A)	Vector (tick)	4–5 days

Disease	Clinical features (agent)	Transmission	Incubation period
Tataguine	Fever and rash (A)	Vector (mosquito)	5–15 days
Tensaw	Encephalitis (A)	Vector (mosquito)	3–12 days
Tetanus	Convulsions (B)	Contamination of abraded skin or umbilicus of newborn	4–21 days
Thogoto	Meningitis (A)	Vector (tick)	4–5 days
Tick-borne encephalitis	(A)	Vector (tick)	4–5 days
Tick typhus	Fever (R)	Vector (tick). Reservoir in ticks	2–10 days
Tinea	Skin infection (F)	Direct, skin contact. Animal contact	4–14 days
Tonate	Fever (A)	Vector (mosquito)	3–12 days
Toscana	Meningitis (A)	Vector (phlebotomine sandflies)	3–6 days
Toxocara	Larva migrans	Ingestion of earth (pica) or vegetables	Weeks–months
Toxoplasmosis	Fever and brain damage (P)	Eating uncooked pork or mutton, earth (pica) or inhalation of oocyst. Transplacental	5–20 days
Trachoma	Red-eye, blindness (B)	Direct or indirect contact with eye discharges from fingers, wipes and clothing. Flies	5–12 days
Trench fever	(B)	Vector (louse)	7–30 days
Trichinosis	Fever and systemic cysts (N)	Food (uncooked pork and other meat)	5–45 days
Trichomonas	Vaginitis (P)	Sexual contact	5–20 days
Trichuris	Diarrhoea (N)	Ingestion of soil (pica) or vegetables contaminated with soil	–
Tropical ulcer	(B)	Contamination of abraded skin by fingers or flies	2–7 days
Tuberculosis	Cough and wasting (B)	Respiratory (droplet). Unpasteurized milk	4–12 weeks
Tularaemia	Ulcer or pneumonia (B)	Vector (*Chrysops*, *Aedes* or ticks). Handling or ingestion of animal tissues. Water-, soil- or dust-borne. Animal bite	2–10 days
Typhoid	Fever and bowel ulceration (B)	Faecal contamination of food and water. Flies	1–3 weeks
Typhus, epidemic	Fever and rash (R)	Vector (louse). Louse faeces scratched in or inhaled	1–2 weeks
Typhus, murine	Fever and rash (R)	Vector (flea). Inhalation of flea faeces	1–2 weeks
Typhus, scrub	Fever and rash (R)	Vector (larval mites). Reservoir in small mammals	1–3 weeks
Usutu	Fever (A)	Vector (mosquito)	3–12 days

Disease	Clinical features (agent)	Transmission	Incubation period
Venezuelan equine encephalitis	(A)	Vector (*Culex* mosquitoes). Reservoir in horses	2–6 days
Wanowrie	Fever and bleeding (A)	Vector (tick)	4–5 days
Warts	Skin growths (V)	Direct contact or inoculation. Possibly indirect (e.g. floors)	2–3 months
Wesselsbron	Fever (A)	Vector (mosquito)	3–12 days
Western equine encephalitis	(A)	Vector (*Culex* mosquitoes). Reservoir in birds	5–15 days
West Nile	Fever (A)	Vector (*Culex* mosquitoes). Reservoir in birds	3–12 days
Wyeomyia	Fever (A)	Vector (mosquito)	3–12 days
Yaws	Skin and bone lesions (S)	Direct contact with lesions and exudates. Indirect or by flies	2–8 weeks
Yellow fever	Haemorrhagic fever (A)	Vector (*Aedes* mosquito). Reservoir in monkeys	3–6 days
Yersiniosis	Diarrhoea (B)	Faecal-contaminated food and water. Faecal–oral. Pig is main reservoir, but also rodents and small mammals	3–7 days
Zika	Fever (A)	Vector (mosquito)	5–15 days

AIDS, acquired immune deficiency syndrome; CNS, central nervous system.

19.2 FURTHER READING

19.2.1 *Epidemiology and Statistics*

Abramson, T.H. (1984) *Survey Methods in Community Medicine*. Churchill Livingstone, Edinburgh.

Anderson, R.M. (1982) *Population Dynamics of Infectious Diseases*. Chapman and Hall, London.

Barker, D.J.P. and Hall, A. (1991) *Practical Epidemiology*. Churchill Livingstone, Edinburgh.

Beaglehole, R., Bonita, R. and Kjellström, T. (1993) *Basic Epidemiology*. World Health Organization, Geneva.

Bennett, F.J. (1979) *Community Diagnosis and Health Action*. Macmillan, Basingstoke.

Bres, P. (1986) *Public Health Action in Emergencies Caused by Epidemics*. World Health Organization, Geneva.

Giesecke, J. (1994) *Modern Infectious Disease Epidemiology*. Edward Arnold, London.

Henderson, R.H. and Sudaresan, T. (1982) Cluster sampling to assess immunization coverage: a review of experience with a simplified sampling method. *Bulletin of the World Health Organization* 60(2), 253–260.

Kirkwood, B.R. (1988) *Essentials of Medical Statistics*. Blackwell Scientific Publications, Oxford.

Last, J.M. (1988) *A Dictionary of Epidemiology*. Oxford University Press, Oxford.

Learmonth, A.T.A. (1981) *The Geography of Health*. Pergamon, Oxford.

Lilienfield, A.M. (1980) *Foundations of Epidemiology*. Oxford University Press, New York.

Lindley, D.V. and Miller, J.C.P. (1952) *Cambridge Elementary Statistical Tables*. Cambridge University Press, Cambridge.

McGlashan, N.D. (1972) *Medical Geography*. Methuen, London.

Smith, P.G. and Morrow, R.H. (1996) *Methods for Field Trials of Interventions Against Tropical Diseases*, 2nd edn. Macmillan, Basingstoke.

Swaroop, S. (1966) *Statistical Methods in Malaria Eradication*. World Health Organization, Geneva.

Vaughan, J.P. and Morrow, R.H. (1989) *Manual of Epidemiology for District Health Management*. World Health Organization, Geneva.

Wellcome Tropical Institute (1987) *Epidemiology, A Nine Part Manual for Distance Learning in Tropical Countries*. Wellcome Trust, London.

19.2.2 Parasitology, Entomology and Microbiology

Cheesbrough, M. (1984) *Medical Laboratory Manual for Tropical Countries*, Vol. 2, *Microbiology*. Butterworth, Sevenoaks.

Cheesbrough, M. (1991) *Medical Laboratory Manual for Tropical Countries*, Vol. 1. Churchill Livingstone, Edinburgh.

Curtis, C.F. (1990) *Appropriate Technology in Vector Control*. Wolfe, New York.

Jeffrey, H.C. and Leach, R.M. (1991) *Atlas of Medical Helminthology and Protozoology*. 3rd edn. Churchill Livingstone, Edinburgh.

King, M. (1973) *A Medical Laboratory for Developing Countries*. Oxford University Press, Oxford.

Montefiore, D.G., Alausa, K.O. and Tomori, O. (1984) *Tropical Microbiology*. Churchill Livingstone, Edinburgh.

Muller, R.L.J. and Baker, J. (1989) *Medical Parasitology*. Mosby, London.

Olds, R.J. (1986) *A Colour Atlas of Microbiology*. Wolfe, London.

Peters, W. and Gilles, H.M. (1995) *Colour Atlas of Tropical Medicine and Parasitology*. 4th edn. Mosby-Wolfe, London.

Service, M.W. (1980) *A Guide to Medical Entomology*. Macmillan, Basingstoke.

Service, M.W. (1996) *Medical Entomology for Students*. Chapman & Hall, London.

19.2.3 Environmental Health

Cairncross, S. (1988) *Small Scale Sanitation*. Ross Institute, London.

Cairncross, S. and Feachem, R. (1978) *Small Water Supplies*. Ross Institute, London.

Cairncross, S. and Feachem, R. (1993) *Environmental Health Engineering in the Tropics*, 2nd edn. John Wiley, Chichester.

Feachem, R., Burns, E., Cairncross, S., Cronin, A., Cross, P., Curtis, D., Khan, M.K., Lamb, D. and Southall, H. (1978) *Water, Health and Development*. Tri-Med, London.

Feachem, R., McGarry, M.A. and Mara, D. (eds) (1978) *Water, Wastes and Health in*

Hot Climates. John Wiley, Chichester.

Feachem, R.G., Bradley, D.J., Garelick, H. and Mara, D.D. (1983) *Sanitation and Disease, Health Aspects of Excreta and Wastewater Management.* John Wiley, Chichester.

Lauria, P.T., Kolsky, P.J., Middleton, R.N., Demke, K. and Herbert, P.V. (1980) *Design of Low-Cost Water Distribution Systems.* World Bank, Washington.

19.2.4 Communicable Diseases

Adams, A.R.D. and Maegraith, B.G. (1989) *Clinical Tropical Diseases.* Blackwell Scientific Publications, Oxford.

Arya, O.P., Osoba, A.O. and Bennett, F.T. (1988) *Tropical Venereology.* Churchill Livingstone, Edinburgh.

Benenson, A.S. (1990) *Control of Communicable Diseases in Man.* American Public Health Association, Washington.

Bryceson, A. and Pfaltzgraff, R. (1978) *Leprosy.* Churchill Livingstone, Edinburgh.

Chambers, R., Longhurst, R. and Pacey, A. (1981) *Seasonal Dimensions to Rural Poverty.* Frances Pinter, London.

Christie, A.B. (1987) *Infectious Diseases.* Epidemiology and Clinical Practice. Churchill Livingstone, Edinburgh.

Cook, G.C. (1988) *Communicable and Tropical Diseases.* Heinemann, Oxford.

Cook, G.C. (1996) *Manson's Tropical Diseases,* 20th edn. W.B. Saunders, London.

Emond, R.T.D., Rowland, H.A.K. and Welsby, P.D. (1994) *Colour Atlas of Infectious Diseases,* 3rd edn. Mosby-Wolfe, London.

Eshuis, J. and Manshot, P. (1978) *Communicable Diseases.* AMREF, Nairobi.

Gilles, H.M. and Warrel, D.A. (1993) *Bruce–Chwatt's Essential Malariology.* Edward Arnold, London.

Jordan, P., Webbe, G. and Sturrock, R.F. (1993) *Human Schistosomiasis.* CAB International, Wallingford.

Lucas, A.O. and Gilles, H.M. (1990) *A New Short Textbook of Preventive Medicine for the Tropics.* Hodder & Stoughton, Sevenoaks.

Macdonald, G. (1973) *Dynamics of Tropical Diseases.* Oxford University Press, Oxford.

Miller, F.J.W. (1982) *Tuberculosis in Children.* Churchill Livingstone, Edinburgh.

Parry, E.H.O. (1984) *Principles of Medicine in Africa.* Oxford University Press, Oxford.

Robinson, D. (1985) *Epidemiology and the Community Control of Disease in Warm Climate Countries.* Churchill Livingstone, Edinburgh.

Stevenson, D. (1987) *Davey and Lightbody's The Control of Diseases in the Tropics.* Lewis, London.

Sturchler, D. (1988) *Endemic Areas of Tropical Infections.* Hans Huber, Toronto.

Warren, K.S. and Mahmoud, A.A.F. (1990) *Tropical and Geographical Medicine.* McGraw Hill, New York.

Wellcome Tropical Institute (1987) *Acute Respiratory Infections, a Manual for Distance Learning in Tropical Countries.* Wellcome Trust, London.

Wood, C.H., Vaughan, J.P. and de Glanville, H. (1981) *Community Health.* AMREF, Nairobi.

Woodruff, A.W. and Wright, S.G. (1984) *Medicine in the Tropics.* Churchill Living-stone, Edinburgh.

World Health Organization (1995) *International Travel and Health.* World Health Organization, Geneva.

World Health Organization Expert Committee Technical Report Series, Geneva:

(1984) *Malaria Control as Part of Primary Health Care,* No. 712.

(1986) *Epidemiology and Control of African Trypanosomiasis.* No. 739.

(1986) *Brucellosis.* No. 740.

(1988) *Rheumatic Fever and Rheumatic Heart Disease.* No. 764.

(1990) *Control of Leishmaniasis.* No. 793.

(1991) *Management of Patients with Sexually Transmitted Diseases.* No. 810.

(1991) *Control of Chagas Disease.* No. 811.

(1992) *Lymphatic Filariasis. The Disease and Its Control.* No. 821.

(1992) *WHO Expert Committee on Rabies.* No. 824.

(1993) *The Control of Schistosomiasis.* No. 830.

(1994) *Chemotherapy of Leprosy.* No. 847.

(1995) *Control of Foodborne Trematode Infections.* No. 849.

(1995) *Onchocerciasis and its Control.* No. 852.

Index